Spiritual Diversity in Psychotherapy

Spiritual Diversity in Psychotherapy

Engaging the Sacred in Clinical Practice

Edited by
Steven J. Sandage and Brad D. Strawn

 AMERICAN PSYCHOLOGICAL ASSOCIATION

Published by
American Psychological Association
750 First Street, NE
Washington, DC 20002
https://www.apa.org

Order Department
https://www.apa.org/pubs/books
order@apa.org

In the U.K., Europe, Africa, and the Middle East, copies may be ordered from Eurospan
https://www.eurospanbookstore.com/apa
info@eurospangroup.com

Typeset in Charter and Interstate by Circle Graphics, Inc., Reisterstown, MD

Printer: Gasch Printing, Odenton, MD
Cover Designer: Gwen J. Grafft, Minneapolis, MN

Library of Congress Cataloging-in-Publication Data

Names: Sandage, Steven J., editor. | Strawn, Brad D., editor.
Title: Spiritual diversity in psychotherapy : engaging the sacred in
  clinical practice / edited by Steven J. Sandage and Brad D. Strawn.
Description: Washington, DC : American Psychological Association, [2022] |
  Includes bibliographical references and index.
Identifiers: LCCN 2021039362 (print) | LCCN 2021039363 (ebook) |
  ISBN 9781433836541 (paperback) | ISBN 9781433838514 (ebook)
Subjects: LCSH: Psychotherapy--Religious aspects. |
  Psychotherapists--Religious life. | BISAC: PSYCHOLOGY / Psychotherapy /
  General | PSYCHOLOGY / Clinical Psychology
Classification: LCC RC489.S676 S644 2022 (print) | LCC RC489.S676 (ebook) |
  DDC 616.89/14--dc23
LC record available at https://lccn.loc.gov/2021039362
LC ebook record available at https://lccn.loc.gov/2021039363

https://doi.org/10.1037/0000276-000

Printed in the United States of America

10 9 8 7 6 5 4 3 2 1

*To Dr. Judith Bunyi, Dr. Micah McCreary, and Dr. Mark Harden,
key mentors who model such vibrant integration of spirituality,
diversity competence, and generativity.*
—STEVEN J. SANDAGE

*To my colleagues and students at the Graduate School of Psychology,
Fuller Theological Seminary, and to my patients who embody the
integration of faith, psychology, diversity, and the continual pursuit
of wrestling with the biggest questions.*
—BRAD D. STRAWN

Contents

Contributors

Neil Altman, PhD, faculty, William Alanson White Institute, New York, NY, United States; honorary member, William Alanson White Society; visiting faculty, Ambedkar University of Delhi, India

Kathryn L. Barrs, PsyD, Clinical Associate Professor/Clinic Director, Military Psychology Specialty, Graduate School of Professional Psychology, University of Denver, Denver, CO, United States

Carrie Doehring, PhD, Clifford Baldridge Professor of Pastoral Care and Counseling, Iliff School of Theology, Denver, CO; Professor, joint doctoral program with University of Denver, Denver, CO, United States

Ruben A. Hopwood, MDiv, PhD, Licensed Psychologist and Founder and Director, Hopwood Counseling & Consulting, LLC, Cambridge, MA; Visiting Researcher, The Albert & Jessie Danielsen Institute, Boston University, Boston, MA, United States

Pilar Jennings, PhD, Psychoanalyst, Private Practice, New York, NY, United States

Shamaila Khan, PhD, Assistant Professor, Boston University School of Medicine; Training Director, Center for Multicultural Training in Psychology; Director, Center for Multicultural Mental Health, Boston Medical Center/Boston University School of Medicine, Boston, MA, United States

Sarah H. Moon, PsyD, Licensed Clinical Psychologist and Diversity, Equity, and Inclusion Consultant, private practice based in Portland, OR, but serving Massachusetts and Oregon residents; Visiting Researcher,

The Albert & Jessie Danielsen Institute, Boston University, Boston, MA, United States

Kenneth I. Pargament, PhD, Professor Emeritus of Psychology, Bowling Green State University, Bowling Green, OH, United States

Steven J. Sandage, PhD, LP, Albert and Jessie Danielsen Professor of Psychology of Religion and Theology, Boston University; Director of Research and Senior Staff Psychologist, The Albert & Jessie Danielsen Institute, Boston University, Boston, MA, United States; Adjunct Faculty in Psychology of Religion, MF Norwegian School of Theology, Religion, and Society, Oslo, Norway

Phillis Isabella Sheppard, PhD, E. Rhodes and Leona B. Carpenter Associate Professor of Religion, Psychology, and Culture, Vanderbilt University Divinity School, Nashville, TN, United States

Karen E. Starr, PsyD, Adjunct Clinical Associate Professor, New York University Postdoctoral Program in Psychotherapy and Psychoanalysis, New York, NY; Clinical Psychologist and Psychoanalyst, Private Practice, New York, NY and Great Neck, NY, United States

Brad D. Strawn, PhD, Evelyn and Frank Freed Chair of the Integration of Psychology and Theology, School of Psychology & Marriage and Family Therapy, Fuller Seminary, Pasadena, CA, United States

Theresa Clement Tisdale, PhD, PsyD, Licensed Clinical Psychologist and Clinical Psychoanalyst, Private Practice, Glendora, CA; Professor of Clinical Psychology, Azusa Pacific University, Azusa, CA, United States

Pratyusha Tummala-Narra, PhD, Professor, Department of Counseling, Developmental and Educational Psychology, Boston College, Chestnut Hill, MA, United States

Acknowledgments

This project was supported by the Center for the Study of Religion and Psychology of The Albert & Jessie Danielsen Institute at Boston University. We are grateful to Executive Director George Stavros and the Danielsen Institute leadership team of Lauren Kehoe, Miriam Bronstein, and David Rupert for their encouragement and input.

We are so very grateful to Barbara Jordan, wife of theologian Merle Jordan, for her enthusiastic and dedicated support to the Danielsen Institute's Merle Jordan Conference, which has served as a creative gathering space for many of the contributors to this book. Over the years, the conference has brought together highly accomplished and diverse scholars, clinicians, and students to advance Merle Jordan's mission for the healing engagement between spirituality and mental health.

Thanks to Dean Emerita Mary Elizabeth Moore and Dean G. Sujin Pak at the Boston University School of Theology, both passionate advocates for the kinds of diversity and social justice values that inspire this book.

A grant project (Number 61603) supported by the John Templeton Foundation on Mental Healthcare, Virtue, and Human Flourishing also provided resources to help integrate virtue and flourishing frameworks into this volume.

—*Steven J. Sandage and Brad D. Strawn*

Spiritual Diversity in Psychotherapy

INTRODUCTION

Spiritual Diversity in Psychotherapy

STEVEN J. SANDAGE AND BRAD D. STRAWN

Ethical mandates within all the professional mental health fields now call for clinician awareness, sensitivity, and skill related to spiritual and religious dynamics in clinical practice. This marks a tremendous shift in recent decades away from the residual antipathy toward religion by such historical figures in psychotherapy as Sigmund Freud and Albert Ellis. Yet these mandates also represent calls for active engagement by clinicians that move beyond the relative neglect of religion and spirituality in many approaches to psychotherapy during the 20th century, when the mental health field was trying to establish itself as an objective science of human behavior. I (S.J.S.) remember being taught in a graduate school psychology class in the 1990s that psychotherapy was "behavioral engineering" (curiously, by a faculty member who was not in clinical practice). The 1990s was a decade in which the multicultural movements in various mental health fields sparked significant changes in training curricula and intensified research on diversity dynamics in treatment. The 1980s to 1990s was also a period of growing empirical research in the areas of (a) spirituality, religion, and mental health; and (b) positive psychology of human strengths, virtues, and flourishing.

https://doi.org/10.1037/0000276-001
Spiritual Diversity in Psychotherapy: Engaging the Sacred in Clinical Practice,
S. J. Sandage and B. D. Strawn (Editors)

For clinicians interested in the roles of spirituality, religion, and related dynamics (e.g., mindfulness) in counseling and psychotherapy, the scientific knowledge base has been rapidly accumulating for at least 30 years into what is now arguably a mainstream set of topics in mental health.

At present, we now have a vast international body of research showing spiritual and religious factors are often positively associated with mental health and well-being (Koenig, 2018). For the majority of people around the world, spirituality or religion, or both, shape meaning systems and practices related to suffering and healing in ways that will impact their views of what counts as effective "health care." However, spirituality and religion are complex phenomena that can emerge from and become embedded in human experiences of trauma and suffering. There is a growing literature on spiritual and religious struggles that shows various forms of struggles with the sacred can be associated with mental and physical health problems (Pargament & Exline, 2021). In addition, some initial evidence suggests both spiritual well-being and spiritual and religious struggles can predict the psychosocial functioning of psychotherapy clients over and above the effects of mental health symptoms (Sandage et al., 2022).

Because spirituality and religion can impact mental health in both positive and negative ways depending on the dynamics and contexts involved, it is encouraging to now see many different treatment approaches that integrate spirituality and religion combined with a growing body of clinical research. A meta-analysis of 97 outcome studies ($N = 7,181$) of spiritually and religiously adapted therapies found these treatment approaches were typically effective for psychological and spiritual outcomes, showing equivalent effectiveness to secular therapies for psychological outcomes and higher effectiveness for spiritual outcomes (Captari et al., 2018). This latter point speaks to the interesting diversity questions related to what gets defined as clinical outcomes and the reality that some clients hold values about spiritual or religious growth that go beyond the simple focus on the alleviation of mental health symptoms that remains dominant in most of Western health care. This means it is increasingly important for clinicians to attend to clients' perspectives on well-being in addition to their reports about symptoms (Jankowski et al., 2020).

Mental health practitioners are expected to respect and respond to client preferences regarding treatment goals and processes, and a considerable body of research over the past 50 years has also investigated individuals' preferences related to spirituality and religion in counseling and psychotherapy (for reviews, see Harris et al., 2016, and Oxhandler et al., 2018). Overall, this research has shown a majority of individuals (a) consider spirituality and religion to be relevant topics in therapy and (b) would prefer to be able to discuss spiritual or religious issues in their own therapy (at least hypothetically). These trends are particularly strong for individuals who score high in spiritual or religious commitment; however this is not exclusively the case. Some clients want to process negative or ambivalent experiences with spirituality or religion, whereas other clients are in a process of spiritual or religious questing (Sandage et al., 2022).

Some research also shows that individuals can be concerned about disclosing their spiritual or religious beliefs with therapists, and the safety to disclose may depend on their perceived spiritual or religious similarity to their therapists or the openness and acceptance communicated by their therapists (Cragun & Friedlander, 2012; Oxhandler et al., 2018). For example, one of our colleagues reported that a client from a Christian Pentecostal tradition "confessed" to him in the second year of treatment that, during prayer, she sometimes tried to hear God's voice of direction for her life. Her adult son, a family practice doctor, had warned her against ever admitting this to a mental health professional because she would likely be put on antipsychotic medication. This therapist had effectively cultivated the client's trust to share her spiritual practice over approximately 18 months of treatment, but we can wonder about cases in which clients' core values and goals remain hidden because of these kinds of fears and reductionistic biases within the power structures of some health care settings.

SPIRITUAL AND RELIGIOUS COMPETENCE

Many of the aforementioned clinical considerations involving spirituality and religion can be related to the development of cultural competence (or multicultural, intercultural, or diversity competence), which involves the skillful and effective application of awareness and sensitivity to cultural diversity. Some have voiced concerns about the term "competence" in terms of clinically navigating diversity considerations for various reasons. We affirm the wisdom of the many excellent scholars and practitioners forming the robust literature on cultural humility (Davis et al., 2018; Hook et al., 2017; Owen et al., 2016), and we see great benefit in holding the themes of cultural competence and cultural humility in a productive dialectical tension. In our view, *cultural competence* suggests a crucial goal of developing capacities to relate effectively across cultural differences and skillful abilities to adapt clinical strategies to the diverse worldviews, values, and practices of clients. *Cultural humility* speaks to the need for a lifelong journey of ongoing learning, critical self-reflection, and accountability to progress in the transformation of power structures toward greater diversity, equity, and inclusion (Tervalon & Murray-García, 1998).

Similar to cultural competence, the emerging literature on spiritual and religious competence in mental health practice emphasizes (a) developing constructive awareness and attitudes about the relevance of spiritual and religious issues in treatment, (b) acquiring relevant knowledge, and (c) cultivating skills to work with clients' spiritual and religious perspectives in treatment (Vieten & Scammell, 2015; Vieten et al., 2016). There is also some empirical evidence that spiritual and religious competence among clinicians is associated with humility and relational maturity (Crabtree et al., 2021). Despite the relevance of spirituality and religion to clinical practice, research findings also suggest this is an area of diversity that is often neglected or absent in clinical training with clinicians frequently reporting the need for more training in this area (Crabtree et al., 2021; Pargament, 2011; Vogel et al., 2013). There are numerous clinical training programs in the United States located in the contexts of religiously affiliated schools, and some of those programs are intentional about seeking to integrate spirituality and religion into training. However, it remains unclear whether clinical trainees from religiously affiliated programs actually fare better, worse, or similar to trainees from secular programs when it comes to effectively engaging spiritual and religious diversity in practice.

The average clinician likely works with clients representing a variety of spiritual and religious traditions and perspectives (including little or no interest in spirituality or religion), and familiarity with a particular tradition or two might not translate into openness and skill in working within a diverse range of client perspectives and traditions. We are also familiar with spiritually or religiously committed clinicians who attended secular training programs in which faculty communicated in various ways that spirituality and religion were unacceptable topics for professional or scholarly discussion. However, trying to compartmentalize those aspects of human experience is not an effective pathway toward spiritual and religious competence (or any form of diversity competence; Sorenson & Hales, 2002).

The development of spiritual and religious competence can also be complicated by the ways the clinical literature on spirituality and religion sometimes uses general definitions of these constructs in an effort at inclusion or eticlike universality. For example, some authors define "spirituality" in positive terms as beliefs or practices that provide a sense of transcendence or meaning. This strategy can seem to offer the efficiency of a generic definition of spirituality that could apply to most people. It has even been suggested that everyone is "spiritual" based on this type of definition, which is actually problematic from a diversity perspective in that some clients do not define themselves as spiritual or religious. These generic definitions of spirituality or religion, typically cast in relatively positive terms, might seem to counter some of the negative views of these constructs in mental health fields. However, overreliance on these kinds of generalizations can be a form of spiritual and religious minimization by focusing on sameness in ways that obscures attention to the vast and meaningful differences in client understandings of spirituality and religion, including positive, negative, and mixed experiences with the sacred (Sandage et al., 2020). Spiritual and religious dynamics can also intersect with other aspects of identity in complex and even painful ways, so we have also emphasized intersectional perspectives in this present volume.

SPIRITUAL, EXISTENTIAL, RELIGIOUS, AND THEOLOGICAL FRAMEWORK

At The Albert & Jessie Danielsen Institute at Boston University, where this project originated, my (S.J.S.) colleagues and I use a spiritual, existential, religious, and theological (SERT) framework in our training program, research, and clinical practice (Rupert et al., 2019; SERT training videos are also available for free viewing; see The Albert & Jessie Danielsen Institute, n.d.). The SERT acronym can remind us of the multiple dimensions involved in the diverse ways individuals orient themselves to sacred and ultimate meaning as well as highlight differing sources of ancient and contemporary wisdom about suffering and healing. Clients and clinicians locate themselves in a variety of ways relative to these SERT dimensions. For example, a client might self-identify as Buddhist and atheist and be matched with a therapist who is Orthodox Jewish, which could involve interesting dynamics as they navigate potential similarities and differences in beliefs, values, and practices. Or, a Sufi Muslim therapist might be working with a couple in which both partners are Evangelical Christian but are conflicted over differing theological beliefs about the legitimacy of getting divorced. This couples therapist might believe it is outside their role to try to arbitrate the couples' theological differences but might consider it relevant to have (a) skills for understanding the relevance of those particular theological issues in the couple relationship and (b) self-awareness of how their own SERT orientation and countertransference reactions might influence their approach to the differences in this case.

Yet another clinical situation can arise with clients who self-define as neither "spiritual" nor "religious" and without obvious commitments to theological traditions but present with concerns about various existential themes, such as loss, death, guilt, despair, or difficult choices in the face of ambiguous outcomes. The existential dimension of SERT might be the most inclusive in referencing human dilemmas of finitude and struggles with meaning that can be found both inside and beyond spiritual, religious, and theological contexts (Sandage et al., 2020; Yalom, 1980). While it is possible for clinicians to interpret existential dimensions of human life quite broadly, it is also important to recognize some clients may hold a pragmatic focus about treatment and a lack of personal interest in any of the SERT dimensions as they understand them (Sandage et al., 2022).

It is also important to note that SERT dynamics can be complicated to negotiate in therapy even when therapists and clients both identify with the same general SERT tradition or orientation (e.g., atheist, Buddhist, Christian). There is diversity within every SERT tradition and orientation. Moreover, it is possible for clinicians to sometimes experience stronger countertransference in working with some clients who hold SERT values closer to their own. This could result from complicated personal feelings and opinions about issues that emerge and greater self-consciousness about trying to manage those responses. But it is worth remembering that a general therapist–client "match" on SERT identifications, like other areas of diversity, will still require therapist self-awareness and diversity competence in navigating SERT issues.

In this edited volume, we did not give the chapter authors specific definitions of SERT dimensions; rather, we asked authors to locate themselves and share the ways particular SERT traditions and values inform their practice of psychotherapy. We sought out a diverse group of clinician-scholars who are intentional about integrating SERT dynamics into psychotherapy to offer insights into the differing forms this can take and illuminate the healing influence of various traditions. In this way, the present volume is intended to complement other resources, such as the *Handbook of Psychotherapy and Religious Diversity* (Richards & Bergin, 2014), by showing some of the differing ways clinicians seek to integrate their particular SERT traditions and values with their preferred theories of psychotherapy into spiritually integrative approaches. We also selected authors who have differing therapy orientations but hold a shared emphasis on interpersonal process and the therapeutic alliance as key sources of gain in psychotherapy, which is a needed area for development in the literature on spiritually integrated psychotherapy.

SPIRITUALLY INTEGRATED PSYCHOTHERAPY

This brings us to the topic of spiritually integrated psychotherapy. To date, the growing literature on spirituality and religion in psychotherapy has tended to focus sizable attention on the use of specific spiritual or religious practices (e.g., mindfulness, other forms of meditation, prayer, forgiveness, yoga, gratitude; see Aten et al., 2011). The consideration of specific practices and clinical techniques or interventions has been a useful pathway toward the integration of spirituality and religion into relatively established treatment approaches. There are also other excellent volumes on related clinical topic areas, such as spirituality and the treatment of trauma (Park et al., 2017; Walker et al., 2015) or spirituality and family therapy (Walsh, 2009, 2019). Pargament (2011) has also been a leader in this field by offering a research-informed model of spiritually integrated psychotherapy that views spiritual and psychological dynamics as mutually interactive for many clients, and he also outlined a coherent theory of therapeutic change that engages both spiritual and psychological dynamics. Pargament's approach to *spiritually integrated psychotherapy* moves beyond specific techniques, modalities, or problem areas toward the integration of (a) psychotherapy theory, (b) in-depth awareness of SERT traditions and values, and (c) specific clinical strategies for intentionally engaging clients' spiritual and religious dynamics in ways that are intended to be theoretically and clinically coherent. Based on this multidimensional definition of spiritually integrated psychotherapy, we note that numerous different models and approaches have been published (e.g., Al-Karam, 2018; Bland & Strawn, 2014; Cashwell & Young, 2014; Frankel, 2003; Jennings, 2010; Johnson, 2013; Jones, 2019; Knabb, 2016; Linehan, 2015; McMinn & Campbell, 2007; Richards & Bergin, 2005; Rosmarin, 2018; Sandage et al., 2020; Sorenson, 2004; Sperry, 2011; Starr, 2008; Worthington & Sandage, 2016). These approaches differ in numerous ways, including (a) varied combinations of theoretical orientations and SERT influences and (b) applications to clients from particular spiritual and religious traditions versus applications to more general client populations.

This consideration of spiritually integrated psychotherapy models and applications invites reflection on the question of whether any approaches to psychotherapy are actually spiritually and religiously neutral. Browning and Cooper (2004) offered rich and insightful interdisciplinary insights into the ways theories in psychology and psychotherapy are built not only on the descriptive sciences of human behavior but also on what they called "metaphors of ultimacy" (p. 15), or ideals of functioning that are actually more ethical and religious than purely scientific. These ideals are sometimes cloaked in scientific language that might seem more palatable to modern sensibilities, but they argued that models of therapy will inevitably rest on certain values and assumptions about human nature that are philosophical or even theological. We share their hermeneutical or late modern view that this is not an inherent problem and that it is more problematic when we who are professional therapists deny or remain unaware of the influence of specific values and ideals on our approaches to our clinical practice. If I am aware of and can articulate my ideals and values, I am in a better position to work at negotiating across differences with clients and colleagues who hold other ideals and values. However, if I pretend that my clinical approach is purely objective and devoid of any connections to particular SERT traditions, principles, or values, I might run the risk of imposing my values and perspectives without awareness of the ways they do not fit for others.

But beyond this problem of bias or SERT microaggression, we want to affirm the benefits of maintaining respectful connections to the deep wisdom on healing and growth to be found in the diverse array of sociocultural and SERT traditions that have been part of efforts at the therapeutic throughout human evolution. The authors of this volume describe a diversity of approaches to spiritually integrative psychotherapy that draw on both ancient and contemporary wisdom, and we think there is great advantage in this kind of reflection and transparency related to SERT dynamics.

PERSON OF THE THERAPIST

Many psychotherapy approaches have emphasized the personal qualities or self of the therapist as central to therapeutic effectiveness. Therapist effects are emerging in psychotherapy research as a significant source of variance predicting outcomes (Constantino et al., 2017). Moreover, there is evidence that therapists do not tend to improve in effectiveness over time combined with concerning findings about risks for burnout (Goldberg et al., 2016). This raises important questions about therapist strengths, virtues, and personal values that might contribute to both effectiveness and resilient capacities to continue to find clinical work meaningful despite chronic exposure to suffering (Jankowski et al., 2020). Psychotherapy is a difficult vocation, and we think it is crucial to understand some of the formative processes and life-giving values that can sustain hopeful practice among different clinicians.

In this book, we invited authors to share some of their personal SERT journeys as they have impacted their clinical approaches. A previous project that tasked master clinicians to reveal connections among their own lives, their SERT values and perspectives, and their clinical work proved to be immensely rewarding through an Albert & Jessie Danielsen Institute conference and a prior edited volume (Stavros & Sandage, 2014). Clinical scholars in this earlier project, including some authors in this present book, have noted it was refreshing to be transparent about the influence of their core values. At this time of extreme polarization and conflict in the United States and many parts of the world, we are encouraged share the work of clinicians who value diversity as a sacred value and are eager to learn from colleagues from diverse SERT traditions.

The meta-analytic review of research on the spiritually and religiously adapted therapies cited earlier (Captari et al., 2018) noted the need for further attention to such therapies (a) with complex "real world" diversity dynamics and "adaptations to other major world religions and spiritual traditions beyond Christianity" (Captari et al., 2018, p. 1948), (b) that are integrated with a variety of theoretical orientations beyond the cognitive behavior models that dominate this research literature, and (c) that illuminate interpersonal process factors that interact with spiritual and religious dynamics. Rather than report original empirical studies, the present volume has a primarily clinical focus. However, as we unpack in the concluding chapter, we hope this project offers clinical models and applications that can serve to advance both research and practice in spiritually integrated psychotherapy in ways that address some of the prior gaps.

OVERVIEW OF THIS BOOK

This book is organized into two main sections. In Part I, eight clinician-scholars articulate the ways their unique approaches to spiritually integrated psychotherapy are shaped by their SERT traditions, values, and experiences as illustrated in clinical case descriptions. Each author shares information on their own SERT background and narrative as it has influenced their clinical approach for engaging the sacred in psychotherapy in the context of human diversity.

In Chapter 1, Pratyusha Tummala-Narra provides an overview of diversity within Hindu spirituality and describes the influences of her Hindu background on her clinical work as illustrated in a case study with a young Indian American man struggling with anxiety. In Chapter 2, Ken Pargament reflects on the influence of both his Jewish background and other SERT traditions on the development of his model of spiritually integrative psychotherapy in the field of psychology, which he applies to case vignettes of individual and couples therapy. In Chapter 3, Pilar Jennings relays her personal journey toward Tibetan Buddhism and her integration of Buddhist traditions into her approach to psychotherapy, including an in-depth case description with a Roman Catholic client. In Chapter 4, Phillis Sheppard describes ways her personal SERT background and move toward womanist traditions have shaped her approach to spiritually integrative psychotherapy, and she offers two contrasting case examples to reveal both clinical struggles and effectiveness. In Chapter 5, Shamaila Khan shares intersections between her multinational background and her Sufi Islam tradition as they influence her approaches to both psychotherapy and international disaster relief work in diverse religious contexts. In Chapter 6, Brad Strawn integrates his evangelical Christian Wesleyan theological tradition with a relational approach to psychotherapy applied to a case with an Eastern Orthodox and Armenian client. In Chapter 7, Karen Starr connects the Jewish mystical tradition of Kabbalah to her clinical approach and view of transformation as illustrated in a case of depressed atheist client. In Chapter 8, Theresa Clement Tisdale offers an integration of Roman Catholic spirituality and theology with psychotherapy applied to a case study of a client struggling with anxiety and interpersonal issues.

Part II focuses on spiritually integrated psychotherapy with specific diversity dynamics. As in Part I, six clinician–scholars share how their SERT traditions and values inform their psychotherapeutic approaches with specific diversity issues. Again, the goal is not for authors to try to describe a generic approach that would fit all clinicians. Rather, the authors seek to convey some of their own unique integration of SERT dynamics, psychotherapy theory and intervention strategy, and case illustrations related to a particular set of intersectional diversity dynamics.

In Chapter 9, Ruben Hopwood considers ways religion and spirituality intersect with nontraditional gender identities in psychotherapy and offers several case applications of his spiritually integrated gender-affirming approach. In Chapter 10, Sarah Moon thematizes authenticity, desire, and power in spiritually integrated psychotherapy with lesbian, gay, bisexual, and queer clients. In Chapter 11, I (S.J.S.) consider religious differences in couples therapy and apply a relational spirituality model to couples cases involving struggles with attachment, differentiation, and intersubjectivity. In Chapter 12, Katy Barrs and Carrie Doehring take an intercultural and process theology approach to spiritually integrated trauma treatment for military moral injury with an in-depth case description of a biracial older adult client. In Chapter 13, Neil Altman reflects on the intersections among spirituality, social class, and diverse understandings of healing as they have impacted his own clinical work in various contexts and in mental health fields, more generally. Our concluding chapter puts forward a set of key themes and clinical dilemmas related to spiritually integrated psychotherapy and diversity that have emerged in this book and highlight future research directions. We also outline a set of considerations and reflection questions for readers who want to pursue growth in spiritual and religious competence and humility.

REFERENCES

The Albert & Jessie Danielsen Institute. (n.d.). *SERT: Spiritual, existential, religious, and theological concerns in clinical practice.* http://www.bu.edu/danielsen/clinical-training-sert-spiritual-existential-religious-theological-groups-for-clinical-practice/

Al-Karam, C. Y. (Ed.). (2018). *Islamically integrated psychotherapy: Uniting faith and professional practice.* Templeton Press.

Aten, J. D., McMinn, M. R., & Worthington, E. L., Jr. (2011). *Spiritually oriented interventions for counseling and psychotherapy.* American Psychological Association. https://doi.org/10.1037/12313-000

Bland, E. D., & Strawn, B. D. (Eds.). (2014). *Christianity & psychoanalysis: A new conversation.* InterVarsity Press.

Browning, D. S., & Cooper, T. D. (2004). *Religious thought and the modern psychologies.* Fortress Press.

Captari, L. E., Hook, J. N., Hoyt, W., Davis, D. E., McElroy-Heltzel, S. E., & Worthington, E. L., Jr. (2018). Integrating clients' religion and spirituality within psychotherapy: A comprehensive meta-analysis. *Journal of Clinical Psychology, 74*(11), 1938–1951. https://doi.org/10.1002/jclp.22681

Cashwell, C. S., & Young, J. S. (Eds.). (2014). *Integrating spirituality and religion into counseling: A guide to competent practice* (2nd ed.). American Counseling Association.

Constantino, M. J., Boswell, J. F., Coyne, A. E., Kraus, D. R., & Castonguay, L. G. (2017). Who works for whom and why? Integrating therapist effects analysis into psychotherapy outcome and process research. In L. G. Castonguay & C. E. Hill (Eds.), *How and why are some therapists better than others? Understanding therapist effects* (pp. 55–68). American Psychological Association. https://doi.org/10.1037/0000034-004

Crabtree, S. A., Bell, C. A., Rupert, D. A., Sandage, S. J., Devor, N. G., & Stavros, G. (2021). Humility, differentiation of self, and clinical training in spiritual and religious competence. *Journal of Spirituality in Mental Health, 23*(4), 342–362. https://doi.org/10.1080/19349637.2020.1737627

Cragun, C. L., & Friedlander, M. L. (2012). Experiences of Christian clients in secular psychotherapy: A mixed-methods investigation. *Journal of Counseling Psychology, 59*(3), 379–391. https://doi.org/10.1037/a0028283

Davis, D. E., DeBlaere, C., Owen, J., Hook, J. N., Rivera, D. P., Choe, E., Van Tongeren, D. R., Worthington, E. L., & Placeres, V. (2018). The multicultural orientation framework: A narrative review. *Psychotherapy, 55*(1), 89–100. https://doi.org/10.1037/pst0000160

Frankel, E. (2003). *Sacred therapy: Jewish spiritual teachings on emotional healing and inner wholeness.* Shambhala.

Goldberg, S. B., Rousmaniere, T., Miller, S. D., Whipple, J., Nielsen, S. L., Hoyt, W. T., & Wampold, B. E. (2016). Do psychotherapists improve with time and experience?

A longitudinal analysis of outcomes in a clinical setting. *Journal of Counseling Psychology, 63*(1), 1–11. https://doi.org/10.1037/cou0000131

Harris, K. A., Randolph, B. E., & Gordon, T. D. (2016). What do clients want? Assessing spiritual needs in counseling: A literature review. *Spirituality in Clinical Practice, 3*(4), 250–275. https://doi.org/10.1037/scp0000108

Hook, J. N., Davis, D., Owen, J., & DeBlaere, C. (2017). *Cultural humility: Engaging diverse identities in therapy.* American Psychological Association. https://doi.org/10.1037/0000037-000

Jankowski, P. J., Sandage, S. J., Bell, C. A., Davis, D. E., Porter, E., Jessen, M., Motzny, C. L., Ross, K. V., & Owen, J. (2020). Virtue, flourishing, and positive psychology in psychotherapy: An overview and research prospectus. *Psychotherapy, 57*(3), 291–309. https://doi.org/10.1037/pst0000285

Jennings, P. (2010). *Mixing minds: The power of relationship in psychoanalysis and Buddhism.* Wisdom Publications.

Johnson, R. (2013). *Spirituality in counseling and psychotherapy: An integrative approach that empowers clients.* John Wiley & Sons, Inc.

Jones, R. S. (2019). *Spirit in session: Working with your client's spirituality (and your own) in psychotherapy.* Templeton Press.

Knabb, J. J. (2016). *Faith-based ACT for Christian clients.* Routledge Press. https://doi.org/10.4324/9781315670744

Koenig, H. G. (2018). *Religion and mental health: Research and clinical applications.* Academic Press.

Linehan, M. (2015). *DBT skills training manual.* The Guilford Press.

McMinn, M. R., & Campbell, C. D. (2007). *Integrative psychotherapy: Toward a comprehensive Christian approach.* InterVarsity Press.

Owen, J., Tao, K. W., Drinane, J. M., Hook, J., Davis, D. E., & Kune, N. F. (2016). Client perceptions of therapists' multicultural orientation: Cultural (missed) opportunities and cultural humility. *Professional Psychology: Research and Practice, 47*(1), 30–37. https://doi.org/10.1037/pro0000046

Oxhandler, H. K., Ellor, J. W., & Stanford, M. S. (2018). Client attitudes toward integrating religion and spirituality in mental health treatment: Scale development and client responses. *Social Work, 63*(4), 337–346. https://doi.org/10.1093/sw/swy041

Pargament, K. I. (2011). *Spiritually integrated psychotherapy: Understanding and addressing the sacred.* Guilford Press.

Pargament, K. I., & Exline, J. J. (2021). Religious and spiritual struggles and mental health: Implications for clinical practice. In A. Moreira-Almeida, B. P. Mosqueiro, & D. Bhugra (Eds.), *Spirituality and mental health across cultures* (pp. 395–412). Oxford University Press.

Park, C. L., Currier, J. M., Harris, J. I., & Slattery, J. M. (2017). *Trauma, meaning, and spirituality: Translating research into clinical practice.* American Psychological Association. https://doi.org/10.1037/15961-000

Richards, P. S., & Bergin, A. E. (2005). *A spiritual strategy for counseling and psychotherapy* (2nd ed.). American Psychological Association. https://doi.org/10.1037/11214-000

Richards, P. S., & Bergin, A. E. (Eds.). (2014). *Handbook of psychotherapy and religious diversity* (2nd ed.). American Psychological Association. https://doi.org/10.1037/14371-000

Rosmarin, D. H. (2018). *Spirituality, religion, and cognitive-behavioral therapy: A guide for clinicians.* Guilford Press.

Rupert, D., Moon, S. H., & Sandage, S. J. (2019). Clinical training groups for spirituality and religion in psychotherapy. *Journal of Spirituality in Mental Health, 21*(3), 163–177. https://doi.org/10.1080/19349637.2018.1465879

Sandage, S. J., Jankowski, P. J., Paine, D. R., Exline, J. J., Ruffing, E. G., Rupert, D., Stavros, G. S., & Bronstein, M. (2022). Testing a relational spirituality model of psychotherapy clients' preferences and functioning. *Journal of Spirituality in Mental Health, 24*(1), 1–21. https://doi.org/10.1080/19349637.2020.1791781

Sandage, S. J., Rupert, D., Stavros, G. S., & Devor, N. G. (2020). *Relational spirituality in psychotherapy: Healing suffering and promoting growth.* American Psychological Association. https://doi.org/10.1037/0000174-000

Sorenson, R. L. (2004). *Minding spirituality.* The Analytic Press.

Sorenson, R. L., & Hales, S. (2002). Comparing evangelical Protestant psychologists trained at secular versus religiously affiliated programs. *Psychotherapy, 39*(2), 163–170. https://doi.org/10.1037/0033-3204.39.2.163

Sperry, L. (2011). *Spirituality in clinical practice: Theory and practice of spiritually oriented psychotherapy* (2nd ed.). Routledge. https://doi.org/10.4324/9780203893876

Starr, K. E. (2008). *Repair of the soul: Metaphors of transformation in Jewish mysticism and psychoanalysis.* Routledge.

Stavros, G. S., & Sandage, S. J. (Eds.). (2014). *The skillful soul of the psychotherapist: The link between spirituality and clinical excellence.* Rowman & Littlefield.

Tervalon, M., & Murray-García, J. (1998). Cultural humility versus cultural competence: A critical distinction in defining physician training outcomes in multicultural education. *Journal of Health Care for the Poor and Underserved, 9*(2), 117–125. https://doi.org/10.1353/hpu.2010.0233

Vieten, C., & Scammell, S. (2015). *Spiritual and religious competencies in clinical practice: Guidelines for psychotherapists and mental health professionals.* New Harbinger Publications.

Vieten, C., Scammell, S., Pierce, A., Pilato, R., Ammondson, I., Pargament, K. I., & Lukoff, D. (2016). Competencies for psychologists in the domains of religion and spirituality. *Spirituality in Clinical Practice, 3*(2), 92–114. https://doi.org/10.1037/scp0000078

Vogel, M. J., McMinn, M. R., Peterson, M. A., & Gathercoal, K. A. (2013). Examining religion and spirituality as diversity training: A multidimensional look at training in the American Psychological Association. *Professional Psychology: Research and Practice, 44*(3), 158–167. https://doi.org/10.1037/a0032472

Walker, D. F., Courtois, C. A., & Aten, J. D. (Eds.). (2015). *Spiritually oriented psychotherapy for trauma* (pp. 29–54). American Psychological Association. https://doi.org/10.1037/14500-000

Walsh, F. (Ed.). (2009). *Spiritual resources in family therapy* (2nd ed.). Guilford Press.

Walsh, F. (2019). Spirituality, suffering, and resilience. In M. McGoldrick & K. V. Hardy (Eds.), *Re-visioning family therapy: Addressing diversity in clinical practice* (3rd ed., pp. 73–90). The Guilford Press.

Worthington, E. L., Jr., & Sandage, S. J. (2016). *Forgiveness and spirituality in psychotherapy: A relational approach.* American Psychological Association. https://doi.org/10.1037/14712-000

Yalom, I. D. (1980). *Existential psychotherapy.* Basic Books.

PART **I**
SPIRITUALLY
INTEGRATED
APPROACHES TO
PSYCHOTHERAPY

1 HINDU SPIRITUALITY AND PSYCHOANALYTIC PSYCHOTHERAPY

PRATYUSHA TUMMALA-NARRA

Public rhetoric and tensions related to religion stand in contrast with silence on religion and spirituality in psychology and psychotherapy. Within psychoanalysis, these issues have long been neglected, even though psychoanalytic inquiry and spiritual inquiry both emphasize meaning making, a growing awareness of the self, and authenticity (Stone, 2005; Tummala-Narra, 2009). These shared goals are met through different conceptualizations and approaches to the human mind. In this chapter, I focus specifically on an approach to spiritually integrated psychotherapy that brings together Hindu and psychoanalytic perspectives.

Emotional suffering, from the perspective of Hinduism, is thought to be a product of karma, and suffering is viewed as an ordinary part of life that is to be endured with the aim of spiritual liberation (Whitman, 2007). There is a core belief in the intricate connection between the mind and body; therefore, healing and recovery involve developing one's control of thoughts and feelings that disrupt well-being. For example, the science and practice of Ayurveda and meditation aim to achieve balance across physical, psychological, and spiritual experiences within the self (Murthy, 2010; Sharma &

https://doi.org/10.1037/0000276-002
Spiritual Diversity in Psychotherapy: Engaging the Sacred in Clinical Practice,
S. J. Sandage and B. D. Strawn (Editors)

Tummala-Narra, 2014). Among many Hindus, psychotherapy is seen as a type of healing that is sought only when spiritual approaches are not effective, even though psychotherapy shares common ground with Hindu spirituality in its emphasis on introspection and understanding of the self in relation to the external world. In this chapter, I describe a framework for integrating spirituality with psychoanalytic psychotherapy. This framework is influenced by my experience as a Hindu Indian American woman who has experienced transformations in the experience of Hindu spirituality since the time of migrating to the United States as a child. I elaborate on the influence of my spirituality on my work with patients in a discussion of theoretical developments in psychoanalysis and through a case illustration.

HINDU SPIRITUALITY

Hinduism is practiced by more than 750 million people across the world (with the majority in South Asia), and North America has an approximately 1.25 million Hindus (Bhagwan, 2012; Sharma & Tummala-Narra, 2014). Across the Hindu diaspora, religion and spirituality hold a wide array of meanings. As such, it is important to consider that interpretations of religious philosophy, traditions, and practices vary across and within regions of South Asia and across and within the diaspora. Furthermore, Hinduism is both an ancient and modern religion that is deeply complex with regard to doctrine whose interpretations are inextricable from cultural context (Sharma & Tummala-Narra, 2014). Therefore, Hindu spirituality is both individually and contextually determined, and it plays a significant role in the everyday lives of many people in the Indian and South Asian diaspora.

Scholars have noted that views of health and wellness continue to be rooted in religious understandings and that spiritual practices are critical to coping with mental illness and emotional issues both within India and within the Indian diaspora (Suchday et al., 2018). In particular, spiritual beliefs in moksha, dharma, and karma often guide understandings of why a person experiences emotional suffering and what makes healing possible. As such, the following section provides a brief overview of these core beliefs within Hinduism.

Core Beliefs of Hinduism

Hinduism encompasses core beliefs, such as the divinity of sacred texts like the *Vedas* (*The Vedas*, ca. 1200 B.C.E./2017); the existence of one supreme being or *Brahman*, or God; the ongoing and endless cycle of creation, preservation, and destruction; the law of cause and effect (e.g., *karma*); reincarnation and *moksha*, that is, liberation of oneself from the cycle of birth, death, and rebirth; the central role of a *guru*, or a spiritual teacher; the sacredness of all life and the practice of *ahimsa*, or nonviolence; and the value of multiple spiritual paths that connect a person with God (Gupta, 2011). Because the complex philosophy of Hinduism is beyond the scope of this chapter, I focus on a few salient aspects that have a pervasive impact on the everyday lives of Hindus.

A central message of the Hindu scriptures (e.g., *Vedas* [*The Vedas*, ca. 1200 B.C.E./2017]; *Upanishads* [*The Upanishads*, ca. 1 B.C.E.–1400 C.E./2001]) is that God or Brahman is one entity that can be observed in multiple forms. Brahman is viewed as an existence without form that has no beginning and no end. The soul, or *Atman*, carries forth from one life to the next in the cycle of birth, death, and rebirth. A central spiritual quest of Hindus is to achieve moksha—liberation from this cycle—through self-realization. The cycle ends when a person is not reborn and the person's soul (Atman) is united with Brahman (Nagpal, 2011). Other conceptualizations of moksha involve liberation from pain and suffering in the present lifetime rather than only in the context of death of the physical body (Mishra, 2013). Ideally, one follows the path of *dharma*, or their duties to self and others, and does so within a framework of achieving moksha (Nagpal, 2011). Seeking moksha entails one's detachment from selfish desire, anger, and greed that result from excessive attachment to material possessions. R. C. Mishra (2013) pointed out that it is common for people in India to pray to Brahman/God before embarking on everyday tasks; for example, a surgeon offers prayers before performing a complex surgery or a businessperson prays before an important meeting or task. These actions reflect the importance of removing the influence of the ego on an individual's spiritual self (Mishra, 2013). In addition, one's actions are related to a belief in karma in which a person is responsible for one's own deeds and their accompanying consequences. In this view, people determine, at least in part, their own fate. Physical and psychological suffering is conceptualized as shaped by karma—not as a punishment but "as a natural and just consequence of the moral laws of the universe for past negative behaviour" (Anand, 2009, p. 818).

Hinduism also values the multiplicity of one's spiritual journey toward moksha and recognizes that people have different personality styles, so they may be more inclined toward a certain spiritual path or yoga. Four paths are described in the Hindu scriptures. One is *jnana yoga*, or the path of knowledge, in which a person contemplates and meditates in a way that moves one from a focus on the personal self to the Divine self. Another path is *bhakti yoga*, or the path of love and devotion, in which a person engages in devotion to Brahman/God as the beloved or love object through chanting of mantras and by holding a specific God image or aspect of God in one's mind and heart. Hinduism places value on the multitude of God images because people vary with respect to the extent to which they can emotionally connect with or admire certain aspects of God. A third path is *karma yoga*, or the path of service, in which a person focuses on service to others without selfish desire or attachment to results of their efforts. A fourth path described in the Hindu scriptures is *Raja yoga*, or the path of experimentation, in which a person engages in inquiry through meditation and experimentation as a way of attaining a deep understanding of human nature beyond what they can assess through their emotions, physical senses, and intellect (Sharma & Tummala-Narra, 2014; Varambally & Gangadhar, 2012). Each of these four paths is thought to result in moksha and unity with the Divine (Brahman). Spirituality among Hindus is further thought to move through four developmental stages: (a) a student who focuses on developing character; (b) a householder who focuses on family, work, and community; (c) a retired individual who moves inward with contemplation of life; and (d) a *sannyas*, that is, an individual who gains spiritual freedom with no attachments or expectations (Sharma & Tummala-Narra, 2014).

Hindu philosophy is traditionally taught through mythological stories about different God forms and through epics. For example, dharma is a concept that is elucidated through epics, such as the *Ramayana (The Rāmāyana of Vālmīki*, ca. 5th century B.C.E./2021) and the *Mahabharata (The Mahābhārata*, ca. 400 B.C.E./2015), which remain as key textual guides to understanding and approaching the complexities of life. The *Srimad Bhagavad-Gita* (n.d.; hereafter, *Gita*), which translates to English from Sanskrit as the "Song of the Lord," is situated within the epic *Mahabharata* in which God, in the manifestation of Krishna, engages in a critical dialogue with Arjuna, a prince who is overwhelmed by grief and confusion in the face of battle against his cousins among other kin. Krishna reminds Arjuna that he is a warrior whose dharma (duty) is to fight in the battle to destroy the power of a treacherous enemy. Krishna also describes the cycle of life, death, and rebirth to Arjuna—specifically, that the Atman (soul) is eternal (Nagpal, 2011) and how karma is the force behind rebirth (Anand, 2009). This dialogue between Krishna and Arjuna reflects the importance placed on the guru (spiritual teacher). The relationship with one's guru is sacred because this relationship is the context in which a disciple receives divine teachings of religious texts, such as the *Gita*. In the *Mahabharata*, Krishna is both a manifestation of God and Arjuna's guru.

My Spiritual Journey

Individual pathways of Hindu spirituality are highly varied and contextually determined. My journey as a Hindu is closely connected with aspects of Hinduism transmitted through my family and community both in India and in the United States as well as with the context of immigration. I emigrated to the United States from India with my family in the 1970s, a time during which there was little access to Hindu temples and to interactions with a large Indian or Indian American community. Before leaving India when I was 7 years old, I had been living in a large city with a diverse population with regard to religion and spirituality. My neighbors and friends were Hindu, Muslim, Christian, and Sikh. Interestingly, the first several years after moving to the United States, I lived in New York City, where I also interacted with people from diverse religious and cultural backgrounds, and I attended a Catholic elementary school. A value of respect for different faith traditions was implicitly and explicitly communicated in my family even while tensions persisted between Hindus and Muslims in India and Christians and Jews in the United States. Relocating to the United States further allowed for an exchange of cultural and religious viewpoints, involving my navigation not only across Indian and American contexts but also across Hinduism (at home) and Christianity (at school). Over the course of my upbringing, I lived in different communities in which I would later have more access to Hindu communities and places of worship.

It is worth considering the role of religion and spirituality in the immigrant context because faith and migration are intertwined for many immigrants. Researchers and clinical theorists have observed the shifts in identity and relationships that take place among different immigrant communities (Akhtar, 2011). Religion and spirituality help many immigrants to imagine their birth countries and "inscribe their memories and worldviews into the physical landscape and built environment" (Vásquez, 2005, p. 238), and they also help immigrants to make meaning of cultural change. In the new country, immigrants integrate religion in everyday life by creating homes with religious and cultural symbols and objects, and through religious organizations and communities, which offer a critical space for spiritual practices, continuity with cultural traditions, and connection with others (Akhtar, 2011; Mazumdar & Mazumdar, 2009).

Religion and spirituality play an essential role for many immigrants in coping with separation from loved ones and with sustaining hope in a new and unfamiliar cultural space. (Abu-Raiya & Pargament, 2015). In some cases, immigrants may adhere even more strongly to religious traditions and practices in the United States than in the country of origin as a way of preserving religious and cultural identity for themselves and for their children (Akhtar, 2011). In both South Asian countries and in the United States, for Hindus, a sense of individual striving for spiritual fulfillment coexists with a collectivistic focus on social cohesion, particularly that within the family (Suchday et al., 2018). Despite the influence of globalization on religion and culture, many first- and second-generation Hindu Americans adhere to a sense of responsibility to family religious and cultural beliefs. Rashmi Gupta (2011), in a qualitative study with Hindu Indian American young adults, middle-aged adults, and older adults, found that all three generations reported believing in Hindu concepts, such as karma, although the extent of engaging in traditional practices varied with immigrant generation. The study highlighted the importance of both retaining religious and cultural identities among all generations of Hindu Indian Americans and recognizing the diversity of religious experience across the three generations. Indeed, in my own experience, Indian cultural identity and Hindu spiritual identity are interconnected and transmitted intergenerationally such that there are distinctions in the way that my grandparents, parents, children, and I experience and practice Hinduism. Nevertheless, across these generations, our Hindu Indian identities are critical to our ability to remain connected to our heritage and the broader Hindu and Indian diaspora.

While recognizing that significant diversity exists in what different Hindu families conceive as core to their religious traditions, I next describe more closely the specific aspects of Hinduism that have guided my spiritual life and my perspective as a psychoanalytic psychologist. Through my parents and grandparents, I learned the importance of prayer and devotion (bhakti yoga) and service to others (karma yoga). As a family, we prayed in our home as well as in a temple. We placed emphasis on others' needs before our own needs, which was connected to the value of serving others. Throughout my childhood and much of my adolescence, I followed the traditions passed on by my parents, such as wearing a *bindi* (a dot—a sacred symbol—worn typically by women in the middle of the forehead); wearing Indian clothing to the temple; and participating in *pujas*, that is, prayer ceremonies. As a young person, I experienced Hindu rituals as both comforting and constricting. For example, hearing prayers sung by my grandparents and great-grandparents helped me to connect with a collective sense of spirituality shared by my family and broader community, and yet other traditions, such as the restriction of women attending temples or pujas while menstruating, felt constricting and discriminatory. These contradictory experiences of being a Hindu posed deeper questions about identity and justice.

As I grew into adulthood, I began to develop a more personal form of spirituality. I immersed myself in reading the *Gita* (n.d.) and other Hindu texts, and I increasingly turned my attention to the philosophical underpinnings of Hinduism. Although I continued to pray and deepen my commitment to the value of serving others, I moved away from some family traditions and rituals, such as wearing a bindi, conducting certain pujas, and observing the restriction concerning menstruation. I also rejected the notion of caste and view it as an oppressive mechanism that diminishes the core of Hinduism, including the view of God as pervading all life, and the value of compassion. I return to a more in-depth discussion of caste in a later section.

Through my immersion in reading Hindu philosophy, I became more interested in the practice of meditation, and paralleling my graduate training in clinical psychology, I engaged more with introspection and self-knowledge. I increasingly attended to the role of self-reflection and of connecting with a spiritual dimension of human life that encompassed something or someone beyond the material world and beyond what may be observable to others. Developing a more personal sense of faith and relationship with God has helped me to feel better grounded and better able to cope with stress and suffering. Exploring this new way of relating to God, distinct in some ways from that of my family, entailed both a connection with the Hindu heritage of my family and a spiritual individuation (Miller, 2013). This individuation process, developed through reading and contemplation, has been essential to forming a religious and spiritual identity unique to my own experiences. My journey has continued to progress over the years with the passage of some Hindu spiritual traditions to my children through the reading of Hindu mythological stories, attendance at spiritual classes, discussion of Hindu beliefs, and prayer at home.

My Hindu spirituality through my early 20s was, at least on the surface level, disconnected from psychology. After completing my training in clinical psychology, I became more attentive to how my spirituality intersected with my desire to understand conflict and alleviate suffering. My Hindu spirituality has shaped my constructions of identity, conflict, and relational life within the context of psychotherapy. Along with psychoanalytic theory, it has shaped my therapeutic approach.

THE ROLE OF PSYCHOANALYTIC THEORY

Historically, religion and spirituality have been largely dismissed by psychoanalysts. Sigmund Freud (1927/1989) conceptualized religious and spiritual experience as an "illusion" and connected this experience with neurosis and with defense mechanisms, such as rationalization, used to cope with suffering. He further linked a belief in God with the Oedipal conflict in which

God representations are reflected in a child's relationship with the father. Although it has been well documented that Freud was unwilling to consider the validity of religious and cultural specifics of human experience, it is interesting to consider that Freud's own Jewish background played a significant role in the development of psychoanalysis, such as the role of interpretation as a technique that parallels the reading of *The Torah* (1962/2015; Aron & Starr, 2013). His commitment to establishing psychoanalysis as a positivistic discipline set the tone for a dominant perspective within psychoanalysis and mental health disciplines more broadly, whereby religion and spirituality would remain largely disconnected from the therapeutic encounter (Tummala-Narra, 2016).

Freud's views of religion have been challenged by psychoanalysts, existential and humanistic theorists, feminists, and multicultural psychologists, among others. Carl Jung (1938), perhaps among the most well-known among early psychoanalysts who emphasized spirituality, developed the concept of the *collective unconscious*, arguing that spiritual experience is a core experience of human beings. However, Jung's views have been criticized for exoticizing Eastern and Native American spirituality (Tummala-Narra, 2009). With respect to the interface between Freud and Hinduism, it is notable that Freud had a long-standing correspondence with Girindrashekhar Bose, a psychiatrist who was developing psychoanalytic ideas in India almost independently of Freud. In 1921, Bose published his book *Concept of Repression* in which he presented his theory of opposite wishes. For Bose, every unconscious wish exists with a counterpart, such as the wish to love coexisting with a wish to be loved. Unconscious conflict is then resolved by engaging with these multiple wishes, developing a compromise formation, or by fulfilling one of the opposing wishes even while the effects of the repressed wish persist (Akhtar & Tummala-Narra, 2005). Bose initiated a correspondence with Freud in 1921 that would last until 1937. While the correspondence was cordial, Freud largely dismissed the points raised by Bose with regard to psychoanalytic concepts, such as castration threat, and how these concepts were experienced differently within the Hindu Indian context (Akhtar & Tummala-Narra, 2005). Although Bose had been developing a theory that was closely tied to Hindu philosophy, Freud questioned the role of religion. This correspondence is one among many illustrations of how the cultural specificity of psychoanalytic ideas became marginalized in Western contexts (Akhtar & Tummala-Narra, 2005).

In Europe, object relations theorists posed new conceptualizations of religion and spirituality in which God representations play a significant role in intrapsychic and interpersonal life. Harry Guntrip (1957), for example, proposed that the ways in which religion is transmitted from one generation to the next shape how God is experienced emotionally—that is, as either a loving being or one who is to be feared. The concept of transitional space proposed by Donald Winnicott (1971) further extended the potential of psychoanalysis with regard to exploring spiritual experience. *Transitional space* refers to subjective experience that lies between internal and external realities, a realm that reflects an individual's own unique subjectivity (Winnicott, 1971). The possibility of subjective experience that lies along this third dimension has served as an impetus for new psychoanalytic conceptualizations of religion and spirituality in Europe and the United States. For example, Ana-Maria Rizzuto (2004), drawing from Winnicott's (1971) concept of transitional space, proposed that God representations are intrapsychically significant (Tummala-Narra, 2009). In addition to the object relations theorists, Erich Fromm and colleagues integrated aspects of Zen Buddhism into psychoanalysis (Fromm et al., 1960). They proposed that psychoanalysis broaden its understanding beyond symptom resolution, character, and psychopathology; they also proposed that Buddhist spirituality offered the ability to transcend the duality of the subject and object such that an object could be seen from the inside (Roland, 2017).

Over the past several decades, psychoanalytic scholars have been increasingly interested in engaging with spirituality from various traditions. Interestingly, however, many of these scholars have noted the conflicts they experienced regarding their ability to write openly about the role of their religious traditions on their psychotherapeutic work. Specifically, they have shared that openly discussing their religious beliefs within the profession has often produced anxiety and conflict because that engagement posed a threat to a secular and scientific approach to psychoanalysis (Aron, 2004; Rizzuto, 2004; Roland, 2006; Safran, 2003). Although silence on religion and spirituality continues to marginalize a core experience for many therapists and clients, these scholars have challenged psychoanalytic therapists to engage with religion and spirituality to develop new conceptualizations and approaches to psychotherapy.

Ana-Maria Rizzuto (2004) wrote about how her experiences as a Catholic and as a psychoanalyst helped her to value self-inquiry, the role of symbolism, and the role of transformation in the context of sharing one's wrong doing and suffering. Lew Aron (2004) explored the impact of the relational aspects of Jewish traditions on his contributions to relational psychoanalysis, particularly the intersubjective nature of ones' relationship to God. Alan Roland (2017) noted that in his therapeutic practice that the phenomenological self, which is typically what is explored in psychoanalysis, intersects with the spiritual self in complex ways. He further described how his practice of meditation has helped him to become more comfortable with ambiguity and the unknown, more sensitive to his patients' feelings and his own feelings, and more intuitive in responding to patients. Importantly, these scholars—Aron (2004), Rizzuto (2004), Roland (2006), and Safran (2003)—have paved the way for ongoing inquiry and development in psychoanalysis, religion, and spirituality.

In my work, I have drawn from the contributions of these scholars and proposed that God representations and spiritual life are revised across the lifespan and that the presence of an "analytic third" (Ogden, 1994, p. 61), that is, God, in psychotherapy facilitates engagement with a spiritual dimension that is interconnected with other aspects of self. I have argued that religion and spirituality do not belong outside of analytic work but, rather, are an inherent part of the therapist's and client's intrapsychic life (Tummala-Narra, 2009). Drawing increasingly from relational psychoanalysis, I emphasize individual subjectivity and the intersubjective nature of relationships as core aspects of both spiritual life and psychoanalysis.

My own personal Hindu spirituality and clinical experience, as well as the contributions of psychoanalytic scholars, have shaped a new framework for culturally informed psychoanalytic psychotherapy. I have argued that attention to sociocultural issues, including religion and spirituality, become a core emphasis of psychoanalytic theory and practice. While scholars have examined specific aspects of identity and sociocultural context, cultural competence has not been included as a core feature of psychoanalytic work. In my view, *cultural competence* is defined from a psychoanalytic perspective as a "process of recognizing, understanding, and engaging with sociocultural context and its influence on intrapsychic and interpersonal processes, including the therapeutic relationship" (Tummala-Narra, 2016, p. 77). I view cultural competence as a dynamic process rather than only an outcome, and I recognize that moving toward cultural competence involves lifelong learning (Sue, 2001).

My framework for culturally informed psychoanalytic psychotherapy includes five areas of emphasis: (a) recognize clients' and therapists' indigenous cultural narrative as well as the conscious and unconscious meanings and motivations accompanying these narratives; (b) recognize the role of context in the use of language and the expression of affect in psychotherapy; (c) attend to how clients' experiences of social oppression and stereotyping influence the therapist, client, therapeutic process, and outcome; (d) recognize that culture is dynamic and that individuals negotiate complex, intersecting cultural identifications in both creative and adaptive ways and in

self-damaging ways; and (e) expand self-examination to include exploration of the effects of historical trauma and neglect of sociocultural issues in
psychoanalysis on present and future theory and practice (Tummala-Narra,
2016). In this framework, the emphasis on sociocultural context is thought
to be inextricable from any other aspect of psychoanalytic work, and, therefore, the therapeutic process must consider how context shapes how therapists and clients engage with each other.

I resonate with Alan Roland's (2017) observation that "our subjectivity
in the psychoanalytic, intersubjective relationship includes the dimension of
a spiritual self underlying our finite personal self" (p. 518). From this view,
psychoanalytic therapists have a responsibility to shift from early psychoanalytic conceptualizations of spiritual life as indicating psychopathology and
move toward recognition of the complexity of spiritual life. Spirituality and
religion encompass beliefs in a presence or absence of God or other non-
material beings, spirits, or forces that shape conscious and unconscious
experiences of self and others. As such, it behooves psychoanalytic therapists
to expand understandings of their clients' and their own religious and spiritual experiences. In my own journey of integrating spirituality in psychotherapy, I have found it helpful to draw on the contributions of relational
psychoanalysis.

Relational psychoanalysis is specifically shaped by interpersonal psychoanalysis, object relations theory, self-psychology, and intersubjective theories,
and it emphasizes individual subjectivity and interrelatedness (Barsness,
2018; Harris, 2011). From the relational perspective, multiple self-states
and shifts in self-states compose identity (Bromberg, 2006). Furthermore,
subjective experience is shaped within a broader social context in which
dynamics of race, gender, religion, social class, and immigration, among other
social locations, are reproduced in the therapeutic relationship (Harris,
2011; Yi, 2014). Relational psychoanalysis is also influenced by *social con-
structivism*, which emphasizes the interaction of the therapist's and client's
subjectivity, thus involving the mutual influence of the therapist and the
client in the co-construction of transference (Harris, 2011). Both here and
now moments in the therapeutic relationship and the repetition of past
experience are important areas of exploration within this perspective. In
integrating religion and spirituality in psychotherapy, both past and current
relational experiences associated with religion or spirituality are explored as
an essential part of identity and psychological well-being. Furthermore, the
therapist and the client each bring to the therapeutic relationship their own
personal religious and spiritual experiences and perspectives, which can be
transformative for both of them.

SPIRITUALLY INTEGRATED PSYCHOTHERAPY: HINDUISM AND PSYCHOANALYSIS

Psychoanalysis and religion have offered me two different lenses through which I can better understand human experience. Although psychoanalysis allows for an in-depth examination of unconscious life, there has been minimal discourse in Western psychoanalysis and psychology about Hindu spirituality. As such, I have found myself engaging in discussions about the unconscious mind with psychoanalytic psychologists that remained largely separated from discussions about Hinduism with friends and family. Nevertheless, psychoanalysis and Hinduism (as other spiritual traditions) share a common purpose of exploring an aspect of the self that lies outside of conscious awareness, developing insight through introspection, and forming a sense of interrelatedness with others.

Psychoanalysis and my Hindu spirituality intersect in my therapeutic work in several ways. The *Gita* (n.d.) has been an important source of self-knowledge for me since I was a young adult, guiding my understanding of conflict, suffering, and identity. As mentioned previously, the *Gita* is set within the context of an impending war among cousins—on one side, the Kauravas, and on the other side, the Pandavas—over the power to rule a kingdom. As the battle is about to start, Arjuna, a Pandava prince, is overcome by grief, anxiety, confusion, and conflict about killing his own family. Krishna, who is his friend and charioteer, and an incarnation of Vishnu, the God of Preservation, reveals his divine self to Arjuna and becomes his spiritual guide. The *Gita* is a dialogue between Krishna and Arjuna in which Krishna teaches Arjuna about the nature of reality and human nature, including the purpose of life, death, and rebirth. In the *Gita*, conflict is seen as a natural part of human life, rooted in bodily senses, emotions, and the intellect. Krishna offers Arjuna a perspective in which a person can free the self of grief, anger, and selfish desire through various paths (e.g., karma yoga, jnana yoga, bhakti yoga). He emphasizes the importance of controlling one's senses and releasing oneself from external gratification (Balodhi & Keshavan, 2011).

Furthermore, Krishna teaches Arjuna practical methods through which he can come to know his spiritual nature, beyond physical senses, feelings, and thoughts. In particular, he emphasizes engaging in meditation; performing selfless service; and seeking guidance from a learned, trusted guru. The guru–disciple relationship is considered to play a critical role in one's spiritual journey. It is important to note, however, that the guru role may be carried forth by a significant person in one's life, such as a parent or an older sibling, and not only necessarily by a formal teacher. In Arjuna's case,

Krishna is his friend, God, and guru. Krishna further models the guru–disciple relationship to Arjuna, allowing the freedom to question and to fully explore his thoughts and feelings. It is through this exploration that Arjuna is able to connect with his spiritual self.

The *Gita's* emphasis on inquiry of the different dimensions of the self resonates with psychoanalytic work. For example, the exploration of affect, in particular, is a core goal of psychoanalytic psychotherapy, as it is within Hinduism. However, although Hindu practices, such as meditation, move one toward a sense of connection to the Divine, psychoanalytic techniques, such as free association and the analysis of dreams and transference, move one toward recognizing affective and cognitive experiences that lie outside of conscious awareness and toward having a deeper understanding of the psychological self. I have found that each dimension of one's whole self (bodily, cognitive or intellectual, emotional, and spiritual) is a critically important area of inquiry in spiritually integrated psychotherapy.

My understanding of the *Gita* and engagement in practices, such as prayer and meditation, have deepened my appreciation for the ways in which these different dimensions interact and shape the psyche. While much of my training as a psychologist focused on conscious and unconscious affective and cognitive processes, my spiritual life has helped me to listen for other dimensions of the self and, more broadly, other perspectives that are less visible in psychology and psychoanalysis. For example, through integrating spirituality in psychotherapy, I am more aware of my clients' spiritual experiences as well as questions about God and the meaning and purpose of their lives. At times, my clients' discoveries regarding these questions are connected with unconscious conflicts related to early life experiences with religion and spirituality, and, in other moments, their discoveries are unrelated to unconscious conflict but, instead, reflect their conscious and unconscious experiences of nearness to or distance from a particular spiritual faith or tradition. Many clients have been taught to keep their spiritual experiences separate from their emotional or psychological concerns and to not speak about their spirituality with people outside of their faith traditions. However, it remains important to invite clients to share these spiritual experiences to create therapeutic space in which they can express all aspects of intrapsychic life more fully.

The freedom to choose one's spiritual path that is extended within Hinduism has further helped me to develop a sense of openness to my client's exploration of the self regardless of whether they practice any particular religious or spiritual tradition. The value of multiple spiritual paths has also helped me to recognize that clients enter psychotherapy at varying points of experience. Specifically, some clients seek help for physical distress (e.g., insufficient basic resources, such as housing and food; symptoms, such as insomnia and poor appetite), and others seek help to cope with overwhelming affect, intrusive thoughts, and loss of meaning and purpose, all of which can be related to loss, grief, and trauma. My Hindu spirituality has been critical to recognizing that each client has not only a unique set of experiences but also a unique pathway to healing.

From a psychoanalytic perspective, these experiences and pathways are linked with past relational experiences that have either expanded or constricted the range of possibilities in connecting with one's true self (Winnicott, 1971). As such, spiritually integrated therapy supports the exploration of the past as related to the present and the role of defenses in coping with emotional suffering, such as disappointment, betrayal, loss, and trauma. Winnicott (1971) suggested that a false self develops as a result of lack of empathy or maternal impingement such that an infant or child accommodates to the conscious and unconscious needs of the mother or the parents (Daehnert, 1998). The false self involves a constriction in spontaneity and creativity that is critical to development. In my perspective, the disconnection that accompanies a false self not only encompasses disconnection from one's own real feelings and thoughts but also an inhibition in the ability to make meaning of one's own experiences (i.e., spiritual self). For example, when clients share that they cannot access what they feel about a loss or a traumatic event, there is an implication that they are struggling with making sense of the experience. In other words, they are unable to connect with their whole self, including the physical, affective, cognitive, and spiritual aspects of the self. This disconnection can further affect how a person experiences God or a particular spiritual tradition, such as when someone questions why God allowed a traumatic loss of a loved one.

In Hinduism, making meaning of life experiences and of approaches to healing from suffering is often rooted in a belief in karma. Although there are multiple interpretations of karma, it typically is interpreted as the belief that every person faces the consequences of one's own actions (positive and negative) either within the present lifetime or in previous lives. This perspective is not fatalistic in the sense that external factors determine one's fate; rather, it places human beings as the drivers of their own fate (Anand, 2009). In Hinduism, Brahman/God is thought to be "a mere overseer of the proper functioning of the Law of Karma" (Anand, 2009, p. 819). Jyothi Anand (2009) aptly pointed out, however, that other interpretations of karma have involved the role of God and gurus in helping to rid one of the consequences of karma through bhakti yoga (i.e., prayer and devotion).

For many Hindus, karma provides an explanation for suffering. Yet, the ways in which individuals interpret their particular karma vary considerably with their unique individual life histories, family narratives, and circumstances. With regard to individual experience, psychoanalysis offers a lens into the internal and external realities that shape how people understand their suffering or suffering of their loved ones. For example, for a client who believes that she has suffered the unexpected death of her spouse because of her karma from a previous life, it would be important to inquire how she developed this understanding. One possibility is that she learned about karma from elders in her family and that karma allows her to make sense of an unimaginable loss through a belief that her spouse's death was meant to occur. Her belief in karma may also involve a belief that her husband's actions in a previous life determined his unexpected death, and therefore, provides comfort in knowing that his purpose in this life was fulfilled. Another potential interpretation is that the husband's good deeds determined a peaceful death even though it was unexpected. This interpretation may also provide a sense of comfort to the client in knowing that her spouse died without prolonged pain or suffering.

Understanding the ways in which clients develop spiritual meanings is highly relevant to psychoanalytic psychotherapy in which past and present intrapsychic and relational experiences influence the meaning of suffering. It is critical that children, adolescents, and adults connect to spirituality that they feel is their own rather than only that which is transmitted by an authority figure. The experience of freedom and creativity is inherent to a personal spirituality. Akin to Winnicott's (1971) transitional experience, a personal sense of spirituality secures a third space in which a person can expand possibilities of meaning making. In childhood and adolescence, spiritual messengers, such as family and members of a religious organization or community, play a significant role in how spirituality is experienced and how meaning and purpose are conceptualized (Miller, 2013). In particular, if a religious tradition or spiritual faith is experienced as being overly rigid rather than providing a holding space (Winnicott, 1971), a person can develop a range of different spiritual experiences that may impede the development of a more personal connection with spirituality. From a psychoanalytic perspective, psychotherapy can provide a holding space for spirituality, a space that may not have been available to a client within a family or community context or within the broader society.

Hindu spirituality is both individual and collective in nature such that personal interpretations and meanings of spirituality coexist with collective beliefs, traditions, and practices. In addition, Hindu communities are diverse with regard to an emphasis placed on individual subjective experience of spirituality versus an emphasis placed on collective practices. An example of how bridging between individual and collective elements of Hinduism occurs is evident in a *satsang*, a gathering of individuals within a Hindu community who engage in dialogue on scriptures, such as the *Gita* (n.d.), sometimes with a teacher or guru. Within a satsang, discussion is encouraged in a way that spiritual aspirants can receive guidance on how to attain liberation, which is a highly personal, individual experience. The satsang can be a particularly critical experience for Hindus when there is an openness to individuals' subjective experiences of God and of spirituality.

Relatedly, in psychotherapy, if a therapist is not open to inquiring about how a client makes meaning of life or connects with spirituality, the therapeutic space becomes more rigid and closed to the possibility of the client's engaging with this dimension of the self and with the dynamic shifts that are inherent to one's spiritual growth across the lifespan. In this sense, the therapist, too, communicates critical messages about the role of spirituality. Furthermore, the therapist may inadvertently close off possibilities not only because of a dismissal of the importance of religion or spirituality but also because of distorted or misguided conceptualizations of a religion of spiritual tradition with which they are unfamiliar. On the other hand, when spirituality is viewed as a source of resilience and is met with curiosity about the client's spiritual life, taking into consideration the dynamic and complex nature of spiritual development, then the client and the therapist can engage in more authentic and creative inquiry.

While it is important for therapists to be informed about general aspects of a client's particular religious or spiritual tradition, it is often a personal relationship with the Divine or personal meaning making that can be especially important to explore in psychotherapy because it reflects the client's unique self. As Lisa Miller (2013) noted, "Central to spiritual individuation is the formation of a felt and personal relationship with the Divine" (p. 343). Individuation in Hindu spirituality can manifest in a number of different ways, such as one's affinity to a specific deity (e.g., Krishna, Shiva, Lakshmi, Ganesha) or to a particular spiritual path (e.g., karma yoga). Because there are many paths to liberation, connecting to one's own personal preferences regarding spiritual practices are accepted among many Hindu families and communities. At the same time, the process of spiritual individuation can have implications for one's relationships with family and religious or spiritual community depending on the degree of acceptance of one's views within these contexts. As such, the relational and communal factors accompanying individuation should be explored in psychotherapy.

An important source of inquiry regarding personal spirituality, from both psychoanalytic and Hindu perspectives, encompasses dreams and myth (Kakar, 1995). In some Hindu texts (e.g., *Upanishads* [*The Upanishads*], ca. 1 B.C.E.–1400 C.E./2001), dream life, like waking and sleep, is seen as a layer of consciousness. The Atman (soul) is the layer of consciousness that is supreme and Divine (Hughes, 2017). Dreams in Hinduism, then, reflect a part of human consciousness, the content of which may carry a variety of different symbolic meanings. Along the same lines, Freud (1927/1989) conceptualized dreams as related to wishes and fears situated outside of one's conscious awareness and as symbols reflecting repressed desires. Freud further connected dreams to myth in his conceptualization of the Oedipal complex based on the well-known myth of Oedipus Rex in Sophocles's play *Oedipus the King*. In both Hinduism and psychoanalysis, a symbolic significance of dreams connects one to emotions and thoughts that lie outside of waking conscious life. While psychoanalysis does not refer here to a spiritual self, dreams and myth are intricately linked with spirituality in Hinduism.

In my approach to spiritually integrated psychotherapy, the exploration of dreams and myths and accompanying narratives are critical points of exploration in psychological inquiry. Hindu mythology played an instrumental role in my upbringing in learning about basic spiritual and cultural beliefs and traditions. For example, stories of different God forms contain messages about family structure and roles that are inextricable from the Hindu Indian context. In my family, the value placed on respect for elders, as well as the deep emotional bonds between parents, and the bonds especially between mothers and their children, were absorbed through listening to my parents and grandparents reciting stories of Ganesha, the elephant-headed God, and his relationship to his parents, Parvati and Shiva.

It is worth noting that people across cultural backgrounds grow up with myths whether these myths are embedded in a specific religion or not. For example, my client, Jordan,[1] who is a 19-year-old agnostic, White (English and Irish descent) college student, spoke of his fascination with the *Star Wars* movie series (e.g., Lucas, 1999), especially how he identified with a character who is torn between choosing good over evil. For Jordan, who has struggled for most of his life with feeling as though he had to please other people at the cost of his own health, watching *Star Wars* helped to articulate an emotional experience that he had repressed because it made him "feel bad." Jordan's experience of *Star Wars* reflects a broader, universal issue

---

[1]The case of Jordan is based on a real client whose identifying details have been changed to maintain their confidentiality.

concerning good versus evil but also a more personal theme of suffering that is unique to his life history and circumstances.

Dreams and myth are further related to the concept of indigenous narrative in psychotherapy. In previous work, I suggested that culturally informed psychoanalytic psychotherapy carefully consider the role of indigenous perspectives (Seeley, 2000) in a way that deepens analysis of how psychological experience is shaped by sociocultural beliefs, sociohistorical conditions, and relational histories (Tummala-Narra, 2016). Both collective narratives of a cultural or religious community and personal narratives of culture, religion, and spirituality are pertinent to indigenous narrative. Within these narratives lie understandings of emotional suffering and pathways to healing. As such, therapists must inquire into indigenous healing methods. In the case of many Hindus, meditation, prayer, yoga, Ayurvedic medicine, homeopathic medicine, and consultation with astrologers are all methods of achieving physical, emotional, intellectual, and spiritual balance. In the Hindu perspective, the body, thoughts, feelings, and Atman are all interrelated; therefore, approaching each aspect of a person as separate may be experienced as incomplete and inauthentic. Interestingly, in my practice, when I ask my clients about other healing practices in which they may be engaged, they typically indicate practices such as Ayurveda and that they hesitate to share this information with their physicians in the United States because of a concern that they will be perceived as less knowledgeable or scientific.

In psychotherapy, the therapist is often faced with the dilemma of conflicting narratives: either that which the client experiences or that between the therapist and the client. In exploring whose narrative is privileged in these situations, it is critical that the client's narrative be articulated and interpreted through the client's own words. Too often, unfortunately, religious, racial minority, and sexual minority clients experience dismissal or overshadowing of their personal and collective narratives by those of therapists who may either impose or distance themselves from a deeper engagement with narrative (Tummala-Narra, 2016). For these clients, the distortion of their indigenous cultural and religious narratives is especially destructive.

Another related aspect of my approach to spiritually integrated psychotherapy involves the area of social oppression and injustice. My commitment to karma yoga, or the path of service to others, has served as a foundation for my interest in issues of social justice, such as those concerning race, immigration, gender, sexual orientation, social class, and disability. Psychoanalytic scholars have contributed significantly to understanding the effects of traumatic experience on one's intrapsychic and interpersonal life. Along with numerous other scholars (Holmes, 2012; Yi, 2014), I have suggested that traumatic experience based on social location and identity (e.g., race, gender) has profound effects on all dimensions of the self and on the self in relation to the external world (Tummala-Narra, 2016). In my practice, many of my clients have shared with me the spiritual damage that sociocultural trauma has imposed on them. For example, Jessica,[2] a Christian, Haitian American woman in her 30s, stated, "I keep my faith, but it's hard when you get beat down by racists, you know, the people that put down Black people. I do wonder sometimes where is God." The consequences of sociocultural trauma are profound and long lasting, and they require careful attention in psychotherapy because many people develop their spiritual identities within the context of constraint even while they are supported by positive spiritual messengers within families and communities.

Families and communities are core sources of spiritual strength for many people. In the case of racial minorities, spiritual communities provide a sense of connection and belonging to individuals and families that are otherwise marginalized in mainstream U.S. society. Among immigrants, these spiritual communities foster a sense of continuity with the heritage culture and religion as well as a sense of extended family in the new or adopted country (Akhtar, 2011; Guzder & Krishna, 2005). At the same time, families and communities may, in some cases, be sources of stress, particularly when an individual develops religious and spiritual beliefs that diverge from others within these contexts. For example, a person who is disowned by family or community based on sexual orientation or gender identity may be told that these aspects of their identity are sinful or deviant as accorded by interpretation of religious interpretation and tradition. From a psychoanalytic perspective, family and community, nevertheless, are core sites for developing safe attachments (i.e., object relations; Bowlby, 1969; Winnicott, 1971).

It is important to recognize that religious identity and spiritual identity are interconnected with other aspects of identity, such as gender, sexual orientation, and race. Multicultural psychologists and feminist psychologists have emphasized the role of intersectionality in the experience of oppression and resilience (Comas-Díaz & Greene, 2013; Espin, 2008). *Intersectionality* involves one's experience of multiple identities and the structural inequalities and injustice that shape privilege and marginalization accompanying these identities (Crenshaw, 1989). The intersections of identity in the context of religion and spirituality implicate questions regarding how people experience different aspects of identity. For example, many Hindu women struggle

---

[2]The case of Jessica is based on a real client whose identifying details have been changed to maintain their confidentiality.

with restrictions placed on their participation in religious rituals based on gender, such as the restriction of entering a temple while menstruating, and inequities, such as being denied the opportunity to become a priest. The images of powerful Goddesses in Hinduism stand in sharp contrast with the ways in which women, particularly those in lower castes, are accorded less power in everyday life (Narayanan, 2014; Navsaria & Petersen, 2007). In a different example, sexual orientation is typically not openly discussed in Hindu families and communities. Hindus who identify as lesbian, gay, bisexual, transgender, queer + (LGBTQ+) often feel unsafe and remain silent about their sexual identity or gender identity. They also struggle with how to develop a sense of connection to their religion and heritage culture when a core aspect of identity is either ignored or marginalized.

Yet another example of injustice within Hindu communities is that related to caste. The caste system was developed in the course of the history of Hinduism, which included a division of professions. *Varna* ("caste" in English) comprises the following groups that are assigned distinct social status: *Brahmanas*, the priests and intellectuals (highest social status); *Kshatriyas*, the warriors and kings; *Vaishyas*, the merchants; and *Shudras*, the laborers (lowest social status; Sharma & Tummala-Narra, 2014; Vallabhaneni, 2015). Gradually, the *Dalits* (previously called "untouchables") were designated as a group outside of the varna system. Varna has increasingly become a rigid social indicator of status, and discrimination and violence against people from lower castes and Dalits have had devastating consequences. Caste has remained integral to how many Hindus view their positions in society with lower castes and Dalits thought to be inferior and even subhuman (Vallabhaneni, 2015). Caste is also transported beyond the boundaries of South Asian countries because it is internalized by people in the South Asian diaspora. As such, caste is often a consideration in who people choose to socialize with and who people marry. Paralleling the concept of race, caste divides human beings into socially constructed categories and links goodness and badness with these categories (Vallabhaneni, 2015).

Having grown up with an awareness of caste and caste discrimination, I recognize the importance of attending to internalized frameworks of discrimination based on a number of different social constructions and their effects on the psyche. In my therapeutic work, I have questioned and explored my clients' and my own constructions of race, caste, culture, and religion that can reflect destructive messages received since early in life. Psychotherapy that integrates psychoanalytic and spiritual perspectives recognizes the contradictory messages that people receive regarding their attitudes toward self and others. For example, on the one hand, we may be taught to be compassionate toward others, and on the other hand, we are encouraged to claim that our own racial, cultural, or religious heritage is superior to that of others.

As I have worked toward integrating my spirituality with my approach to psychoanalytic psychotherapy, I have increasingly recognized the intersections of my own identities and in which contexts I experience privilege and marginalization based on these identities. I value a conceptualization of the therapist as one who bears mutual influence (Mitchell, 1988) with the client and carries forth a responsibility to inquire about the multiplicity of life experiences, worldviews, and spiritual paths. Spiritually integrated therapy invites inquiry into these various dimensions of the client's psyche and recognizes the influence of the therapist on the nature and process of this inquiry. It is critical to be mindful of the diversity within any particular spiritual tradition and for the therapist to inquire about how a particular client has experienced their religious or spiritual traditions and the ways that the client, the client's family, and community make meaning of significant events in their lives (Tummala-Narra, 2016). We cannot rely on only broad knowledge regarding a particular religion of culture; rather, in spiritually integrated psychotherapy, we attend to both unconscious and conscious meanings of personal and collective religious or spiritual experiences. In addition, spiritually integrated psychotherapy involves an in-depth understanding of resilience in the face of suffering, and the recognition that resilience is embedded in cultural and religious narratives and beliefs. Therefore, attending to transference and countertransference related to culture and spirituality is essential for this engagement.

An important element of spiritually integrated psychotherapy entails humility. Specifically, cultural humility has been defined as both intrapersonal and interpersonal:

> Intrapersonally, cultural humility involves a willingness and openness to reflect on one's own self as an embedded cultural being, being aware of personal limitations in understanding the cultural other and guarding against forming culturally unfounded, automatic assumptions; interpersonally, cultural humility involves being open to hearing and striving to understand aspects of the other's cultural background and identity. (Watkins & Hook, 2016, p. 490)

Cultural humility is essential to avoiding overgeneralizations of people and communities as well as to deepening engagement with religious and spiritual experiences and the role of intersectionality in identity development. As such, the therapist takes a position of curiosity, guided by existing knowledge and by an openness to expanding this knowledge. This therapeutic stance aims then to expand understanding of the self and one's relation to the external world.

Hindu spirituality aims to help a person move toward an understanding of the purpose of life, and a component of this knowledge concerns one's purpose in relation to others. For example, seeking to help others in need without expecting personal rewards and finding ways to reduce one's anger, greed, and selfish desire are Hindu values that are central to the purpose of life and to a path of liberation. Psychoanalytic psychotherapy facilitates the exploration of conscious and unconscious feelings and motivations that underlie interactions with others. Exploring both psychological and spiritual dimensions is necessary to gain a more complete understanding of how people interact with others and how they are affected by and affect others. Both Hindu spirituality and psychoanalytic psychotherapy value a sense of curiosity and humility in the process of achieving self-understanding.

CASE EXAMPLE: DINESH

This case example[3] provides a glimpse into spiritually integrated psychotherapy. Although a full description of the case is not possible, I focus on specific aspects of Hindu spirituality and psychoanalytic theory relevant to my psychotherapeutic work with one particular client.

Dinesh is a 25-year-old single, Hindu Indian American heterosexual cisgender man. He has been suffering from anxiety that has gradually escalated to a point at which he can no longer concentrate on tasks at work. He works as a paralegal in a law firm, and his employer referred him to psychotherapy.

Dinesh was born and raised in a small city in the United States, and his parents and older sister emigrated from a large city in Southern India to the United States a few years before his birth. He has a close relationship with his parents and his sister, and, growing up, attended a Hindu temple and spiritual and language (Hindi) classes every weekend in a nearby suburb. Most of his friends both within and outside of his school were of South Asian origin. He developed a strong connection with Hindu traditions, such as participating in pujas and praying at home with his family. At school, though, Dinesh experienced significant bullying, particularly in elementary and middle schools. Some of his White peers used slurs, such as "terrorist," "sand n__," and "brownie" to refer to Dinesh. His Hindu and South Asian communities provided a sense of security and comfort in the face of this bullying, particularly because little intervention was provided by his teachers or administrators at school.

---

[3]The case of Dinesh is based on a real client whose identifying details have been changed to maintain their confidentiality.

In his senior year of high school, Dinesh suffered an injury from a car accident when his parents' car was hit by another driver who had lost control of his malfunctioning car. The accident left Dinesh with significant injuries, and, ultimately, he was unable to participate in activities, such as sports. He often experienced a great deal of physical pain while attending college in a geographic area that was distant from his family's home. Dinesh continued to cope with ongoing intermittent physical pain when I first met him in psychotherapy, although homeopathic remedies were helpful to an extent.

After graduating from college, Dinesh decided to pursue a career in law, securing a job as a paralegal. At his workplace, he felt increasingly isolated from his coworkers and as though he did not belong with them. He felt as though they looked down on him, and at times, felt invisible in his office. As a college student, he had connected with the Hindu Student Council on campus, where he met his girlfriend whom he dated for the following 2 years. The relationship ended when he learned that his girlfriend was interested in dating someone else. Since the ending of this relationship, Dinesh was reluctant to become seriously involved with anyone else, and he continued to struggle with trusting a potential partner.

When Dinesh began psychotherapy, he had increasingly felt disconnected with his spiritual faith. Early in our work together, he stated,

> Being a Hindu is important to me, but sometimes I think that it's become a thing to do, like go to temple, but I don't feel anything. When I was younger, I used to feel something special about God, like he would always help me.

He proceeded to tell me about how his physical pain from the injuries and the ending of his relationship in college felt overwhelming to him even though he "managed to get through."

As he discussed his loss of his relationship and the physical pain, I asked Dinesh about his loss of connection to God. He responded, "God isn't giving me a break. Maybe it's not real or maybe not the way my parents taught me how to think about God." I posed questions, such as, "When you were younger, how did you imagine God?" and "How do you imagine God now? Tell me more." Dinesh described his younger vision of God as one that was connected mostly to mythological stories of Krishna and Rama, forms of the God Vishnu, who manifested in human form to help those who were most vulnerable. In one session, he recalled an incident of racist bullying in middle school. He remembers silently praying to Krishna when he was bullied in school, being called a "brownie"; afterward, his older sister came by and walked him away from the bully. He stated, "I thought God was actually listening to me. Maybe he was. I don't know. I don't feel protected now. The world is crazy. People disappoint you." I responded, "I can see why you are wondering about God, whether he is real or not. It seems like you worry a lot about being disappointed." Through this engagement, Dinesh revealed that he often felt anxious about someone hurting him and about being disappointed with himself for not defending himself. Specifically, in revisiting his hope of Krishna saving him in the face of a bully, he had wished that he was more like Krishna, the savior, rather than the victim who needed to be saved. In sharing this with me, he said, "I don't know that I was ever really aware of that before."

Gradually, Dinesh was able to talk in more depth about his experience of being bullied, which he had kept hidden from most of his family and friends. He also spoke about ongoing racism that he faced in the workplace and in the broader U.S. context. Furthermore, he had hoped that dating a Hindu Indian woman would help him feel more secure and safe as he had felt within his community while growing up. When he was betrayed by her, he became unsure about what and who he could count on to feel safe. He wondered if these disappointments were a result of his own actions or karma. He had been struggling to make sense of why these negative experiences seemed to follow him.

After several weeks of working together, I asked Dinesh whether he was unsure about whether working with me, a Hindu Indian American woman, and if he worried that I may disappoint him as well. He replied by telling me that he wanted to trust me and hoped that I would validate his experience but that there were times when he worried that I may do something to disappoint him. He also shared with me that he sometimes viewed me as someone who is knowledgeable about Hinduism and other times, as someone who may be more identified with Western culture, and that he was engaged in a parallel process in which he was discovering what he truly believes and does not believe, distinct from his family.

We continued to talk about the ambivalence he felt toward his spiritual faith and significant people in his life that both supported and challenged his sense of faith. About a year after starting psychotherapy, he joined a local *Gita* (n.d.) reading group (i.e., satsang) specifically for younger adults. There, he began to reconnect with discussions regarding Hinduism in a collective context. In psychotherapy, our conversations about his Hindu identity involved his feelings about being an Indian American man and others' perceptions of his racial and cultural backgrounds. Our discussions about the intersections of his identity became critical in his exploration of his spiritual self. He stated,

> I feel like I need to pull apart all of these different parts of myself so that I can really know who I am and what I believe. I don't want to just believe something because someone tells me that I should.

This case vignette highlights the ways in which spirituality is linked with multiple layers of experience, self-states, and intersections of identity (Bromberg, 2006; Crenshaw, 1989). It also underscores the importance of the interaction of traumatic events and losses as well as one's connection and disconnection with the spiritual self. It was clear that Dinesh was engaged in forming a personal spirituality distinct from his family (e.g., spiritual individuation) while maintaining a connection with his family and a spiritual community. As he explored new possibilities, he started to revisit and integrate his childhood experience of Hindu epics, such as the *Mahabharata* (*The Mahābhārata*, ca. 400 B.C.E./2015) and *Ramayana* (*The Rāmāyana of Vālmīki*, ca. 5th century B.C.E./2021). In doing so, he was able to imagine a new relationship with God (Krishna).

Psychotherapy can be a powerful space in which the therapist's and the client's conscious and unconscious experiences related to spirituality can be explored. Dinesh's experiences of being bullied are distinct from my own personal experiences of discrimination. We share an Indian American identity that intersects with our own unique set of experiences of Hinduism. While we were both raised as Hindus, we each carry distinct developmental histories that shape each of our subjectivities as Hindus. My Hindu spirituality played a role in how I listened to Dinesh, as it would with other clients who are not Hindu. However, with my Hindu clients, it is also important that I recognize the sameness and difference between my own perspective and that of the client. For example, at times, there were differences between us with regard to interpreting a Hindu mythological story, and these differences largely centered around the contexts in which we each learned these stories. In some sessions, we would share and explore each of our interpretations, which allowed for a deeper examination of his subjectivity.

In addition, when Dinesh described his positive experiences of being a Hindu and his traumatic experiences of being bullied, I found myself struggling with how he makes meaning of the contradictory messages about his identity that he received throughout his school experiences and with my own feelings of anger and frustration concerning the racism that he faced. I did share with him that I found the bullying outrageous and pointed out how unfair it was to him. At the same time, I recognized that it was important for Dinesh to have the space to experience and express his feelings without having to manage my reactions. It was critical to hold and explore the tension produced by the presence of my Hindu spirituality, Indian heritage, and experience of discrimination as juxtaposed against the exploration of his experience of spirituality, culture, and race. It was our shared willingness to bear this tension that helped him to eventually discover and connect with his authentic, spiritual self.

REFERENCES

Abu-Raiya, H., & Pargament, K. I. (2015). Religious coping among diverse religions: Commonalities and divergences. *Psychology of Religion and Spirituality, 7*(1), 24–33.

Akhtar, S. (2011). *Immigration and acculturation: Mourning, adaptation, and the next generation*. Jason Aronson.

Akhtar, S., & Tummala-Narra, P. (2005). Psychoanalysis in India. In S. Akhtar (Ed.), *Freud along the Ganges* (pp. 3–28). Other Press.

Anand, J. (2009). Psychological healing and faith in the doctrine of Karma. *Mental Health, Religion & Culture, 12*(8), 817–832. https://doi.org/10.1080/13674670903020889

Aron, L. (2004). God's influence on my psychoanalytic vision and values. *Psychoanalytic Psychology, 21*(3), 442–451. https://doi.org/10.1037/0736-9735.21.3.442

Aron, L., & Starr, K. (2013). *A psychotherapy for the people: Toward a progressive psychoanalysis*. Routledge. https://doi.org/10.4324/9780203098059

Balodhi, J. P., & Keshavan, M. S. (2011). Bhagavadgita and psychotherapy. *Asian Journal of Psychiatry, 4*(4), 300–302. https://doi.org/10.1016/j.ajp.2011.10.005

Barsness, R. E. (Ed.). (2018). *Core competencies of relational psychoanalysis: A guide to practice, study, and research*. Routledge.

Bhagwan, R. (2012). Glimpses of ancient Hindu spirituality: Areas for integrative therapeutic intervention. *Journal of Social Work Practice, 26*(2), 233–244. https://doi.org/10.1080/02650533.2011.610500

Bose, G. (1921). *Concept of repression*. Sri Gouranga Press.

Bowlby, J. (1969). *Attachment and loss*. Basic Books.

Bromberg, P. M. (2006). *Awakening the dreamer: Clinical journeys*. Analytic Press.

Comas-Díaz, L., & Greene, B. (2013). *Psychological health of women of color: Intersections, challenges, and opportunities*. Praeger.

Crenshaw, K. W. (1989). Demarginalizing the intersection of race and sex: A Black feminist critique of antidiscrimination doctrine, feminist theory and antiracist politics. *University of Chicago Legal Forum, 1989*, 139–167.

Daehnert, C. (1998). The false self as a means of disidentification: A psychoanalytic case study. *Contemporary Psychoanalysis, 34*(2), 251–271. https://doi.org/10.1080/00107530.1998.10746361

Espin, O. M. (2008). My "friendship" with women saints as a source of spirituality. In C. A. Rayburn & L. Comas-Díaz (Eds.), *Womansoul: The inner life of women's spirituality* (pp. 71–84). Praeger.

Freud, S. (1989). The future of an illusion. In P. Gay (Ed.), *The Freud reader* (pp. 685–722). W. W. Norton & Company. (Original work published 1927)

Fromm, E., Suzuki, D. T., & De Martino, R. (1960). *Zen Buddhism and psychoanalysis*. Harper & Row.

Guntrip, H. (1957). *Psychotherapy and religion*. Harper and Brothers Publishers.

Gupta, R. (2011). Death beliefs and practices from an Asian Indian American Hindu perspective. *Death Studies, 35*(3), 244–266. https://doi.org/10.1080/07481187.2010.518420

Guzder, J., & Krishna, M. (2005). Mind the gap: Diaspora issues of Indian origin women in psychotherapy. *Psychology and Developing Societies, 17*(2), 121–138. https://doi.org/10.1177/097133360501700203

Harris, A. E. (2011). The relational tradition: Landscape and canon. *Journal of the American Psychoanalytic Association, 59*(4), 701–736. https://doi.org/10.1177/0003065111416655

Holmes, D. E. (2012). "Why can't we simply treat people's problems, not their race (or physical disability, or sexual orientation)?!": A psychodynamic approach to the therapeutic relevance of multiple minority identities. In R. Nettles & R. Balter (Eds.), *Multiple minority identities: Applications for practice, research, and training* (pp. 187–205). Springer.

Hughes, J. F. (2017). Dreams, myth, and power. *Dreaming, 27*(2), 161–176. https://doi.org/10.1037/drm0000055

Jung, C. G. (1938). *Psychology and religion.* Yale University Press.

Kakar, S. (1995). Clinical work and cultural imagination. *The Psychoanalytic Quarterly, 64*(2), 265–281. https://doi.org/10.1080/21674086.1995.11927452

Lucas, G. (Director). (1999). *Star wars: Episode 1—The phantom menace* [Film]. Lucasfilm; 20th Century Fox.

The Mahābhārata (Vols. 1–10; B. Debroy, Trans.). (2015). Penguin Random House India. (Original work published ca. 400 B.C.E.)

Mazumdar, S., & Mazumdar, S. (2009). Religion, immigration, and home making in diaspora: Hindu space in southern California. *Journal of Environmental Psychology, 29*(2), 256–266. https://doi.org/10.1016/j.jenvp.2008.07.004

Miller, L. (2013). Spiritual awakening and depression in adolescents: A unified pathway or "two sides of the same coin." *Bulletin of the Menninger Clinic, 77*(4), 332–348. https://doi.org/10.1521/bumc.2013.77.4.332

Mishra, R. C. (2013). Moksha and the Hindu worldview. *Psychology and Developing Societies, 25*(1), 21–42. https://doi.org/10.1177/0971333613477318

Mitchell, S. A. (1988). *Relational concepts in psychoanalysis: An integration.* Harvard University Press.

Murthy, R. S. (2010). Hinduism and mental health. In P. J. Verhagen, H. M. van Praag, J. J. Lopez-Ibor, J. L. Cox, & D. Moussaoui (Eds.), *Religion and psychiatry: Beyond boundaries* (pp. 159–179). Wiley-Blackwell. https://doi.org/10.1002/9780470682203.ch9

Nagpal, A. (2011). A Hindu reading of Freud's beyond the pleasure principle. In S. Akhtar & M. K. O'Neil (Eds.), *On Freud's "beyond the pleasure principle"* (pp. 230–249). Karnac Books.

Narayanan, A. (2014). Ambivalent subjects: Psychoanalysis, women's sexuality in India and the writings of Sudhir Kakar. *Psychodynamic Practice, 20*(3), 213–227. https://doi.org/10.1080/14753634.2014.916839

Navsaria, N., & Petersen, S. (2007). Finding a voice in *Shakti*: A therapeutic approach for Hindu Indian women. *Women & Therapy, 30*(3/4), 161–175. https://doi.org/10.1300/J015v30n03_12

Ogden, T. H. (1994). *Subjects of analysis.* Karnac Books.

The Rāmāyana of Vālmīki: The complete English translation (Vols. 1–7; R. P. Goldman & S. J. Sutherland Goldman, Eds. & Trans.). (2021). Princeton University Press. (Original work published ca. 5th century B.C.E.)

Rizzuto, A.-M. (2004). Roman Catholic background and psychoanalysis. *Psychoanalytic Psychology, 21*(3), 436–441. https://doi.org/10.1037/0736-9735.21.3.436

Roland, A. (2006). Across civilizations: Psychoanalytic therapy with Asians and Asian Americans. *Psychotherapy, 43*(4), 454–463. https://doi.org/10.1037/0033-3204.43.4.454

Roland, A. (2017). Erich Fromm's involvement with Zen Buddhism: Psychoanalysts and the spiritual quest in subsequent decades. *Psychoanalytic Review, 104*(4), 503–522. https://doi.org/10.1521/prev.2017.104.4.503

Safran, J. D. (2003). *Psychoanalysis and Buddhism: An unfolding dialogue.* Wisdom Publications.

Seeley, K. M. (2000). *Cultural psychotherapy: Working with culture in the clinical encounter.* Jason Aronson.

Sharma, A. R., & Tummala-Narra, P. (2014). Psychotherapy with Hindus. In P. S. Richards & A. E. Bergin (Eds.), *Handbook of psychotherapy and religious diversity* (2nd ed., pp. 321–345). American Psychological Association. https://doi.org/10.1037/14371-013

Srimad Bhagavad-Gita. (n.d.). Bhagavad-Gita Trust. https://bhagavad-gita.org/

Stone, C. (2005). Opening psychoanalytic space to the spiritual. *Psychoanalytic Review, 92*(3), 417–430. https://doi.org/10.1521/prev.92.3.417.66545

Suchday, S., Santoro, A. F., Ramanayake, N., Lewin, H., & Almeida, M. (2018). Religion, spirituality, globalization reflected in life beliefs among urban Asian Indian youth. *Psychology of Religion and Spirituality, 10*(2), 146–156. https://doi.org/10.1037/rel0000161

Sue, D. W. (2001). Multidimensional facets of cultural competence. *The Counseling Psychologist, 29*(6), 790–821. https://doi.org/10.1177/0011000001296002

The Torah: The five books of Moses (3rd ed.). (2015). The Jewish Publication Society. (Original work published 1962)

Tummala-Narra, P. (2009). The relevance of a psychoanalytic perspective in exploring religious and spiritual identity in psychotherapy. *Psychoanalytic Psychology, 26*(1), 83–95. https://doi.org/10.1037/a0014673

Tummala-Narra, P. (2016). *Psychoanalytic theory and cultural competence in psychotherapy.* American Psychological Association. https://doi.org/10.1037/14800-000

The Upanishads (Swami Paramananda, Trans.). (2001). The Pennsylvania State University. (Original work published ca. 1 B.C.E.–1400 C.E.)

Vallabhaneni, M. R. (2015). Indian caste system: Historical and psychoanalytic views. *American Journal of Psychoanalysis, 75*(4), 361–381. https://doi.org/10.1057/ajp.2015.42

Varambally, S., & Gangadhar, B. N. (2012). Yoga: A spiritual practice with therapeutic value in psychiatry. *Asian Journal of Psychiatry, 5*(2), 186–189. https://doi.org/10.1016/j.ajp.2012.05.003

Vásquez, M. A. (2005). Historicizing and materializing the study of religion: The contribution of migration studies. In K. I. Leonard, A. Stepnick, M. A. Vásquez, & J. Holdaway (Eds.), *Immigrant faiths: Transforming religious life in America* (pp. 219–243). Rowman & Littlefield.

The Vedas: The saṃhitās of the R̥ig, Yajur (white and black), Sāma, and Atharva Vedas (R.T.H. Griffith & A. B. Keith, Trans.; J. W. Fergus, Ed.). (2017). Kshetra Books. (Original work published ca. 1200 B.C.E.)

Watkins, C. E., & Hook, J. N. (2016). On a culturally humble psychoanalytic supervision: Creating the cultural third. *Psychoanalytic Psychology, 33*(3), 487–517. https://doi.org/10.1037/pap0000044

Whitman, S. M. (2007). Pain and suffering as viewed by the Hindu religion. *The Journal of Pain, 8*(8), 607–613. https://doi.org/10.1016/j.jpain.2007.02.430

Winnicott, D. W. (1971). *Playing and reality.* Routledge.

Yi, K. (2014). From no name to birth of integrated identity: Trauma-based cultural dissociation in immigrant women and creative integration. *Psychoanalytic Dialogues, 24*(1), 37–45. https://doi.org/10.1080/10481885.2014.870830

2 HARVESTING RELIGIOUS FRUITS IN SPIRITUALLY INTEGRATED PSYCHOTHERAPY

Personal Reflections of a Jewish Psychologist of Religion

KENNETH I. PARGAMENT

This is the first time I have ever used the term "reflections" in a title of one of my chapters or papers, and I think it's a reflection (pardon the pun) of the fact that I'm aging. But the later years in a career are a particularly apt time to take a step back and reflect on oneself, one's own work, and the state of the field. (Of course, it's not a bad idea to do that when you're younger, too.)

In this chapter, I reflect on how my own approach to spiritually integrated psychotherapy has been implicitly shaped by my own identity as a Jew and how it's been shaped as well by my encounters with other faiths. I've never spoken so directly to these issues before; what I'm really doing here is making something that has been implicit more explicit. This process of moving from implicit to explicit, I believe, is particularly important in spiritually integrated therapy.

A few assumptions underlie this chapter that I'd like to highlight. The first assumption is that we cannot disconnect our approaches to psychotherapy from who we are as human beings, including our own gender, ethnicity, race, sexual orientation, and, yes, spiritual and religious orientation. I like the way Stanton Jones (1994) put it: "One cannot intervene in the fabric of

https://doi.org/10.1037/0000276-003
Spiritual Diversity in Psychotherapy: Engaging the Sacred in Clinical Practice,
S. J. Sandage and B. D. Strawn (Editors)

human life without getting deeply involved in moral and religious matters" (p. 197). The notion that the therapist can be a tabula rasa, a blank slate to write on, is not borne out by the empirical evidence or the realities of clinical experience. To put it more bluntly, complete neutrality on the part of the therapist is impossible. In a classic paper written in 1980, Allen Bergin warned us that in the effort to remain neutral and personally detached, we are likely to become hidden or subtle influencers in therapy. Being more explicit about our own distinctive identities, then, offers an important corrective to this potential bias.

The second assumption is one grounded in an empirical reality: The world is becoming increasingly pluralistic religiously. In this age of the internet and remarkable mobility, adherents of faith traditions are exposed to the exceptional diversity within and between religious groups. In 1991, Anderson and Hopkins captured this dynamic in the United States: "[Here] Hindu yogis teach next door to South American shamans, and Congregationalist churches share their space with Buddhist and Taoist communities. Jewish men and women become Zen masters and Catholic priests learn Japanese forms of meditation and purification" (p. 122). As a result of this movement toward pluralism, it is now a misnomer to speak of "the" Protestant, Catholic, Muslim, Buddhist, Hindu, Jewish, or, for that matter, atheist client. People have become more spiritually eclectic, picking and choosing from what Reginald Bibby (1987) once described as an à la carte menu of religious choices of beliefs and practices that can be found within and across religions.

This leads to the third assumption: Psychotherapy is essentially a meeting of worlds—the world of the client and the world of the therapist. To conduct effective spiritually integrated psychotherapy, therapists must learn about and respond respectfully to the distinctive religious world of the client while remaining well-aware of the worlds they, as practitioners, bring to psychotherapy and how their own worldviews may shape the therapeutic encounter in desirable or undesirable ways.

With these assumptions in mind, let me begin by providing a little background on myself as a Jewish psychologist of religion.

DISCOVERING MY OWN RELIGIOUS IDENTITY

From my earliest years, I knew that I was Jewish, but I didn't realize that I was *really* Jewish until sometime in my twenties. I was born and raised in a conservative Jewish community in Washington, DC. Like most of my Jewish friends, much of my education in Judaism was geared to preparing me for my rite of passage into adulthood, my Bar Mitzvah, at the ripe old age of 13. I learned to read Hebrew quite well but without understanding what I was reading. I learned to participate in Jewish customs and rituals without understanding their underlying meaning. I did a very nice job at my Bar Mitzvah, as I was told. But when that was completed, like most of my friends, I stopped my formal Jewish education. My parents didn't offer complaints; while Judaism permeated our home through customs, holiday meals, and occasional attendance at synagogue, we didn't speak about the meaning of being Jewish. Don't get me wrong, I *felt* deeply Jewish. I just wasn't sure why.

In my 20s, I read a book that profoundly affected me. It was written by Irving Howe (1976) and entitled *World of Our Fathers*: *The Journey of the East European Jews to America and the Life They Found and Made*. As the title conveys, the book presents the stories of Jews who emigrated from Europe to the United States in the late 19th and early 20th centuries. Listening to the rich descriptions of their lives, I saw, heard, and experienced myself in their vigilance, indeed, hypervigilance to a world that could come crashing down on them at any time; in their sense of a flawed universe and broken world in desperate need of repair; in a skepticism to external authority and even their own understanding of the world; in a love for deep thinking about questions that were so meaningful to me—most importantly, why we're here and how we should live our lives—and in a sense of humor that absolutely refuses to let suffering and tragedy have the last word. One of my favorites whose origins are unknown: Three Jews have been condemned to death in the Russian gulag. Before they are about to be shot, their guard and executioner asks them if they want a blindfold. The first two accept, but the third says no emphatically. The second Jew leans over to the third one and says, "Take the blindfold. Don't make trouble" (Aish.com, n.d.). I realized then that I was Jewish in a way that went well beyond whether I attended synagogue, followed all of the 613 commandments of the Hebrew Bible, or even believed in God. Jewishness was an inseparable part of my personality, my character, and my approach to life and the world. This was only a starting point for me; I was just beginning to understand how I was Jewish, and I wanted to learn more.

Around the same point in time, I was pursuing studies of psychology. I went into psychology because I thought it would provide insights into what makes people (including me) tick, what the key is to a life of meaning and purpose, and how we might make the world a better place. But I was disappointed by what I was learning. I only semi-joke that my first client, Walter, was a three-pound pigeon. I met and cared for Walter in my class on operant conditioning, and Walter did in fact teach me valuable principles of reinforcement and punishment that came in handy when I worked with children or people with disabilities. But when it came to the big questions— Why are we here? What's the meaning of it all? How can we deal with suffering in the world?—Walter had very few words—actually, no words at all. The other major therapeutic paradigm of my time—psychodynamic— struck me as very dark and pessimistic. Not that this child of the Holocaust had to be persuaded of the darkness and evil in the world, but how, I wondered, could we help other people whose feet are stuck in the muck and mire of life when we we're standing with one foot in quicksand ourselves?

I began to wonder whether religious thought and practice might offer a way to deepen psychology. Even though I didn't agree with many of their answers, my sense was that the religions of the world shared my interest in the big questions that had drawn me to psychology. I started to take a closer look at religious life. Early on, though, I decided I didn't want to focus exclusively on Judaism. I wanted to learn about the religions of the world more generally. I also found myself less interested in theological matters and more interested in the very concrete ways religion expressed itself in peoples' lives, particularly in the most pivotal times of life. So, I began to go to churches, temples, congregations, mosques, and synagogues and talk to people about how religion affected them for better or worse. Initially, this was a pretty scary thing to do; after all, what was a Jewish guy doing in a church? I was always welcomed though, albeit sometimes with the hopes, I think, that I'd become a convert. And I saw what a powerful role religion played in peoples' lives: often helpful it seemed but, at times, harmful.

The field of psychology, I quickly learned, had its own "issues" with religion. Freud and Skinner, for instance, were not huge fans of religious life, to say the least. However, I felt that there was much to be gained by bridging the two domains of psychology and religion, and over the years, I came to the conclusion that we can enhance our effectiveness as practitioners when we integrate the distinctive resources of various religions into treatment. Spiritually integrated psychotherapy, as I have written about it (Pargament, 2007), rests on that premise. It draws on the fruits of many religious traditions.

With this background in mind, let me shift to the main focus of this chapter. I discuss two fruits that I have tried to harvest that are deeply rooted in (although not exclusive to) my own tradition: Judaism. I then go on to consider how we can enrich our work as therapists by harvesting the fruits of other religious traditions and adding them as vital ingredients into the recipes of our clinical work. I conclude this chapter with the recommendation for greater sharing of religious resources in therapy in ways that remain sensitive to and respectful of clients' particular religious identification and commitments.

HARVESTING THE FRUIT OF SANCTIFICATION

The first fruit I plucked from Judaism was sanctification. Let me quickly state this fruit can also be harvested from other religious trees. And, in fact, my collaborator in much of this work on sanctification, Annette Mahoney, is a liberal Christian psychologist. We defined *sanctification* as a process of perceiving seemingly ordinary elements of life as being reflective of God or higher powers and/or as possessing extraordinary or divine qualities (Pargament & Mahoney, 2005). However, my own awareness of and interest in harvesting sanctification for psychotherapy was, I'm sure, implicitly embedded in Judaism.

Let me try to make the implicit more explicit here as I talk about sanctification. At the risk of overgeneralizing, I'd say that, in comparison to Christianity, Judaism is less concerned about direct encounters with God. Although I haven't seen data on this, I'd guess that Jews report fewer personal experiences with the divine than Christians. In the Hebrew Bible, God tells Moses to warn the Jewish people not to gaze directly at the Lord "lest many of them perish" (Harkavy, 1951, Exodus 19:21–22).

Within Judaism, it is more common to have what Peter Berger (1969) called "signals of transcendence" (p. 52), or, as Samuel Karff (1979) put it, "intimations" of God's presence through ordinary this-worldly experiences (p. 113). Judaism is very concerned with the connection between "heaven and earth." It teaches that a divine presence can be found in everyday life; in fact, we are told to look for it. How?

One way is through prayer. Twice a day, Jews recite a prayer of sanctification: "Kdosh, kdosh, kdosh, Adonai tsevahot, melot kol ha'aretz kvodo. Holy, holy, holy is God, master of legions, the whole world is filled with his glory" (*The Art Scroll Siddur*, 1990).

A second way is through Jewish laws and customs. Jewish commandments, all 613 of them, are about treating every aspect of life as sacred—how we eat; how we work; how we rest; how we treat animals; how we act toward family, friends, strangers, and even enemies. In each of these activities, Jews are reminded of God's presence. There are blessings for everything from waking to going to sleep, from welcoming a baby into the world to departing the world, from going on a trip to coming home. The central message of these blessings is that God's hand is in all of life, and that all of life is a divine blessing.

A third way is through rituals. In the simple acts of lighting candles, eating a special meal, and taking a ritual drink of wine and sharing challah, we are encouraged to see the world in a new light. The transitions rituals— Bar and Bat Mitzvah, weddings, circumcision, and funerals—are more than opportunities for gift-giving and celebration. They are rites of passage, what Edwin Friedman (1985) described as "hinges of time" (p. 164) that offer windows into the deeper flow and currents of the universe and the eternal truths of existence—when we move from childhood to adulthood, when we join our lives together in marriage, when new lives are welcomed into our community, when life comes to an end. These rituals insist that we sit up and take note of a deeper dimension to our lives.

In short, Jews are asked to make sacred, to sanctify the world, to see the world through a sacred lens. My interest in sanctification came to me in a subtle, subterranean way through my lifelong exposure to this perspective so deeply embedded in Judaism.

Again, I want to stress that sanctification is not exclusive to Judaism. Other religions of the world also encourage their adherents to see the sacred in various aspects of life. For example, within the *Upanishads*, Hindus read: "Filled with Brahman are the things we see, Filled with Brahman are the things we see not, From out of Brahman floweth all that is: From Brahman all—yet is he still the same" (*The Upanishads*, ca. 1 B.C.E.–1400 C.E./1975, p. 80). And Christians are taught: "Now there are varieties of gifts, but the same Spirit; and there are varieties of service, but the same Lord, and there are varieties of working, but it is the same God who empowers them all in every one" (*The Holy Bible,* 2006, English Standard Version, 1 Corinthians 12:4–6).

We can find rich examples of sanctification in Judaism and other traditions as well. For example, Judaism sanctifies time and the day of rest, or Sabbath, in particular. Abraham Heschel (1955) described the Sabbath this way:

> What is the Sabbath? The presence of eternity, a moment of majesty, the radiance of joy. The Sabbath is an assurance that the spirit is greater than the universe, that beyond the good is the holy. The Sabbath is holiness in time. (p. 417)

Protestant theologian and minister Frederick Buechner (1992) spoke beautifully of seeing all of life as sacred:

> Taking your children to school and kissing your wife goodbye. Eating lunch with a friend. Trying to do a decent day's work. Hearing the rain patter against the window. There is no event so commonplace but that God is present within it, always hiddenly, always leaving you room to recognize him or not to recognize him, but all the more fascinatingly because of that, all the more compellingly and hauntingly. . . . Listen to your life. See it for the fathomless mystery that it is.

> In the boredom and pain of it no less than in the excitement and gladness: touch, taste, smell your way to the holy and hidden heart of it because in the last analysis all moments are key moments, and life itself is grace. (p. 2)

It is important to add that the process of sanctification may also be experienced by atheists. Although they may reject beliefs in God or labels of being religious or spiritual, they, too, can imbue aspects of life with qualities often associated with the divine, including transcendence, boundlessness, and ultimacy, as we can hear in the words of a Swedish atheist coping with cancer:

> Whatever happens in the world for me or others, nature is still there, it keeps going. That is a feeling of security when everything else is chaos. The leaves fall off, new ones appear, somewhere there is a pulse that keeps going. . . . It is a spiritual feeling if we can use this word without connecting it to God, this is what I feel in nature. (Ahmadi, 2006, p. 134)

Sanctification is not at all a rarity or an experience of only the devoutly faithful—if national surveys are to be believed. For instance, in one such survey, 78% of the sample agreed that they see signs of God in nature and creation, and 76% agreed that they experience life as more sacred and more than material (Doehring & Clarke, 2002).

A number of us have been studying sanctification for several years now, and our findings appear to underscore its potent role in our lives (Pargament, 2013; Pomerleau et al., 2016; Wong & Pargament, 2017). Let me highlight a few of these implications. First, whatever we perceive as sacred seems to act as a magnet, drawing us forward, giving us something to strive for in life. Several years ago, I saw a 45-year-old woman who had come into therapy after being diagnosed with glioblastoma, a malignant brain tumor that left her with the prognosis of only 2 more years of life. In talking about what she might like to accomplish in therapy, I asked her what matters most to her in her life, what she held sacred. She responded quickly, "My children. They're sacred to me." A Jewish woman and mother of four boys, she said she wanted to live to be present for her youngest 9-year-old son's Bar Mitzvah. And she asked for my help in coping with the difficult treatment ordeal she would have to go through to reach that goal. And that is what we did. It was an onerous treatment, but I believe she endured it with such courage because she was motivated by a sacred mission. She defied the odds and lived to celebrate her son's Bar Mitzvah and most of his progress through high school. To paraphrase Viktor Frankl (1959), she had a "why" to live for.

Second, we are motivated to preserve and protect whatever we sanctify in our lives; after all, it is sacred. In one study, led by Annette Mahoney, we examined the degree to which college students perceived their physical bodies to be sacred temples of the holy spirit (Mahoney et al., 2005). Those who did, we found, took better care of their bodies, ate better, exercised more, got enough sleep, and were less likely to use drugs and alcohol.

Third, what we sanctify tends to become a "precious object," a potent resource for health and well-being. A few years ago, I taught a small graduate class and asked my students to bring in and share an object each held sacred. Some students brought in crucifixes; others brought in special objects that had been given to them by loved ones. One student, a Buddhist, held up a small pendant that she always wore around her neck. Noting that her father had died when she was only 8 years old, she said the pendant contained a small part of his ashes, and by wearing the pendant, she was able to keep him close to her heart. This was her most precious object and a source of loving memory that gave her support, strength, and solace.

The flip side of these points is that an inability to sanctify may pose problems for people. Harold Kushner (1989) spoke to this point:

> A world without [the sacred] would be a flat, monochromatic world, a world without color or texture, a world in which all days would be the same. Marriage would be a matter of biology, not fidelity. Old age would be seen as a time of weakness, not of wisdom. In a world like that, we would cast about desperately for any sort of diversion, for any distraction from the emptiness of our lives, because we would never have learned the magic of making some days and some hours special. (p. 206)

We believe this work on sanctification also has clinical application for people from diverse religious and spiritual backgrounds. One example comes from work I was involved in with Brian McCorkle and his colleagues at The Albert & Jessie Danielsen Institute (McCorkle et al., 2005). Our focus was on people seeking treatment for social anxiety disorder. We conceptualized social anxiety as, in part, a disorder arising from an inability to place anxiety within a larger background, a background of greater meaning and sacredness. To use the example of figure–ground illusions from Gestalt psychology, social anxiety involves getting lost in the foreground of a picture. We developed a group treatment program in which we taught people with social anxiety to see sacredness in the many dimensions of their lives: in nature, in loving relationships, and in ordinary events. We had some success in teaching people to see sacredness as measured by pre- and post-ratings of levels of social anxiety and of sacredness.

In short, sanctification is a fruit that I plucked from the tree of Judaism, but it grows on other trees as well. And once harvested, it can add an important spiritual ingredient to the recipe of psychotherapy.

HARVESTING THE FRUIT OF SPIRITUAL STRUGGLES

Years ago, when I first began my studies of religious and spiritual coping with stressful life situations, it became clear to me that while most people saw their faith as a support to them in stressful times, others were experiencing struggles with their faith, struggles that were magnifying the effects of their encounters with stress and trauma. They were feeling punished by God; they were feeling a sense of divine betrayal or abandonment; they were questioning their most basic religious beliefs; they were having conflicts with friends, family, and religious institutions about spiritual matters; they were feeling that they had failed to live up to their spiritual values and beliefs; and they were questioning what, if any, ultimate meaning their lives held. I resonated strongly with these struggles because they were so familiar to me as a Jew.

Elie Wiesel, survivor of Auschwitz and winner of the Nobel Prize in Literature, once said, "What is Jewish history if not an endless quarrel with God" (Wiesel, 1978, p. 6). In Wiesel's (1979) play *The Trial of God*, God stands accused and is ultimately convicted of the pogroms in Chmielnicki in which 100,000 Jews were murdered. Wiesel reportedly based the play on an actual small trial of God he witnessed in Auschwitz, where God was also accused by a small group of inmates of crimes against humanity. There, too, God was found guilty.

Although the very idea of putting God on trial may be shocking, even blasphemous, to some, expressions of struggle such as this one are nothing new within Judaism. Sacred Jewish literature is replete with examples of exemplary figures engaged in passionate arguments with God. Moses complains about God's mistreatment of the Israelites, Jeremiah feels betrayed and deceived by God, and Job angrily calls God to task for his suffering:

> Does it seem good to you to oppress, to despise the work of your hands and favor the schemes of the wicked (Job 10:3). . . . Why do you hide your face and count me as your enemy? Will you frighten a windblown leaf and pursue dry chaff? (*The Holy Bible*, 2006, English Standard Version, Job 13:24–25)

In short, I found myself quite at home in hearing about spiritual struggles. That is a very personal reason why I so eagerly plucked the fruit of spiritual struggles from the Jewish tree. You might wonder how spiritual struggles could be a fruit; they may seem to be more of a weed. But again, from a Jewish perspective, spiritual struggles are not a sign of pathology or weakness. Questioning, disputing, debating, arguing, and struggling are built into the Jewish method of studying *The Torah* (1962/2015). At the risk of overgeneralizing once again, I'd say that struggles may be just as interwoven into the ways Jews deal with each other and the wider world. Struggle, for Jews, is a way of facing the brokenness within oneself and the world and trying to repair some of the damage.

As with sanctification, though, spiritual struggles are a fruit that can be picked from many religious trees. Consider just a few examples. Before he became the Buddha, Siddhartha Gautama had to struggle with the demon, Mara, who presents him with the greatest worldly temptations from lust to pride (*Buddhist Legends*, 1921). In Jesus' final words on the cross, we hear his struggle with feeling abandoned: "My God, my God, why hast thou forsaken me?" (*The Holy Bible*, 2006, English Standard Version, Matthew 27:46).

There is no shortage of modern-day accounts of spiritual struggle. I received the following note from an undergraduate student after I had given a lecture on this topic. She wrote,

> I'm suffering, really suffering. My [bipolar] illness is tearing me down, and I'm angry at God for not rescuing me, I mean really setting me free from my mental bondage. I have been dealing with these issues for 10 years now, and I am only 24 years old. I don't understand why he keeps lifting me up, just to let me come crashing down again.

I began my work in the area with studies of positive and negative religious coping. I have shifted from the language of "negative religious coping" to "spiritual struggles" because the latter term better captures the possibility of positive transformation and growth through spiritual tensions, strains, and conflicts (Pargament, 1997). For several years now, Julie Exline and I, along with our colleagues, have been collaborating on further studies of spiritual struggles. We have defined *spiritual struggles* as tensions, strains, and conflicts about sacred matters (Exline, 2013; Pargament et al., 2005), that can occur within oneself, with others, or with the divine. We developed a brief measure of spiritual struggles through the Brief RCOPE (Religious Coping; Pargament et al., 2011) and a more extensive measure that assesses divine struggles, demonic struggles, interpersonal struggles, moral struggles, religious doubt struggles, and struggles of ultimate meaning (Exline et al., 2014).

Our surveys showed that spiritual struggles are not uncommon. We surveyed a sample of 17,000 adults and asked them whether they had experienced each of our six types of spiritual struggles in the past few weeks (Exline et al., 2014). Of the sample, 31% to 49% reported experiencing the six types of spiritual struggle. The percentages rose to even higher levels, from 39% to 88%, when we asked a national sample about whether they had ever encountered each type of struggle at any point in their lives (Pargament & Exline, 2022).

Spiritual struggles involve deep questions about core beliefs, practices, connections, and values. They can shake us to the core. Perhaps unsurprisingly, they are often a source of distress and disorientation. For example, in her book *Scarred by Struggle, Transformed by Hope*, Joan Chittister (2003) described her experience as a sister in the Roman Catholic church. She had won entrance into the prestigious Iowa State writer's workshop, fulfilling a dream she had long held of becoming a writer. A few days before she was going to leave, the head of her order told her, without explanation, that she could not attend the workshop. Here's how Chittister (2003) wrote about the ensuing spiritual struggle:

> Suddenly without warning . . . I would find myself swimming in a sea of black, my arms and legs heavy and lifeless, tears in my eyes. The frustration of it all swept over me like waves on a beach, pulling me under, upending me in deep water, washing me out away from a firm emotional shore. Day after day, the struggle raged. (p. 91)

Chittister is not alone in her experience. A number of empirical studies have documented robust links between spiritual struggles and signs of psychological distress. For example, in a study of a nationally representative sample of American adults, Abu-Raiya, Pargament, Krause, and Ironson (2015) found that all types of spiritual struggles were tied to depression, generalized anxiety, and less life satisfaction and happiness, even after controlling for demographic variables, neuroticism, social isolation, and religious commitment. Similar findings have emerged from studies across diverse religious groups and cultural contexts (e.g., Abu-Raiya, Pargament, Exline, & Agbaria, 2015; Abu-Raiya et al., 2016; Pedersen et al., 2013; Ramirez et al., 2012).

Spiritual struggles have also been linked to more serious problems, including suicidality (Currier et al., 2017), serious pathology (Berzengi et al., 2016), physical symptomatology (Sherman et al., 2005), and even greater risk of mortality (Pargament et al., 2001). For example, in a study of veterans from the Iraq or Afghanistan wars, higher levels of spiritual struggles were strongly tied to greater suicidality (Currier et al., 2017). For each point of increase on the spiritual struggles measure, the veterans were 1.44 times more likely to have discussed a plan to commit suicide with a desire to die and 1.51 times more likely to attempt suicide in the future. It is important to add that suicidality was not predicted by any of the other variables in the study, including the number of deployments, combat-related exposure, moral injury experiences, depression, and posttraumatic stress disorder symptoms. Spiritual struggles were uniquely predictive of suicidality.

These findings present a pretty dark picture of spiritual struggles. Questions can be raised, though, about whether this picture is complete. After all, we often tell our clients that their struggles and trials can be a source of growth and transformation. Each of the world's great religious figures experienced struggles in life, from Moses and Jesus to Buddha and Muhammad. But each also experienced growth and transformation through these struggles. And there is no shortage of narrative accounts describing growth through spiritual struggles. Chittister (2003) went on to write: Spiritual struggle "gives life depth and vision, insight and understanding. It not only transforms us, it makes us transforming as well" (p. 82). On the other hand, a few empirical studies have examined the relationship between spiritual struggles and reports of growth, and, surprisingly, the findings have been uneven (e.g., Chan & Rhodes, 2013; Gall et al., 2011; Park et al., 2017). Given the robust relationships between spiritual struggles and distress, disorientation, and serious problems, it seems clear that we have to avoid a sentimental view of spiritual struggles as inevitable sources of growth and transformation. Growth through struggles may be possible, but it is not a foregone conclusion. It may take quite a while for people to realize fundamental change. Moreover, people may need help to move from the pain and despair of spiritual struggles to a more positive trajectory. We are working now to identify and mobilize those qualities of wholeness that may facilitate growth and positive transformation (Pargament et al., 2016).

These findings underscore the importance of addressing spiritual struggles within the context of psychotherapy. But how? Here are a few suggestions. First, assess for spiritual struggles in therapy. Just as we ask how the clients' problems affect them emotionally, behaviorally, socially, and physically, we can and should ask how they affect them spiritually. That simple question can open up the door to an important conversation about spiritual struggles. Second, we can draw on our basic clinical skills in conversations about spiritual struggles. Simply listening with compassion and without judgment can be a gift to clients who may be feeling shame that their struggles are a sign of spiritual weakness or fearing punishment from others or the divine about their struggles. Third, we can normalize spiritual struggles as a natural part of the spiritual journey, drawing on the wealth of empirical data to say this is, in fact, the case. If we have the training, we can help clients broaden and deepen their spirituality in ways that foster growth. For example, Nichole Murray-Swank (2003) developed a promising spiritually integrated therapy to address the spiritual struggles of women who have been sexually abused. Her program, Solace for the Soul, helps women discuss the ways their abuse has impacted their understanding of and relationship with God. Many can no longer worship a male representation of God—it is simply too fraught with memories of the trauma and powerful negative emotions. As a result, they have disconnected from their religious traditions. Murray-Swank helps these clients consider other images. In one of her exercises, she has her clients visualize God in gender-neutral terms:

> Picture God as a waterfall within you . . . pouring down cool, refreshing water . . . the waters of love, healing, restoration throughout your body . . . a cool, refreshing waterfall washing down over your head, your face, your shoulders, your neck, out through your arms, down your legs, out through your toes, refreshing bringing life, quenching thirst . . . renewing, refreshing, restoring. (Murray-Swank, 2003, p. 232)

I have highlighted two of the fruits harvested from a Jewish tree, but not exclusive to Jewish trees, that have shown real value in spiritually integrated psychotherapy. As important, though, are the fruits that we can harvest from religious trees that come from other fields. Let me briefly consider how therapists from a variety of religious backgrounds can draw on these fruits.

HARVESTING RELIGIOUS FRUITS FROM OTHER RELIGIOUS TRADITIONS

The ability to draw on the richness of other traditions rests on a pluralistic understanding of religion. This perspective is nonexclusivist. It assumes that every religion may be a container of important truths, but these truths come to us through the hands and voices of human beings who, great as they are, are also frail, fallible, and flawed. Every religion is, as a result, limited. As a group, however, religious traditions may complement each other with each bringing distinctive sources of wisdom to the therapy process. It follows that practitioners can, in their therapeutic roles, partake of not only the fruits from their own traditions but those of others. There is, however, a danger here of communicating a misunderstanding or superficial understanding of these fruits, unfamiliar to the therapist, to clients. To avoid these risks, practitioners must be willing to develop a deeper understanding of these fruits before bringing them to the therapeutic table.

Let me give a personal example. For many years, I found myself frustrated in my clinical work with couples. Oftentimes, they came to therapy with a litany of complaints about each other that they had accumulated over the years. They were, in short, grudge-collectors, looking to me as the judge who might be persuaded by the weight of their grievances to rule in their favor. Working from a communications perspective, I helped them share their complaints with each other, doing my best to make sure they were speaking clearly and listening carefully to each other. I found, though, that this approach could make matters worse rather than better. Airing their grudges more articulately and paying closer attention to those of their partners seemed only to inflame their feelings of anger and resentment.

One day, as another meeting with a grudge-collecting couple was winding down, I asked them, more out of my own frustration than any clinical wisdom, whether either had thought about forgiving their partner. That stopped the finger-pointing conversation in its tracks. After a lengthy pause, both admitted that they had never given the idea of forgiveness any thought at all. This was as much a turning point for me as it was for the couple.

Like the couple, I had given little thought to forgiveness as a resource for psychotherapy. My lack of attention to forgiveness, in part, reflected my understanding of this concept from a Jewish perspective. Within Judaism, forgiveness is described as a relational process. The individual is obligated to forgive transgressors when they have taken responsibility for their mistakes and made proper amends (Rye et al., 2000). Although forgiveness can be offered as an act of charity, there is no obligation to do so on the part of the injured party. This can leave the victim essentially at the mercy of the instigator, holding on to feelings of anger, bitterness, and resentment until the transgressor has done their part. With the couples with whom I was working, each partner was stuck, essentially waiting for the other to go first.

In my conversations with colleagues, I learned that within Christianity, forgiveness is more of a psychological than a relational process. Intrigued, I wanted to learn more. So, I agreed to coedit a book with Michael McCullough and Carl Thoresen on forgiveness (McCullough et al., 2000). And I was able to harvest a fruit from another religious field. In Christianity, I discovered, forgiveness is possible and encouraged regardless of whether the offender is repentant; as a result, the injured party is freed from any dependence on the acts of the perpetrator. Empirical studies also demonstrated the emotional, social, and physical benefits of forgiveness, understood and measured as a psychological process (e.g., Worthington, 2005).

Although it comes from a different religious tree than my own, the Christian fruit of forgiveness has proven helpful in my clinical work. Let me give an example based on my work with a real client whose identifying details have been changed to maintain her confidentiality. Several years ago, I saw Mary, a 30-year-old Roman Catholic woman in therapy who presented with anxiety and depression related to repeated failures in romantic relationships. She had hoped to marry early and have a large family, but she was continually disappointed in her relationships with men, and the older she got, the more she felt her dream fading away. In exploring her history of relationships, I learned that Mary entered each new relationship with high hopes. Within the first date or two, she was imagining the wedding she would have and what their children would look like. Inevitably, however, her potential partner would act insensitively, commit a blunder, or hurt Mary's feelings. Mary would then angrily and abruptly end the relationship and isolate herself for months at a time, stewing in bitterness and resentment until she felt "her biological clock" ticking and once again entered the world of dating.

Much of our time in the early sessions was devoted to Mary's extensive list of complaints against her former partners. A pivotal point occurred in therapy when I asked Mary whether she had ever considered forgiveness of the men who had hurt her. I told her that, although Jewish myself (as Mary knew), I understood that forgiveness was an important value within her own religious tradition. Mary responded by saying that she knew, as a Catholic, she should forgive, but had never been very good at it. She was, however, willing to take a closer look. The focus in therapy shifted then to whether and how Mary might be able to let go of some of her anger and resentments and take a more empathetic and compassionate attitude toward her former partners, even though they were, as she put it, "clueless." We explored Mary's understanding of forgiveness and drew on readings from her Roman Catholic tradition. This was productive work, and Mary was able to make peace within herself about her former partners.

Now the question was whether Mary could apply her new insights to ongoing relationships. I spent several sessions with helping Mary normalize and anticipate the blunders and hurt feelings that would likely arise in forming a new romantic relationship. Rather than end the relationship in a huff, though, we discussed the possibility of responding to these transgressions by sharing feelings and concerns, making concrete efforts to improve the relationship, and cultivating an attitude of forgiveness. Again, this was new territory for Mary, but she was an eager and motivated client. When Mary began dating again, she was able to apply these insights and work through the problems that inevitably arose—but this time, in a spirit of forgiveness that was less a felt obligation and more a deeply felt value. I still receive occasional cards from Mary; she is now married with five children.

It's important to stress that adding the Christian fruit of forgiveness to my recipe of therapeutic ingredients complemented rather than clashed with other fruit I have harvested from Judaism. This is only one example. Psychotherapy can be enhanced by many other fruits growing in still other religious fields.

CONCLUSION

Spiritually integrated therapy is not simply the application of current psychotherapies to religious or spiritual clients. As the name indicates, it involves the integration of spiritual resources and concerns into the context of psychotherapy and, in the process, adds a vital dimension to treatment (Pargament, 2007). However, as yet, relatively little explicit attention has been given to how the therapists' own religious and spiritual orientation may express itself in spiritually integrated psychotherapy. In this chapter, I have tried to address this deficit in a small way by offering personal reflections on how, to some extent consciously and to some extent unconsciously, I have taken fruit from my own religious tradition, Judaism, in therapy. I have also described how I harvested fruit from other religious trees in my work.

Integrating spirituality into psychotherapy in the ways I have illustrated here is not without its challenges. To conclude this chapter, I want to reflect briefly on some key questions that arise. One question is whether therapists should help clients explore religious and spiritual resources that come from traditions other than the therapist's own. For example: Should a therapist who is Christian help a Hindu client explore resources embedded in Hinduism? The answer, I believe, is: It depends. It depends on whether the therapist either has or is willing to develop some familiarity with Hinduism. Of course, few of us have the time or inclination to become expert comparative religionists, mastering the religions of the world. However, therapists are obligated to become conversant enough with the client's religion to engage in a meaningful dialogue about spiritual matters. If not, then the client should be referred to a practitioner better suited to their needs. Having said that, it is important to emphasize that even when therapist and client come from the same religious background, they will undoubtedly differ in some religious respects. As I mentioned earlier, there is no such thing as "the" Protestant, Catholic, Buddhist, Muslim, Hindu, Jewish, or atheist client. Thus, there may be no way around the need for therapists to become more knowledgeable about and engage the particular religious orientation of the individual client. Hospital chaplaincy provides a useful model for therapists in this regard. While rooted in their own faith traditions, chaplains are also well versed in multiple religious worldviews and able to offer sensitive and respectful counsel to religiously diverse patients.

A second key question is whether it is appropriate for therapists to help clients explore religious resources that lie outside the client's own tradition. To use the metaphor of this chapter, Should therapists help clients look into the fruits that come from other religious fields? Mental health professionals are ethically obligated to respect their clients' core beliefs and values, including their religious beliefs and values. For clients who are deeply and exclusively committed to their own tradition, it would be insensitive and inappropriate to suggest that they explore other religious resources and options. Of course, therapists can encourage clients to learn more about resources within their own tradition that they may be unaware of. There are clients, though, who come to us uncommitted to a particular religious identity or committed to their tradition but are nevertheless interested in exploring a variety of religious and spiritual alternatives. In these instances, therapists can facilitate the clients' spiritual quest. Doing so could pose a challenge to therapists who work for a religiously based mental health organization. It is important to remember, however, that the primary obligation of the clinician is to foster mental health while remaining respectful of the client's own autonomy, identity, worldview, and values, even if they do not conform to those of the therapist or the therapist's home institution.

A final key question focuses more on the potential impact of spiritually integrated therapy on the spiritual lives of therapists: Can practitioners explore religious traditions other than their own in therapy while remaining committed to their own religious or spiritual perspective? To some, the idea of learning about other religious worlds may feel disloyal or even an act of betrayal to one's own faith commitments. However, from my own experience, engaging in other religious worlds has not threatened my beliefs and practices. To the contrary, I think my personal spirituality has been enriched and deepened by my contacts with other traditions. Here, I return to my belief that every religion contains important truths, and each may have a distinctive contribution to make to the larger truths we seek in the search for the sacred. It follows that we may have much to gain by drawing from the wisdom of diverse wisdom traditions, but that does not require us to move out of our own spiritual homes. This is admittedly a difficult thing to do, but we may ask no less of clients grappling with diverse attitudes, beliefs, and practices among people in their own families, communities, and cultures.

Each of the key questions I have raised calls for self-reflectiveness on our part as therapists—a keen awareness of how our own approach to religion and spirituality shapes our values, worldview, and clinical practice. In this chapter, I have tried to share some of my self-reflections. Self-awareness can be fostered in other ways as well, for example, by writing a spiritual autobiography, consulting and collaborating with colleagues who come from diverse religious traditions, and taking advanced training in spiritually integrated psychotherapy.

So let me conclude this way: There are many religious fruits ripe for picking. By harvesting these fruits from our own traditions as well as those growing in other religious orchards, we can enrich the lives of our clients, our work as therapists, and spiritually integrated therapy as a whole.

REFERENCES

Abu-Raiya, H., Pargament, K. I., Exline, J. J., & Agbaria, Q. (2015). Prevalence, predictors, and implications of religious/spiritual struggles among Muslims. *Journal for the Scientific Study of Religion, 54*(4), 631–648. https://doi.org/10.1111/jssr.12230

Abu-Raiya, H., Pargament, K. I., Krause, N., & Ironson, G. (2015). Robust links between religious/spiritual struggles, psychological distress, and well-being in a national sample of American adults. *The American Journal of Orthopsychiatry, 85*(6), 565–575. https://doi.org/10.1037/ort0000084

Abu-Raiya, H., Pargament, K. I., Weissberger, A., & Exline, J. J. (2016). An examination of religious/spiritual struggle among Israeli Jews. *The International Journal for the Psychology of Religion, 26*(1), 61–79. https://doi.org/10.1080/10508619.2014.1003519

Ahmadi, F. (2006). *Culture, religion, and spirituality in coping: The example of cancer patients in Sweden.* Acta Universitatis Upsaliensis.

Aish.com. (n.d.). *Blind spot.* https://www.aish.com/j/j/477641713.html

Anderson, S. R., & Hopkins, P. (1991). *The feminine face of God: The unfolding of the sacred in women.* Bantam Books.

Berger, P. L. (1969). *A rumor of angels: Modern society and the discovery of the supernatural.* Anchor Books.

Bergin, A. E. (1980). Psychotherapy and religious values. *Journal of Consulting and Clinical Psychology, 48*(1), 95–105. https://doi.org/10.1037/0022-006X.48.1.95

Berzengi, A., Berzengi, L., Kadim, A., Mustafa, F., & Jobson, L. (2016, August 8). Role of Islamic appraisals, trauma-related appraisals, and religious coping in the posttraumatic adjustment of Muslim trauma survivors. *Psychological Trauma: Theory, Research, Practice, and Policy, 9*(2), 189–197. https://doi.org/10.1037/tra0000179

Bibby, R. W. (1987). *Fragmented gods: The poverty and potential of religion in Canada.* Irwin.

Buddhist legends. (E. W. Burlingame, Trans.). (1921). Harvard University Press.

Buechner, F. (1992). *Listening to your life: Daily meditations with Frederick Buechner.* Harper.

Chan, C. S., & Rhodes, J. E. (2013). Religious coping, posttraumatic stress, psychological distress, and posttraumatic growth among female survivors four years after Hurricane Katrina. *Journal of Traumatic Stress, 26*(2), 257–265. https://doi.org/10.1002/jts.21801

Chittister, J. D. (2003). *Scarred by struggle, transformed by hope.* William B. Eerdmans.

The complete ArtScroll siddur. (1990). (N. Scherman, Trans.). Mesorah Publications.

Currier, J. M., Smith, P. N., & Kuhlman, S. (2017). Assessing the unique role of religious coping in suicidal behavior among U.S. Iraq and Afghanistan veterans. *Psychology of Religion and Spirituality, 9*(1), 118–123. https://doi.org/10.1037/rel0000055

Doehring, C., & Clarke, A. (2002, August 22–25). *Perceiving sacredness in life: Personal, religious, social, and situational predictors* [Paper presentation]. 110th Annual Convention of the American Psychological Association, Chicago, IL, United States.

Exline, J. J. (Ed.). (2013). Religious and spiritual struggles. In K. I. Pargament, J. J. Exline, & J. W. Jones (Eds.), *APA handbook of psychology, religion, and spirituality: Vol. 1. Context, theory, and research* (pp. 459–476). American Psychological Association. https://doi.org/10.1037/14045-025

Exline, J. J., Pargament, K. I., Grubbs, J. B., & Yali, A. M. (2014). The Religious and Spiritual Struggles Scale: Development and initial validation. *Psychology of Religion and Spirituality, 6*(3), 208–222. https://doi.org/10.1037/a0036465

Frankl, V. E. (1959). *Man's search for meaning.* Washington Square Press.

Friedman, E. H. (1985). *Generation to generation: Family process in church and synagogue.* Guilford Press.

Gall, T. L., Charbonneau, C., & Florack, P. (2011). The relationship between religious/spiritual factors and perceived growth following a diagnosis of breast cancer. *Psychology & Health, 26*(3), 287–305. https://doi.org/10.1080/08870440903411013

Harkavy, A. (1951). *The holy scriptures: Revised in accordance with Jewish tradition and modern Biblical scholarship.* Hebrew Publishing Company.

Heschel, A. J. (1955). *God in search of man: A philosophy of Judaism.* Farrar, Straus & Giroux.

The Holy Bible. (English Standard Version). (2006). Crossway.

Howe, I. (1976). *World of our fathers: The journey of the East European Jews to America and the life they found and made.* New York University Press.

Jones, S. L. (1994). A constructive relationship for religion with the science and profession of psychology: Perhaps the boldest model yet. *American Psychologist, 49*(3), 184–199. https://doi.org/10.1037/0003-066X.49.3.184

Karff, S. E. (1979). *Agada: The language of Jewish faith.* Hebrew Union College Press.

Kushner, H. (1989). *Who needs God.* Fireside.

Mahoney, A., Carels, R. A., Pargament, K. I., Wachholtz, A., Leeper, L. E., Kaplar, M., & Frutchey, R. (2005). RESEARCH: "The sanctification of the body and behavioral health patterns of college students." *The International Journal for the Psychology of Religion, 15*(3), 221–238. https://doi.org/10.1207/s15327582ijpr1503_3

McCorkle, B. H., Bohn, C., Hughes, T., & Kim, D. (2005). "Sacred moments": Social anxiety in a larger perspective. *Mental Health, Religion & Culture, 8*(3), 227–238. https://doi.org/10.1080/13694670500138874

McCullough, M. E., Pargament, K. I., & Thoresen, C. E. (2000). *Forgiveness: Theory, research, and practice.* Guilford Press.

Murray-Swank, N. A. (2003). *Solace for the soul: An evaluation of a psychospiritual intervention for female survivors of sexual abuse* (Publication No. 3114946) [Doctoral dissertation, Bowling Green State University]. ProQuest Dissertations and These Global.

Pargament, K. I. (1997). *The psychology of religion and coping: Theory, research, practice.* Guilford Press.

Pargament, K. I. (2007). *Spiritually integrated psychotherapy: Understanding and addressing the sacred.* Guilford Press.

Pargament, K. I. (2013). Searching for the sacred: Toward a nonreductionistic theory of spirituality. In K. I. Pargament, J. J. Exline, & J. W. Jones (Eds.), *APA* handbook of psychology, religion, and spirituality: Vol. 1. Context, theory, and research (pp. 257–273). American Psychological Association.

Pargament, K. I., & Exline, J. J. (2022). Working with spiritual struggles in psychotherapy: From research to practice. Guilford Press.

Pargament, K. I., Feuille, M., & Burdzy, D. (2011). The Brief RCOPE: Current psychometric status of a short measure of religious coping. Religions, 2(1), 51–76. https://doi.org/10.3390/rel2010051

Pargament, K. I., Koenig, H. G., Tarakeshwar, N., & Hahn, J. (2001). Religious struggle as a predictor of mortality among medically ill elderly patients: A 2-year longitudinal study. Archives of Internal Medicine, 161(15), 1881–1885. https://doi.org/10.1001/archinte.161.15.1881

Pargament, K. I., & Mahoney, A. (2005). Sacred matters: Sanctification as a vital topic for the psychology of religion. The International Journal for the Psychology of Religion, 15(3), 179–198. https://doi.org/10.1207/s15327582ijpr1503_1

Pargament, K. I., Murray-Swank, N. A., Magyar, G. M., & Ano, G. G. (2005). Spiritual struggle: A phenomenon of interest to psychology and religion. In W. R. Miller & H. D. Delaney (Eds.), Judeo-Christian perspectives on psychology: Human nature, motivation, and change (pp. 245–268). American Psychological Association. https://doi.org/10.1037/10859-013

Pargament, K. I., Wong, S., & Exline, J. J. (2016). Wholeness and holiness: The spiritual dimension of eudaimonics. In J. Vittersø (Ed.), Handbook of eudaimonic well-being (pp. 379–394). Springer International Publishing. https://doi.org/10.1007/978-3-319-42445-3_25

Park, C. L., Smith, P. H., Lee, S. Y., Mazure, C. M., McKee, S. A., & Hoff, R. (2017). Positive and negative religious/spiritual coping and combat exposure as predictors of posttraumatic stress and perceived growth in Iraq and Afghanistan veterans. Psychology of Religion and Spirituality, 9(1), 13–20. https://doi.org/10.1037/rel0000086

Pedersen, H. F., Pedersen, C. G., Pargament, K. I., & Zachariae, R. (2013). Coping without religion? Religious coping, quality of life, and existential well-being among lung disease patients and matched controls in a secular society. Research in the Social Scientific Study of Religion, 24, 163–192. https://doi.org/10.1163/9789004252073_008

Pomerleau, J. M., Pargament, K. I., & Mahoney, A. (2016). Seeing life through a sacred lens: The spiritual dimension of meaning. In P. Russo-Netzer, S. E. Schulenberg, & A. Batthyany (Eds.), Clinical perspectives on meaning (pp. 37–57). Springer. https://doi.org/10.1007/978-3-319-41397-6_3

Ramirez, S. P., Macêdo, D. S., Sales, P. M. G., Figueiredo, S. M., Daher, E. F., Araújo, S. M., Pargament, K. I., Hyphantis, T. N., & Carvalho, A. F. (2012). The relationship between religious coping, psychological distress and quality of life in hemodialysis patients. Journal of Psychosomatic Research, 72(2), 129–135. https://doi.org/10.1016/j.jpsychores.2011.11.012

Rye, M. S., Pargament, K. I., Ali, M. A., Beck, G. L., Dorff, E. N., Hallisey, C., Narayann, V., & Williams, J. G. (2000). Religious perspectives on forgiveness. In M. E. McCullough, K. I. Pargament, & C. E. Thoresen (Eds.), Forgiveness: Theory, research, and practice (pp. 17–40). Guilford Press.

Sherman, A. C., Simonton, S., Latif, U., Spohn, R., & Tricot, G. (2005). Religious struggle and religious comfort in response to illness: Health outcomes among stem cell transplant patients. *Journal of Behavioral Medicine, 28*, 359–367. https:// doi.org/10.1007/s10865-005-9006-7

The Torah: The five books of Moses (3rd ed.). (2015). The Jewish Publication Society. (Original work published 1962)

The Upanishads: Breath of the eternal. (S. Prabhavananda & F. Manchester, Trans.). (1975). Mentor Books. (Original work published ca. 1 B.C.E.–1400 C.E.)

Wiesel, E. (1978). *A Jew today.* Random House.

Wiesel, E. (1979). *The trial of God (as it was held on February 25, 1649 in Shamgorod): A play in three acts* (M. Wiesel, Trans.). Random House. (Original work published 1987)

Wong, S., & Pargament, K. I. (2017). Seeing the sacred: Fostering spiritual vision in counseling. *Counseling et Spiritualité, 36*(1–2), 51–69. https://doi.org/10.2143/ CS.36.1.3285226

Worthington, E. L., Jr. (Ed.). (2005). *Handbook of forgiveness.* Routledge.

3

THE HEALING TRUTH OF EMPTINESS

Tibetan Buddhism in the Clinical Space

PILAR JENNINGS

In all the great healing traditions, both religious and psychological, there is the suggestion that something new can emerge—and with it, our capacity for well-being. Whether it's a new experience of God's love, an increased capacity to remember the power of ancestral care, or an awakened feeling of trust in a spiritual mentor or therapist, these changing experiences can transform our sense of who we are and the world we inhabit. Implicit in each tradition is the conviction that nothing is as solid or permanent as it seems—no suffering, no state of hopelessness or resignation. For this reason, trust in a future happiness and relief from suffering are warranted.

In Tibetan Buddhism, my spiritual lineage, this foundational insight is called *emptiness*, or *sunyata* in Sanskrit (*tongpanyi* in Tibetan). This enlivening teaching was originally evoked in the *Heart Sutra* (*Buddhist Wisdom*, ca. 100 B.C.E.–600 C.E./2001), when, in the Buddha's time, the legendary Shariputra, the Buddha's disciple, asked Avilotikeshvara, the great bodhisattva of compassion, how to understand and implement the wisdom found in teachings known as *Prajnaparamita Sutras* (*Perfect Wisdom*, ca. 100 B.C.E.–600 C.E./1993). This was his answer: "Form is emptiness, emptiness is form;

https://doi.org/10.1037/0000276-004
Spiritual Diversity in Psychotherapy: Engaging the Sacred in Clinical Practice,
S. J. Sandage and B. D. Strawn (Editors)

emptiness is not other than form, form too is not other than emptiness. Likewise, feelings, perceptions, mental formations, and consciousness are all empty" (Gyatso, 2005, p. 60; see this work for full prayer and commentary).

This prayer is now recited daily in many Buddhist communities as a means of orienting toward a shared understanding of reality. It is a remarkably helpful and psychologically relevant teaching on nondualism that suggests our most entrenched or troubling realities also hold the potential for deepest insight, awakening of compassion, and freedom from suffering—that no experience or moment lacks the potential to be filled with illuminating truth, an awareness, or bare attention that offers needed understanding. It points toward a way of living that finds the sacred in the conventional, the profound in the tangential. It is suggesting that we are not other than a Buddha, an awakened being resplendent with wisdom and compassion; a Buddha is not other than us. No trauma, either personal or collective, has the power to undo this basic truth.

On a first, or even second or third, hearing, this teaching, which undergirds the so-called 84,000 teachings given by the historical Buddha Shakyamuni, can seem ethereal and illusive, and, for some, nihilistic. It seems to suggest that everything we experience as powerfully real—ourselves, our bodies, feelings of love and attachment, memories of our childhood, and so forth—are purely imaginary and insubstantial.

This response is understandable: In Buddhist spirituality, practitioners are encouraged to hold their attachment to experience more lightly, to know that everything we live into is by its nature prone to change in subtle and dramatic ways. Therefore, what gives happiness in one moment can easily become fodder for frustration or vexing pain in another. Conversely, the very things that cause us pain—and for this reason, seem inherently painful—can transform into critically needed aspects of a future happiness. These teachings on attachment are informed by the central Buddhist teaching that everything is empty of anything fixed in nature, enduring from its own side, and thus inherently has the capacity to defy the truth of impermanence and endless transformation.

Another way of describing this, most relevant to our conversation in this book, is that we are relational, and nothing about us exists outside this pervasive relational field. Thus, all phenomena, including our most entrenched interpersonal experiences, are empty of anything that won't be impacted by changing causes and conditions that we are in dynamic relationship with as well as by the inevitable passage of time that will influence the psyche and its inevitable changes.

MY SPIRITUAL BEGINNINGS

I was first exposed to these teachings in adolescence. Having grown up without a religious affiliation, but with a spiritually curious parent, I was exposed to numerous places of worship. As I child, I attended Presbyterian, Unitarian, and a range of services in the conservative and reform Jewish traditions. I also went to my first Buddhist meditation course with my mother and felt a resonance and sense of belonging that stayed with me. In particular, I was struck by the healing impact of quiet reflection; even though it looked like we were all hanging out doing nothing, internally, there was a maelstrom of activity and depth of experience. Our minds were actively sorting through the fullness of life, attempting insight, experimenting with contentment.

As I grew into adolescence, I began to read more about Buddhist spirituality. What I found struck me as revelatory—that the complexity of life, and especially unforeseen adversity, could be experienced with a curious, steady, and nonreactive state of mind. By extension, our internal experience shaped our external one, and not the other way around, as was tempting to imagine. This perspective and the methods supporting it seemed to offer a needed ballast for life's tumult: the ability to stay anchored to a part of the mind that is able to remain open and reflective even when faced with painful circumstances or exciting ones that stir their own flavor of storminess. It seemed to me this was a way to navigate life and to be in the world with integrity.

I continued to contemplate these spiritual teachings, all circling around the ability to cultivate *mindfulness*, a nonreactive and nonjudgmental curiosity that is sustainable in all circumstances. From a Buddhist perspective, this capacity to remain relatively steady internally and to tap into a ready feeling of buoyant receptivity was ultimately informed by wisdom or a visceral insight into the nature of reality. In the Buddhist religious tradition, to be mindful was something that had much deeper and more complex psychospiritual roots than was popularly suggested. The ability to settle the mind and hold one's focus nonreactively was ultimately informed by key insights into the human condition that support this focus.

After years of practice and study of this underlying insight, called sunyata or emptiness, it seemed to me there was something deeply freeing proffered. As a spiritually curious teen who was growing keenly aware of the pervasive and complicated suffering that seemed endemic to the human experience, I began to appreciate how this perspective directly challenged the feeling of being hemmed in by life without needed choices or opportunities for liberation.

PSYCHE BRIDGING THE EMPTINESS

When, years later, I became a psychoanalyst informed by relational, Jungian, and intersubjective perspectives, what I discovered in clinical theory and practice struck a deep chord with my spiritual exploration. I sought out analytic training, in particular, for its emphasis on the unconscious and appreciation for psychological complexity. It seemed to me that these key components could be brought into lively conversation with central Buddhist teachings that appealed to the ameliorative impact of increased consciousness. Early in my training, I noticed that in the patients I worked with, invariably there seemed to be a part of the psyche that pushed for freedom and disentanglement from the most ornate psychic knots (see Ulanov, 2014, for a discussion of entrenched complexes). Even when mired in suffering, there was a part that expressed hope for an altered experience, even if only tacitly and unconsciously conveyed by pursuing a healing process in therapy. It was for this reason that the emphasis on multiplicity and self-states in a relational analytic perspective seemed beautifully resonant with a Buddhist understanding of mind. In both traditions, there was recognition of internal psychic resources that may be well camouflaged but accessible when sought out.

I also appreciated the relevance of Jung's (De Laszlo, 1959) archetypal paradigm through which he identified the origins of multiplicity. Jung understood this push as inherited parts that seek truth and do so while forging one's own way, empowered by the ability to work out and heal persistent and vexing wounds. I would add to this that there seemed to be a part, even in people consciously expressing hopelessness, that is determined to live into a new experience, perhaps sensing that this is not only possible but unavoidable. Unconsciously, we know that change is coming and often seek to ward off unfavorable change or a dashed hope for positive change with a defense against this ineluctable truth.

In my Buddhist studies of sunyata, reinforced by my clinical work, I was struck by the radical suggestion that nothing about our history or psychospiritual development will necessarily bring us to a fated and ossified future. Building on this insight was the growing and felt awareness that favorable childhood circumstances, while a precious resource, were not ultimate sources of healing and well-being, nor, for that matter, were optimal experiences of romantic partnership, something held out in most cultures as a primary healing source. This was an initial awakening, a sense that Buddhist teachings were attempting to challenge thinking and feeling about one's personal reality that lacked the truth of how dynamic we are and how susceptible we are to change, regardless of our origins and imprinting.

Undergirding this insight was the suggestion that what is most needed for feelings of genuine well-being reside within one's own mind. This idea, of course, was picked up and reinforced by Freud and his reverence for intrapsychic experience some 2,000 years later.

Throughout the initial years of my analytic work, it soon became clear that a central part of human suffering is the tendency to impute too rigid notions of oneself and the world one inhabits onto a personal and collective reality that is highly dynamic. I say this with a pointed awareness that it is also critically important to acknowledge the forms of suffering that seem to change so slowly as to render the changes imperceptible—for example, the collective and deeply entrenched ills of racism, misogyny, and xenophobia. Most of my patients have personally suffered the impact of these biases and the pain of feeling and being insufficiently seen or known because of entrenched racial, gendered, and class-based prejudice.

Yet, even with this larger reality in mind, I have observed that the experience of oneself and one's relational dynamics remaining stuck is more often than not fueled by narratives and expectations of self and other that have grown too fixed in meaning and thus are prone to be repeated in all subsequent experience. These are the stories we often tell ourselves about who we are that become a form of unconscious mantra, a scary bedtime story that we become attached to hearing despite the terror it fuels. One could think of this story as an adult Brothers Grimm fairy tale that transfixes and scares into submission. To use Bob Stolorow, Bernard Brandchaft, and George Atwood's (1995) idea, these stories function as organizing principles that set in during a prereflective, presymbolic time in development. They cause suffering by reinforcing distorted and usually negative feelings about oneself but also provide a needed sense of orientation, a psychic road map from which to navigate the tumult and terror of relationship.

The teaching of emptiness could be viewed as another organizing principle—but one meant to challenge all fixed ideas about all principles, including the principle of emptiness. It is sometimes described as the antidote to all rigidified concepts.

This teaching points to the protective tendency to reduce meaning through recognizing only one aspect of a much fuller truth. It suggests that when we suffer, the mind tends to conflate the suffering into one part of an expansive whole. The mind gets rigid, putting aspects of experience into narrow categories of good and bad, pleasurable and unpleasant. And it is this dualism that ultimately keeps the suffering alive. You might rightly ask: Can this teaching be used to dodge or minimize the truth of suffering? Might it put a too positive spin on the truly dreadful realities mentioned earlier—whole groups of people systematically maltreated and exploited for the benefit of the most privileged among us? These are, indeed, pitfalls that I might describe as spiritual bypassing. But I would also suggest that in any healing tradition, the methods and teachings can be used to protect against a more full and complex truth. This is as true of psychotherapy as it is of all religious traditions.

EMPTINESS IN SESSION

As a psychoanalyst, I find myself orienting my clinical work around this teaching of sunyata. Although the methods and teachings of Buddhism are pervasive in my clinical approach, it is this spiritual perspective that most foundationally informs my work as a Buddhist psychoanalyst. With patients, this may feel subtle or overt depending on what is unfolding in the treatment. But in all treatments, I find that this nondual perspective holds us both gently in a place of unknowing where something generative can emerge. More specifically, for the patient, it supports them in a process in which they can first come to know the self-states, or parts, or introjects, that have taken on absolute and fixed meaning, and then enter a place of uncertainty about who they are and who they might become. Potentially, this nondual perspective can usher them into the experience of feeling and claiming more of who they are, inclusive of the parts they dislike—the parts resembling those who have caused them pain and suffering, and what I would describe as their most sacred internal resource of Buddha-nature. Neville Symington (1993) described this part I call Buddha-nature as the "life-giver" (p. 41), the part that decides to turn toward reality rather than its protective disavowal. And, interestingly, he suggested that even the infant chooses this direction of entering into or away from its relational experience.

In the *Abhidharma* (Frauwallner, 1963/1996), the primary text on Buddhist psychology, *Buddha-nature* is described as a place in the psyche below the level of the repressed unconscious, a place of clarity, luminosity. It is the part of the psyche that holds with equanimity all the mental content we are conscious of that tends to run us ragged: the stormy feelings, personal memories, unrelenting fears and desires, and our many protective defenses. These are all thought to camouflage our most useful, sacred internal resource like a thick psychic cloud cover behind which a brilliant sun remains. This Buddha-nature is the part of the mind that can see what we live through with steady curiosity, a willingness to understand more, even to appreciate with some friendly feeling that all of our reality warrants our efforts at care, understanding, and a skillful and compassionate response.

But often, in my personal and clinical experience, some visceral sense of the truth of emptiness is first needed to feel that there is any healing value in building contact with this curious, nonreactive part of the mind. The semiconscious logic goes something like this: If I am fated to pain and suffering, what good would there be in bearing witness consciously? Why not find ways to distract or protect, to seek refuge in mental states of excitement or dissociation? In all clinical work, it soon becomes clear that patients often come into treatment with a dread that past suffering will remain perennial only to be recreated at every turn despite one's best efforts and intentions, even as Stephen Mitchell (1993) wisely suggested there is invariably somewhere in the heart and mind a well-guarded hope that this might not be the case. Mitchell reminded clinicians that, in this way, hope and dread go together.

Optimally, in the unfolding experience with the therapist, a patient may come to find that how they expect to be treated will change because of a sufficiently reliable and good-enough interpersonal experience, and, perhaps over time, their very sense of self will similarly change. In the therapeutic process, they may come to discover that even their history can change as their understanding about what transpired augments to illuminate more full and complex truths. Nothing exists from its own side—even our critical and earliest stages of development. This is good news for patients, something that must be felt and experienced before it can be accepted as another more liberating organizing principle.

BUDDHISM AND DEVELOPMENTAL ANALYTIC THEORY

The Buddhist teaching of emptiness resonates with most contemporary analytic developmental theories that posit a fluid, multiple, or cocreated self and self–other experience. This is likely because of a shared relational emphasis.

In developmental analytic theory, explored, in particular, by Daniel Stern (1985), Jessica Benjamin (2004), and Beatrice Beebe (Beebe et al., 2005), we find our always growing and changing self through being found by another. In this way, our evolving self grows within the shifting currents of a relational matrix (Beebe et al., 2005). In the mother–infant research conducted by these analysts, the baby slowly discovers their own mind through their mind and its potential, first being held in the mind of the mothering one. The baby's sense of themselves as a viable person separate from the mother yet still safely connected in a way that can allow for their authentic differences grows steadily stronger with the gift of the mother's attunement and recognition of who this particular child is and is becoming.

Before this research, analysts such as Winnicott (1958/1992) and Kohut (1984) wrote with reverence for the impact of feeling emotionally held in the mind of an attuned and empathic other, an interpersonal holding that allows the child this gift of spontaneous and fluid development. It is an early experience that spares a growing child the suffering of feeling stuck or fated to be or feel something that cannot change without undue risk of loss. It also protects needed psychic resources in the developing infant's physical and emotional "feel" for the world they are in relationship to.

Benjamin (2004) evoked the blessing of an attuned other by emphasizing the child's resulting and growing capacity for mutual recognition: to both see the other and be seen by the other—not one, not two but both subjects and with a third reality that grows between them. This mutual recognition is a constantly renewed commitment. When it's lost, the work is done for repair to restore the balance of seeing and being seen. It is interesting that, for this very reason, in spiritual practice of all types, we affirm our own sacredness *and* the sacredness of the other—lover, stranger, enemy—over and over again.

In the Buddhist tradition, to support this effort, we practice cultivating *equanimity*, the visceral sense that all beings, whether we personally know them, like them, or find ourselves in their perception of us, wish to be well and freed from all forms of suffering. Without this renewed awareness and commitment, the part of us that feels fundamentally and concretely separate and thus in need of vigilant protection easily creeps in and takes over. That third and generative space that Benjamin (2004) described is easily lost, an insight recognized and directly addressed by all religious traditions.

What I have come to find is that in both Buddhist psychology and contemporary analytic theory, emptiness undergirds and supports trust in subjective and intersubjective healing. We enter into relationship with our patients with faith (now backed by copious interpersonal neurobiological research) that both patient and therapist are changed by the experience of being in this relationship. Therapists may notice this in the unexpected evolution from initial and powerful transference and countertransference that can grip us with the feeling of absolute truth. Maybe we feel it as a compelling conviction of being inadequate for a particular patient that is perhaps confirmed by a patient's rage about our inadequacies; or, conversely, we feel it through an early warm and loving transference that convinces us of our more esteem-enhancing qualities, all of which seem to dissolve or radically change as the work deepens as one or both of us risk greater honesty, speaking hard but necessary truths that may destabilize us but also illuminate formerly hidden parts of who we are and how we are changing together (Hirsch, 2008).

In Buddhist traditions, the student–teacher dyad works together with a similar understanding that who the student is in their fullness of being can emerge, shift, and grow when in close relationship to a spiritual mentor who seeks to find hidden resources of compassion, insight, and wisdom in the student's mind. Traditionally, this has been referred to as *mind-to-mind transmission* rather than transference (Richmond, 2012). It is not as mystical as it sounds. In my experience, mind-to-mind transmission more closely mirrors the analytic encounter with two people getting to know each other in the spirit of honest communing, respect, and appreciation for what will arise from this encounter. This intimate exchange makes room for a bidirectional idealizing transference that is felt consciously and invited in, and where fixed or delimiting notions of who the student is, will likely shift to make room for who and what the teacher is recognizing in the student (see Jennings, 2013, for an exploration of needed room for the Buddhist teacher's experience).

Nevertheless, even with these compelling parallels, there are some interesting differences in the traditions and in how they posit entry into fullness of self and relational experience. Here's one: In the Mahayana tradition, which includes Zen and Tibetan Buddhism, the primary credo is that we find ourselves through finding another. This is symbolized by the bodhisattva who has achieved fullest awakening and could thus opt to leave the endless cycle of life and death but is determined to stay in this world until all beings are freed from suffering. And through this process of finding others, responding skillfully and swiftly to their suffering and their need to feel well, the bodhisattva reinforces their own deepest nature of wisdom that generates compassion. The bodhisattva orients toward their clear-seeing that we are inherently relational beings—that we are empty of any fundamentally discrete or separate nature. We are empty of anything that won't be affected by others or by our changing experience.

We find ourselves through finding others. And the primary agent for healing in this whole endeavor resides deep within one's own psyche. It doesn't reside solely in the analyst, or in the guru, or in a devout partner, or even in favorable life circumstances. These are resources but not of ultimate healing power. It is Buddha-nature, a mind of clear-seeing that is the agent for well-being.

As I mentioned earlier, in developmental theory and in most contemporary analytic theories, in contrast, we find ourselves through being *found* by another. While there has been increasing emphasis on the bidirectional impact of mothers (or mothering ones) and infants (Beebe et al., 2005) and the coconstruction of relational experience in all relationships (Hoffman, 1998), there has nevertheless been an implicit emphasis on what the mother or therapist can facilitate in the child or patient's experience. In the Buddhist tradition, as referenced earlier, there's a comparable appreciation for the importance of having a mentor, someone to midwife to the mind's foreground our extraordinary and shared inner resources. But just as there's an implicit privileging of the mentor's role in the analytic tradition, there's an implicit suggestion in Buddhism that we are already capable of being a mentor; what's needed is already in place. So, we see that the emphasis on what ushers in fluid but sufficiently cohesive self and self–other experience is not incompatible but different.

Not surprisingly, some of my Buddhist friends take issue with the dependency need proposed in developmental theory. It seems, to them, to bypass the primary internal agent for change and too dependent on another to locate this agent within the growing child. And some of my analytic friends take issue with the absence of this early relational need in Buddhist spirituality. And it's true: Interestingly, there is no dharma (Buddhist teaching) of early childhood. But I don't think that's solely because of the historical Buddha's own unconscious relationship to his early childhood, although I would imagine that's in the mix. What I imagine is that this has more to do with the internal orientation in the Buddha-dharma that does not minimize the impact of our circumstance and relational history. Rather, it suggests what is most needed is the direct experience of emptiness—that nothing is fixed in meaning—supported by contact with one's Buddha-nature, the part that sees one's reality with abiding, nonreactive curiosity and a freeing awareness of sunyata.

In my clinical experience, it is typically people who have had some—albeit fleeting—contact with this part who come in for treatment. This might be because they have lifted to awareness what it would be like to live from this part and therefore know the suffering of losing contact with it. There is the sense of needed psychic air having been taken in then lost. While such patients might not articulate their experience in this way, I sense them asking themselves before treatment, How much aliveness, how much awareness can I stand? How radically will my life have to change if I risk this aliveness?

As a side note, but one that feels important to name, these are often the patients, at least in my clinical experience, whom Dan Shaw (2014), in his excellent work on narcissism, would describe as having suffered the cumulative developmental trauma of being raised within a relational matrix by someone who cannot tolerate their separate subjectivity. Of course, such patients have strong narcissistic currents, too, and can be deeply disappointing to others as a result, but typically they are in treatment to somehow make sense of and heal from the active destruction of their authentic and fluid subjectivity, a shaming of their dependency needs, and a simultaneous and crazy-making demand for unquestioned loyalty.

Such patients come to treatment with an insufficient sense of their own viable subjectivity—as if their very personhood were an affront to the absolute reality of others and their absolutely essential need for perfect mirroring and accommodation. And if they are Buddhists, and many of my patients are at least curious about Buddhism, this gnawing, although usually only semiconscious sense of needing more room for their own subjective reality, can be cause for an additional layer of confusion and guilt. They ask, Isn't the whole point to let go of self, to hold everything lightly?

What is not yet clear to them is that just as the mythical Narcissus was frozen by the image of himself, they get frozen in a mirroring position, the mythical Echo's stance. Both are stuck in self-experience that lack the suppleness for anything new or life-giving to emerge.

I'll tell you a little about a patient who closely matches this description and our evolving work together.

CASE EXAMPLE: EDDIE

The Beginning: Ease and Empathy

When we began working together, Eddie[1] was in his early 50s, a well-educated, highly intelligent Latino man with a gentle demeanor who had aspired to be a sculptor. He was raised by parents of Colombian descent in a traditional Roman Catholic home with religious values that were rigidly adhered to. While he described himself as a lapsed Catholic with a subtle interest in Buddhist spirituality, the religious values of his youth were deeply entwined with his sense of self. In the early stages of our work, he seemed very dear to me: tender hearted, kind, and clearly hurt. His elderly mother had recently died, a loss that seemed to consume him in a haunting way. And his father, then 92 years old, was left alone. His two older siblings were not participating in their father's care, something that seemed to cause Eddie endless confusion.

Slowly, we explored Eddie's family history in a working-class town outside of Los Angeles. His brother and sister were 10 and 12 years older, respectively. Because he was the sole caretaker of his elderly father, who still lived in his childhood home across the country from his New York City apartment, Eddie was traveling back and forth once a month. It was knocking him out,

---

[1]Identifying details of the client have been changed to maintain their confidentiality.

he said. He'd exhale as if he'd just returned from Mt. Everest, no words matching the feeling of total depletion.

Over time, it came out that his father was riddled with anxiety and became irate when faced with any minor unforeseen change or irritant—for instance, the need for a new toaster or a new eyeglasses prescription. He would endlessly repeat to Eddie the impossibility of this new catastrophe and always imply that Eddie should have been able to protect him from those untenable stressors. When I'd suggest that his father's behavior sounded quite challenging, Eddie would shrug and follow with, "It's nothing a real person wouldn't be able to deal with."

I soon came to understand that Eddie did not consider himself to be a real person. He was, in his words, "a zero, a nonperson. A total nonstarter."

In the early stages of our work, I felt a palpable empathy for Eddie. I, too, had an elderly father whom I cared for and wanted to help, but, at times, I feared losing myself in this caretaking. I could easily image Eddie's painful dilemma. There were occasional moments in our sessions when I felt him relaxing into some auxiliary empathy for himself.

Given my temperament and spiritual training, this empathy felt clinically "right" and comfortable. It was an intuitive and accessible way to restore Eddie's capacity to care for and hold his own suffering.

But, with each new stressor faced in his caregiving, the merciless nature of his self-condemnation disturbed me. I quickly found myself consumed with an uncomfortable and burning anger, mostly toward his father. When I tried to offer a reality check that his father's eruptions and chronic suggestion that Eddie's efforts were insufficient or were the cause for these various unavoidable snafus distorted the truth of what transpired, he'd shake his head as if my interpretations were up against his father's unquestionable validity. He continued: "My siblings are not around, so clearly I'm the common denominator. I'm the nonperson. The failure." The unquestioned brutality of his self-attack was painful to witness and feel.

I tried to help Eddie think about his siblings and the various reasons they had both suffered a rupture with the father. We talked about the contempt they were all up against: the father's rageful eruptions in their childhood seemingly without provocation, his alcoholism that worsened over time and had gone untreated, his severe anxiety that manifested as unbearable efforts at control. Eddie would shake his head again as if to undo the dots of light in our conversation. In these moments, I was grateful for Bion's (1959) pithy phrase: "attacks on linking." Increasingly, I began to feel Eddie's struggle to let my perspective meet or impact his own. This disrupted link between our thoughts and feelings reflected a deeper internal disruption between his own authentic feelings and perspectives and those of his internalized family members.

So, too, I felt in a visceral way how Bion's (1959) description of ultimate reality, interestingly symbolized by *O*, and the determined defense against it, were powerfully in the room in our sessions. It was as if Eddie were actively warding it off for fear that whatever truth and ensuing aliveness he accessed would once again remain maddeningly elusive or would usher in over-whelming grief about what hadn't yet been possible. In this way, the hope and the dread were so intimately bound that each moment felt increasingly painstaking and treacherous.

Covert Longings

Soon, we began to talk about his mother. When the treatment began, Eddie's mother had been deceased for a little over 1 year. He would sink into an undertow of turgid despair during these conversations, something I initially attributed to the proximity of this loss. But, before too long, he described a quality of closeness that unnerved me. Eddie was the "special one" in his mother's eyes, the one she held close. It became Eddie's job to meet her needs perfectly, something he would devote himself to accomplishing.

There were other memories that suggested another layer of enforced merger, of staying close physically and in ways that were not unusual in childhood but stirred uncomfortable and "weird" feelings in Eddie. In the first 2 years of our work, these memories would resurface and clobber Eddie. This was his logic: If they were true and he'd allowed for too much close-ness, then he was a wuss, a coward for not having escaped as his siblings had managed to. If these events hadn't happened and he was overdramatizing what had happened, then he was drumming up self-pity and was, therefore, pathetic.

I felt stymied by the madness and cruelty of this inner critic and would point out the presence of this critical protector part, the part that indicted him for his suffering. Again, he'd shake his head "no" as if my perspective were an intrusion on the absolute and fixed reality that he had failed at his job to comply perfectly with his parent's needs and expectations. This was the program, and his suffering indicated his failure to successfully complete it.

All throughout his childhood, his father's behavior and alcoholism wors-ened, and Eddie felt pulled ever closer to the mother. He said it felt like they were dating. At the dinner table, after his elder siblings left for college, the father sneered at Eddie, exuding hatred toward him. In a quiet way, he knew he'd been the chosen one, the special one, but also, as a result, the one who would never become a real person. His job was to join with the mother, to mirror her perfectly, and to gratify her every unmet need. All this meant splitting off his sexuality so much so that he says he had no conscious sexual feeling until he was well into adulthood.

Eddie had read most of Freud's work and was well aware of his Oedipal theories. This embarrassed him, reinforcing his sense that he should have been able to avoid something "so cliché." With a powerful shame always hovering in the background, Eddie courageously told me about memories that filled him with toxic shame: being at parties or work events and meeting people, both men and women, whom he grew curious about but could never pursue romantically. There was the sense that these longings must be put away, were somehow, by their very nature, unseemly. But he feared that somehow the people who stirred his interest could sense his curiosity, and, in a way, that burdened them.

In the session, Eddie cried, knowing that he communicated needs indirectly, the way his mother did and that his bisexuality, which he had begun to grapple with when he was 40, and his overarching sexuality, pushed into the unconscious, seeped out despite his very best efforts. He'd spent years writing lists of every woman he'd ever met, trying to convince himself that one of them could be attractive to him. In his traditional Catholic home in which acceptable gendered roles and expressions of sexual desire were tightly bound to heteronormative tradition, and with the libidinally charged relationship with his mother, Eddie came to recognize his bisexuality as carcinogenic. If he were openly gay or bi, this difference would shatter his role as the mother's mirror.

It was during these sessions that I noticed Eddie occasionally staring at me with a hunger that felt devouring and invasive. There was the sense of Eddie wanting me to be his—not a separate person. He struggled to leave each session and often cried as the session was coming to an end, usually leaving in tears and once telling me, "I don't know how you can let me go like this."

I knew what he meant. He was grief stricken and depressed, and was wading through enormous complexity. In such moments, my spiritual training was especially helpful in noticing and working with the strength of my countertransference in real time. With mindfulness offering needed support, I noticed my own strong feelings of entrapment and the chronic gnawing sense that I could not adequately help him. The vague awareness of sunyata during these times helped me relax into a deepening exploration of this countertransference. I sensed more fully that I was experiencing, as I imagined he did with his mother, the overwhelming presence of his perpetual need that I couldn't possibly meet but must keep trying to do so—that his needs had an absolute and overarching reality that required a correct response. For the time being, I made efforts simply to notice this parallel process and slowly to explore with Eddie the burden of attempting to meet an expectation that can never be met without relinquishing one's own vitally needed separate reality.

New Loss: New Gains?

Five years into the treatment, Eddie's father died. He was 96 years old. Just minutes before he died, he apologized to Eddie and thanked Eddie for having helped him. He told Eddie how much he loved him and felt grateful for his love and care. It felt real, genuine, as if he was seeing his son with an affection Eddie could trust for the first time. This moment was deeply meaningful for Eddie but also painful because his father had no contact with his other children before he died.

A part of me hoped that perhaps a new space would open in Eddie's life for him to cultivate a more meaningful relationship with himself outside the asphyxiating narcissistic matrix that had run his life. For 56 years, he had suffered a severe ensnarement of caretaking with too little room for him to develop a new and potentially healing relational experience. But, instead, he now felt that "it was over." Meaning, he was over.

This was a difficult time in the treatment for us both. He seemed unable to begin mourning what had not yet been possible and was instead collapsing into a swamp of melancholia I worried he may be drowning in. At times, I also felt him refusing the work of therapy but instead unconsciously waiting for a new history and therefore a new life. It would take me several more years to appreciate the ways in which this dynamic sustained his fantasy of a "do-over." If he accepted more fully what he had suffered with his family and what hadn't been possible, he would be giving up any efforts at retroactive control.

In one session, when he wept about my summer break after having taken it, and after my father's sudden death, he admitted to googling me, having found my father's obituary online, and having read about him and my family. He risked telling me directly that our session before the break had been unhelpful and stirring when he most needed time to prepare for my time away—that, with all these mobilized feelings, he'd found a way to feel connected. I felt simultaneously moved by his trust in me that allowed for this honest and direct communication and invaded. I said,

> I understand that it upsets you when I when I tend to my own needs that don't align with yours. It's true: There *are* limits to what I can offer you. But, here, you can experience being in a relationship where we can talk directly about

what you need and where there is room for us to have separate, even conflicting needs. Even our stories can be different.

He nodded, weeping, lingering at the door, and left my office begrudgingly. During this time, I tried to sustain awareness of how stuck I felt in repetitive dynamics with Eddie and inadequate to meet his needs. I also made efforts to let my awareness land in this feeling directly—and for fleeting moments to know that, as stuck as I felt, as stuck as Eddie felt, we were experiencing something rife with meaning and highly dynamic. Almost immediately following this awareness, Eddie told me that with his mother, he often had the feeling of "trying to shake her off." He felt his mother staring into him, needing him relentlessly. It never stopped.

These moments of awareness brought needed air into our sessions. They were moments of reality that broke through his own entrenched narcissistic defenses and mine. He even admitted that he would no longer be attending my various public talks on Buddhism and clinical work because he knew that doing so fed his fantasy and also reinforced his feeling and belief that the best he could do was be a psychic host, to sidle up to people he admired and get some feeling of romantic closeness. It's all he would allow for, but he had begun to feel that it was better to interrupt that cycle, to feel what he hungered for more consciously. I deeply respected Eddie's willingness to divulge this struggle and to attempt to work it through with me directly. I pointed out that as risky as that exposure must have been, it ushered in a mutually held boundary that would give him a needed feeling of safety. He nodded, seeming to take this in.

NEEDED METHODS BEYOND THE CLINICAL

I have found that with Eddie and most patients who have suffered getting caught in this vexing relational web, I have needed more than my clinical training to do this work. Often what helps me stay the course, to feel into it directly without getting swallowed whole while holding some awareness for what might shift, even in subtle ways and slowly, are the methods and teachings I've explored in my religious life. Awareness of the unconscious and its many complex protective mechanisms are invaluable but, for me, only one critical dimension of a full and meaningful treatment.

I say this with awareness that a psychodynamic approach to human suffering can usher in extraordinary compassion for the suffering patient. We clinicians keep chambers of the heart open for what has been protectively defended against in the patient, at times, over the course of decades.

However, with complex developmental trauma, the work tends to be slow going and can easily tug on the protective defenses in the clinician. So, too, as described earlier, enactments are likely to develop and require capacities in the clinician that I would suggest transcend psychodynamic methods. With Eddie, I felt the presence of my spiritual training in every session, specifically, the skillful means, or *upaya*, that include patience, joyous effort, and concentration. Throughout the treatment, as I've explored in this chapter, I felt the potential to lose myself in the overwhelm of countertransference. But with these skillful means and, centrally, the teaching of emptiness, I also felt able to take note of the experience with a witnessing part able to access sufficient patience to wait for and imagine how my experience and Eddie's might shift over time.

It is my hunch that analytic training alone did not bolster the very resources that have protected the unfolding work with Eddie. I have needed to recognize and orient toward his Buddha-nature, the part of him that can access awareness of a fuller truth with compassion and respect for his profound suffering. So, too, the skillful means have offered me support as I continue reconnecting with this part of Eddie when my own anxiety or doubt obfuscate a deeper trust in the healing potential of our work. And I have needed to orient toward my awareness that no aspect of Eddie's history would render him incapable of recognizing his own deepest value beyond anyone's limiting judgment. This might be a slower process than either of us would wish for, but with the skillful means of patience and joyous effort, there is a spaciousness provided to work toward and live into this new experience.

It is also my sense that our work has been informed to some degree by the intersection of our respective religiously informed values. Eddie had internalized a sense of absolute right and wrong, sin and sinner that permeated his sense of self, of not being the "right" kind of man to garner love and care from his family. And while such absolutes can be unknowingly absorbed in all faith traditions, I felt him receiving comfort from the concept of emptiness. This was and remains a slow process, but the Buddhist practice of recognizing that nothing is imbued with inherent qualities of good or bad but is infused with multiple and always dynamic conditions was opening some small space in his psyche to hold the parts of himself he'd come to feel were inherently unlovable.

Of course, it's possible that if we'd both been Roman Catholic, such spaces would still have emerged, perhaps informed by my notions of God's love, or grace that stirred his own less conscious relationship to these spiritual blessings. However, I continued to sense that our spiritual differences were needed, and, I hope, ultimately generative.

NEW PERSPECTIVES, NEW AWARENESS

Several months later, Eddie and I were coming to the end of a session. He was describing an upcoming social event that filled him with overwhelming anxiety. The opportunity for him to not be who they needed him to be was endless, treacherous. In such moments, the needs of others took on absolute meaning, something defying reflection, something fixed in its very essence.

I asked, "Is there any part of you that might want something from the experience that's separate from the need to accommodate your friends' expectations?" He looked at me, both perplexed and with a sense of knowing more fully that the web he'd been caught in, had been raised in, could be thought about, considered—even challenged.

Eddie knew I was a Buddhist and had come to talks I'd given on the conversation between Buddhism and psychoanalysis. In my office, just above him, was a painting of Green Tara, the bodhisattva of swift compassionate action. I pointed it out to him, something I'd never done before. I mentioned that this female Buddha had one foot extended outward, symbolizing her commitment to joining others in their experience, and one tucked inward, symbolizing her ongoing commitment to nurturing her own deepest well-being—not one or the other, but both.

Eddie stood up and stared at it, seemingly struck by this image of a woman committed to her own well-being without suffering catastrophic rupture or condemnation. Tara Buddha, interestingly referred to as the Mother of All Buddhas, looked so unconflicted. "Ha," he exclaimed. "Interesting," he said quietly while bopping his head back and forth as if to say, "I'll think about it." He left my office with an uncharacteristically relaxed and mirthful expression.

This painting of Tara Buddha is what I see while working with my patients. I often feel that this symbol of my own Buddha-nature reminds me that we are all forever working out this effort to feel fully and dynamically in relationship to ourselves and others. Tara Buddha is described as being in a dancing pose, as if this simultaneous relationship to her own awakened mind that can tolerate and enter into reality alongside her efforts to recognize others and their awakened mind requires a readiness to be dynamic, fluid, not stuck in any one position.

Her pose also has me considering that just as we need to be dynamic interpersonally, holding that empty and generative space that can nurture the birth of something new, we also need to dance between and with contrasting healing traditions. Perhaps there is no one tradition that necessarily has the capacity to ensure a person who has taken refuge in a rigidly protective position will find what's needed to extricate themselves. Healing traditions are empty, too, and receive what participant and dyad bring to the experience. The healing is not inherent in the method.

I would like to suggest that experiencing the healing truth of emptiness involves, for patients and therapists, the necessary challenge of thinking beyond what we've previously thought or been taught to think, of letting our thoughts make direct contact with feelings that we haven't previously felt, and risking a quality of aliveness that may come with the terror of all things new. And, as we do this radical work, we may come to find that no one is left out of the generative space that's created, a space that can heal the protective currents that thwart fullness of living. This is the great gift of our own spiritual and psychological work: coming to find that it is an ever-expanding and reliable space that can hold all parts of who we are and all beings who compose our world.

REFERENCES

Beebe, B., Knoblauch, S., Rustin, J., & Sorter, D. (2005). *Forms of intersubjectivity in infant research and adult treatment*. Other Press.

Benjamin, J. (2004). Beyond doer and done to: An intersubjective view of thirdness. *The Psychoanalytic Quarterly, 73*(1), 5–46. https://doi.org/10.1002/j.2167-4086.2004.tb00151.x

Bion, W. R. (1959). Attacks on linking. *The International Journal of Psychoanalysis, 40*, 308–315.

Buddhist Wisdom: The Diamond Sutra and the Heart Sutra (E. Conze, Trans.). (2001). Vintage Books. (Original work published ca. 100 B.C.E.–600 C.E.)

De Laszlo, V. S. (Ed.). (1959). *The basic writings of C. G. Jung*. The Modern Library.

Frauwallner, E. (1996). *Studies in Abhidharma literature and the origins of Buddhist philosophical systems* (S. F. Kidd & E. Steinkellner, Trans.). SUNY Press. (Original work published 1963)

Gyatso, T. (2005). *Essence of the heart sutra: The Dalai Lama's heart of wisdom teachings* (G. T. Jinpa, Ed. & Trans.). Wisdom Publications.

Hirsch, I. (2008). *Coasting in the countertransference: Conflicts of self interest between analyst and patient*. Analytic Press.

Hoffman, I. Z. (1998). *Ritual and spontaneity in the psychoanalytic process: A dialectical–constructivist view*. Analytic Press.

Jennings, P. (2013). Knowing our teachers: Intersubjectivity and the Buddhist teacher/student dyad. In N. Cater & P. Young-Eisendrath (Eds.), *Buddhism and depth psychology: Refining the encounter* (Vol. 89, pp. 79–89). Spring Journal.

Kohut, H. (1984). *How does analysis cure?* The University of Chicago Press. https://doi.org/10.7208/chicago/9780226006147.001.0001

Mitchell, S. A. (1993). *Hope and dread in psychoanalysis*. Basic Books.

Perfect wisdom: The short Prajnamaramita texts (E. Conze, Trans.). (1993). Buddhist Publishing Group. (Original work published ca. 100 B.C.E.–600 C.E.)

Richmond, L. (2012, July 30). *Commentary: Three levels of transmission.* Lion's Roar. https://www.lionsroar.com/commentary-three-levels-of-transmission/

Shaw, D. (2014). *Traumatic narcissism: Relational systems of subjugation.* Routledge.

Stern, D. N. (1985). *The interpersonal world of the infant.* Basic Books.

Stolorow, R. D., Brandchaft, B., & Atwood, G. E. (1995). *Psychoanalytic treatment: An intersubjective approach.* Routledge.

Symington, N. (1993). *Narcissism: A new theory.* Karnac Books.

Ulanov, A. B. (2014). *Knots and their untying.* Spring Journal Books.

Winnicott, D. W. (1992). *Through paediatrics to psycho-analysis: Collected papers.* Brunner-Routledge. (Original work published 1958)

4

NAVIGATING DEEP WATERS

Spirituality and Religion in the Womanist Psychodynamic Space

PHILLIS ISABELLA SHEPPARD

Thanks to You, source of all being, life giving wisdom, and Holy Spirit.
As it was with the ancestors, in the beginning, is now, and in faith, we believe,
it shall ever be.

—P. I. Sheppard

When I began my clinical training, first at the Center for Religion and Psychotherapy of Chicago (CRPC) and later at the Institute for Psychoanalysis in Chicago ("the Institute"), there was a great deal of excitement in psychoanalytic circles, especially in the still relatively early days of Heinz Kohut's self psychology. It was in this context that I began to theorize religion and spirituality in the clinical space. In the late 1980s and early 1990s, I began the first leg of my training in psychoanalytic psychotherapy at the CRPC. The faculty and clinical staff were composed primarily of clergy, former pastors, and chaplains who discerned a revised vocation that moved them beyond the pulpit and the office of congregational care to pastoral psychotherapy. Given these roots, one would think that developing a clinical appreciation

https://doi.org/10.1037/0000276-005
Spiritual Diversity in Psychotherapy: Engaging the Sacred in Clinical Practice,
S. J. Sandage and B. D. Strawn (Editors)

for spirituality and religion would be straightforward and uncomplicated. However, in my experience, the CRPC was actually somewhat ambivalent about the place of religion as an aspect of clinical work. It was not unusual to hear in our case conference the question "What does it mean?" "It" referred to religion, because "it" could never be just religion. There was, in my view, an undercurrent of suspicion—possibly therapeutic suspicion, but suspicion nevertheless—when it came to religion. As much as religion was at the center of our personal life orientation, as clinicians, our desire to be truly psychoanalytic would often override an openness to exploring religion *as religion*. The fact that we were several blocks south of the Institute—founded in 1932 and the second oldest psychoanalytic training institute established in the United States—surely fueled our image, fantasy, and practice of what psychoanalytic psychotherapy should be. Under these competing forces, religion was never uncomplicated. In 1989, I entered clinical training already inclined to read religion as complicated, complex, and yet powerful. In part, that was because of an early experience that resulted in me learning the complicated feelings my parents brought to religious experience. While eavesdropping on a heated conversation between my parents, I learned that my father had relatives who practice "roots."[1]

It seems that my mother was referencing the power of roots spirituality to do harm, and this, in my 10-year-old's mind, unnerved my father. Upon further reflection, I think it is possible my father was familiar with roots practices. The accusation of having family members who practiced roots could also have been a reference to the religious practice's proximity to African spiritualities and, therefore, in conflict with the Sheppard side of the family's public identification as Christian and Baptist. My parents had converted to Roman Catholicism early in their marriage and, seemingly, did not experience any loss. They could not imagine that these relatives could be both Christian and root workers simultaneously. I did not know what root practices were, but I was fascinated that something about religion could evoke such strong reactions in both of them.[2] Perhaps this powerful family memory drove my education and training. At the CRPC, and later at the Institute, the excitement in psychoanalytic circles, especially in the still relatively early days of Heinz Kohut's self psychology, affirmed my sense that religion and spirituality had a place in the clinical setting.

---

[1]"Hoodoos" and "root workers" were the most common vernacular expressions that depicted persons believed to be able to manipulate unseen forces or "work the spirits." "Root doctors" was a prevalent euphemism describing persons who practiced healing only. "Conjure doctors" could include those who possessed the power to do harm as well as to heal (Chireau, 2003/2006, p. 21).

[2]This story from my childhood was previously discussed in Sheppard (2017).

SELF PSYCHOLOGY AND RELIGION AT THE CENTER FOR RELIGION AND PSYCHOTHERAPY

The CRPC, founded in 1965, is a psychotherapy and pastoral counseling, as well as a clinical training program. Several of the clinical faculty had been analyzed by self psychologically oriented psychoanalysts, and this perspective became integral to the curriculum and clinical practice at CRPC.

Heinz Kohut (1977) developed his self psychology primarily in response to his psychoanalytic patients who did not present with oedipal concerns. These patients were more likely suffering from frequent bouts of diminished self-esteem, fluctuations between grandiosity and depression, and a lack of sustained purpose. In other words, their narcissistic equilibrium was difficult to maintain. These patients were not struggling with competitive rivalry in their relational lives, but instead they were arrested in their development along self-development lines. According to Kohut, he shifted his focus from the Freudian instinctual models, because his patients experienced Oedipal interpretations as an empathic failure and did not improve. Kohut did not discount the value of the Oedipal model, but he surmised that the radical shifts in the cultural milieu related to the patient's parenting. Specifically, Kohut argued that the shift in the middle-class Victorian model of intense parental involvement in children's lives to one of increased distance brought on by the changes in family and work life after World War II subjected children to significant periods of emotional and/or physical parental absence. The psychological needs for mirroring, recognition, kinship, and idealizing figures were sporadically met or in some cases, were completely neglected. The "self" Kohut theorized was subject to experiences of alienation—from self, intersubjective, and cultural experience (Kohut, 1985a; see also Asante, 2009; Bonovitz, 2005; Gehrie, 1980; Miliora, 1997).

Throughout my training, and later, as I deepened my understanding, I came to believe/realize/be persuaded that Kohut never fully linked these three, but close readings of his essays on culture, idealization, and courage do create a red thread between the formation of the self and the broader sociocultural context (Kohut, 1985). It is a thread that he could have given more clinical consideration. However, Kohut maintained his strong interest in cultural experience—especially in the arts and their psychological meaning for affinity groups' self-formation, which he saw as comparable to the individual self. As such, groups also experienced self-enhancement and diminishment in self-esteem and their self-state (cohesive, fragmented, vulnerable). This led him to postulate the notion of a group self (Kohut, 1985a, 1985b). The group self was and is a concept still subject to debate and contestation, because "the group" does not have "an" intrapsychic dimension (except as individual members of groups share similar experience)—although it must be recognized that it is unlikely that any two individuals experience the same phenomenon exactly in the same manner and with the same psychological impact.

Central to his theory is the concept of self-object experiences. Basically, a self-object in Kohut's theory is the interior experience of someone who sustains our feeling of selfness—we feel whole and emotionally stable (Baker & Baker, 1987). A mirroring self-object, for instance, enhances our sense of importance, self-worth, and intrinsic value. An idealizing self-object, a connection to a deeply admired person, group, or ideology, infuses us with a sense of strength and aliveness, and even commitment. Kinship self-objects are those experiences that make us feel a part of a group; it may be a family, cultural group, or religious body. The important dimension to these self-object experiences is the affect they have on one's sense of self. According to Kohut (1985a), we need self-objects throughout life, but, as we mature, the demands for these experiences are modulated and we find multiple ways of fulfilling them.

Along these same lines, Kohut also conceptualized a cultural self-object— distinct from but having functions related to mirroring, idealization, and kinship. Again, Kohut did not give fulsome attention to the clinical dimensions of the group self or cultural self-object. This left cultural and group experiences related to religion—as well as race, ethnicity, gender, and sexuality, with rare exception—underdeveloped in psychoanalytic self psychology.[3]

These views were important to my introduction to the subject of self psychology and psychoanalytic clinical work; however, between 1995 and 1997, I was also writing my dissertation (Sheppard, 1997), where I placed self psychology and womanist theology in dialogue. Womanist practical theology centers Black women's experiences and cultural symbols—literature, music, religious expressions, art, and language intergenerational relational styles. Womanist theo-ethical social analysis, strategies, and praxis are aimed at dismantling the interior-social dimensions of oppression, while also drawing upon Black women's cultural knowledge, practices, and spiritual wisdom accessed flourishing. In so doing, any engagement or use of theories and practices are held accountable to multiple discourses but, foremost, to their efficacy for shaping change to society and for Black life. Therefore, in my work, self psychology is subject to this kind of critical read.

It was clear that self-object experiences and development were affected and informed by broader sociocultural realities of—and the convergence

---

[3]The most cogent attention to these ideas is given in Kohut (1985a).

of—race, gender, class, and sexuality. Kohut (1985b) stressed, for instance, the necessity of mirroring self-object experiences for the maintenance of self-esteem and self-regard; however, sociocultural factors, such as racism and sexism, are systematically embedded and operative in the self-object milieu and, for those subjected to sustained exposure to them, counteract self-enhancing experiences. At first glance, Kohut's theorizing of cultural self-objects would seem to promise a solution. However, Kohut continued to privilege the individual psyche; as such, most self psychologists failed to capitalize and expand his theories of the group self, cultural self-objects, and group self-object. To the degree that Kohut's early followers considered these ideas, they often ultimately discarded their usefulness for the clinical milieu. In part, the contestation of these concepts was due to Kohut's tendency to be less than clear and consistent in their usage.[4]

Kohut (1985a, 1985b) postulated that the group collective has a group self with self-object functions and needs met by the group. Strozier (1985) summarized as follows: "A group self, that aspect of common psychological experience of individual people in a group, maintains its cohesion in a confirming merger with leader self-objects" (p. xxix). Obviously, such a merger can be, for the individual in the group or the whole group, defensive and vulnerable to grandiose expectations or rage when the group fails to live up to the fantasies. Institutional religion, for instance, in denominations, sects, and intentional communities are reoccurring sites for the development and breakdown of the group self and the individuals making up the group. In the 2019 annual meeting of the Evangelical Covenant Church, the denomination of the seminary where I was on faculty for 11 years, the vote on the denomination's position on LGBTQ members resulted in a congregation being excommunicated and two pastors having their ordination revoked because their theology was out of harmony with the denomination's stated theological position. The emotional turmoil for the denomination and the excommunicated has been palpable. Most striking to me was the way in which those who identified as open and affirming of LGBTQ members held two competing ideas: (a) the vote would be negative and their colleagues would be excommunicated; and (b) the denomination (leadership and voting delegates) would make a 180-degree shift and affirm these ministers. Since the time of the vote and excommunications, more members have left (or threatened to leave) the denomination. In my view, what is noteworthy from the perspective of self psychology and religion is the repeated call by some to begin a new

---

[4]For an excellent discussion of the shifting conceptualization of self-object, see Goldberg (1998).

denomination built on the historic values of the current denomination. The urgency of the demand seems to be based upon the experience of rage and fragmentation induced by the denomination's refusal to maintain cohesion in allowing for multiple point of views and pastoral practices in relation LGBTQ (i.e., the denomination determined that ordained clergy may not pray or read scripture at or celebrate marriages of LGBTQ members—even if the marriages occur among family members—and that church buildings may not host these marriages). As such, those who remain feel the theological ground crumbling along with their religious identity as members of the denomination, which many can trace back several generations—some even to the beginning of the denomination.

The merger with the denomination and its religious culture has failed this part of the group, but, for the majority in harmony with the denomination's position, the merger remains intact. The call to immediately create a new denomination is likely a futile attempt to slow down the rage and depression that accompanies such disappointments; it is most likely that, as clinicians, we will encounter those for whom the idealization and merger with the religious group have failed.

My involvement in these matters as consultant and friend to those advocating an open and welcoming position repeatedly led me to articulate a view informed by my training at CRPC. My perspective on this recent example was influenced, in part, during a formative time in my training at CRPC. Three faculty members, Randall Mason, Constance O. Goldberg, and Lallene Rector, each informed my understanding of conceptualizing religion and religious experience in the therapeutic space, and this also pushed me to think about them in public and religious spaces. The works of these faculty members—Mason (1980), Goldberg (1996), and Rector (1996)—looked at conceptualizing religion and religious experience in the therapeutic space during this formative time in my own training. It was Mason who was instrumental in the founding of the CRPC and in fostering its relationship to Kohut. Mason was drawn to self psychology theory and the clinical interventions and saw potential for its efficacious appropriation in pastoral psychotherapy. In his 1980 article, "The Psychology of the Self: Religion and Psychotherapy," Mason argued for the conceptualization of clinical religion, where religion as a clinical phenomenon accelerated self-psychological perspectives. In this early work, Mason was concerned with demonstrating the influence and contribution of Kohut's psychology of the self for understanding of religion and pastoral psychotherapists' commitment to the intrapsychic exploration of the self in treatment. In other words, Mason wanted a pastoral psychotherapy grounded in psychoanalytic theory that would welcome religious experience and not assume pathology as the source of religious or cultural experience.

But just as important to Mason was the need to engage in research of clinically observed religion. Specifically, he sought to observe and to define religious phenomena that were specifically located and observable in psychotherapy. This specific expression of religion that was observed in the therapeutic encounter led him to the idea of clinical religion—religious phenomena that was specific to, and emerged in, the therapeutic space. In order to make the claim that clinical religion was religious *and* psychological phenomena, Mason required a definition of religion that (a) privileged the psyche over and against the rules and regulations provided by institutional religions, and (b) privileged the clinical milieu. Mason (1980) argued that religion

> has to do with a valuing affirmation of a transcending reality that has the power to define the Good Life, expresses itself in ritual and celebration, and results in norms for achieving the Good Life. Such a definition is more useful in the area of psychotherapy than defining religion as belief in God or by reference to the traditional major religions, or by borrowing definitions from other disciplines. It permits inclusion of the secular religions and may even include the individual system of paranoid schizophrenia.
>
> Despite outward difference, such diverse religions appear to serve as psychic equivalents, and their inclusions in one definition begins to clarify a category of psychic phenomena for observation and study . . . these religions, despite outward variations, deal in similar fashion with basic psychological issues such as cohesiveness and fragmentation. (p. 410)

Therefore, Mason's basic argument is that religion serves to meet self-object functions resulting in cohesive self and/or restores episodes of self-fragmentation. It is not based in defense, resistance, or regression; it contributes to the stability of the self. Given that the state of the self, in this self-psychological perspective, is always on the front burner, Mason's argument makes clinical sense from a Kohutian perspective. It is worth noting that, although Mason stresses the nomenclature "clinical religion," his attention to the state of the self in relation to religion, it can be argued that clinical religion is no different from other clinical phenomena revealing the structure or state of the self, unmitigated self-object needs, and the import of ideological convictions to promote and sustain a sense of cohesiveness.

What may be most important about Mason's perspective is his insistence that the client's point of view of what is religion, and why it is or is not important, remain the points of departure for grasping a deep, experience near, understanding of the client—and not the understanding of religion. Mason's article set the stage for how religion would be thought about at the CRPC, and his immersion into the developing work of psychoanalytic self psychology was shaped by the early theorists, in particular, Kohut and Arnold Goldberg, resulting in a functional, though self-psychological, approach to religion in the clinical space. This is particularly evident in the Goldberg (1996) and Rector (1996) articles that followed Mason's work. Although Goldberg's self-psychological approach does look at religion with the suspicion and assumption of pathology that we see in Freud's work (like other functionalist approaches), in the clinical context, Goldberg listens for the psychological needs that religion satisfies. In particular, one can readily hear similarities to Erik Erikson (1950, 1958) and Carl Jung (1963, 1952/1973), who argued that religion could foster the psychological well-being of individuals and social groups.

The psychoanalyst D. W. Winnicott (1953, 1971) located religion and the arts in the transitional space of infants' earliest movement toward engaging the world. This makes religion part of a developmental move toward healthy adulthood. As such, religion, although viewed positively, primarily serves psychological and social needs. Post-Freud, however, most functionalist psychological models of religion see religious experience in terms of its contribution to, or disruption of, psychological development (Erikson, 1950, 1958; Jung, 1963, 1952/1973; Meissner, 1992; Winnicott, 1953, 1971; see also Freud, 1907/1976, 1927/1961, 1930/1962). Goldberg's functional model based on self psychology is distinct, however, because self psychology is concerned with the self and its state in relation to religion. In other words, does religion foster the coherence of the self as opposed to its fragmentation?

In addition to Mason, I was deeply influenced by Goldberg. She served on CRPC faculty for over 30 years, was my supervisor during my last year of clinical training at the CRPC, and then she was one of my primary clinical consultants for the next 5 years. In her article "The Privileged Position of Religion in the Clinical Dialogue," she wrote that, due to her proximity to religious professionals and her own experience growing up in a religious home, she was frequently referred clients who wanted a therapist who would be sensitive and even welcoming of their religiosity:

> I have had referred to me several active, as well as former, religious professionals. Because of this association, and because of my own experience of being raised in a religious home, other patients who have felt that I would be understanding of and sympathetic toward the framing of their experiences in religious terms have come to me for psychotherapy. (Goldberg, 1996, p. 126)

In this article, Goldberg (1996) argued that the clinician was not infrequently impeded in the work by "significant countertransferences . . . in therapy when the religious dimension of the patient's life experience is the focus" (p. 130). She conceptualized three possibilities for understanding religious experience as part of the clinical exchange: (a) the metaphorical, (b) the foundational, and (c) the functional.

Goldberg's metaphorical model is the one least likely to evoke consciousness of one's countertransference. In this listening stance, Goldberg argued that the clinician hears in the patient's religious description language that is, for the patient, evocative and poetic. As such, for many clinicians, the language is resonant and, in my view, more palatable, because it does not make a demand of the therapists to believe or reject a conviction that the patient holds dear. As therapists, "in fact, we are relieved that the patient is content to use imagery" without the expectation that the therapist shares the language or beliefs that may be intertwined (Goldberg, 1996, p. 130).

The foundational model involves the patient who is devotee of a specific religious ideology that structures important life experience. Or, as Goldberg (1996) put it, "foundational—that which gives grounding—to the patient's life" (p. 131). As such, the patient may explicitly or unconsciously believe that the therapist relates to religion in the same essential way. What is interesting to me about this model is that Goldberg ultimately argued that foundational religious experience (i.e., religious experience that gives grounding to their life) cannot be analyzed, even though the therapist accepts the patient's framing of religion and its place in life. The psychic importance or even the necessity of religion gives rise to "the pull toward treating the religious matrix as foundational (that which we will seek no further understanding of)" (Goldberg, 1996, p. 132). It could be argued here that Goldberg's foundational model is essentially, although implicitly, a developmental model of religion, where religious belief is understood as a developmental arrest except when belief is relegated to a value system. In a vignette used to represent the foundational model, Goldberg (1996) hears in a prayer that the patient reads every morning a childhood/like longing

> for an omnipotent, all-caring parent. . . . When the patient above read the phrase—"and you will never leave me to face my perils alone," I thought of her as a five-year-old who decided, . . . in the absence of parental action, to walk to the nearest school and enroll herself in kindergarten. (p. 132)

Goldberg seems to be suggesting that the therapist should avoid analyzing religious experience, because it is foundational to the preservation of the self. Religion of this sort is inextricable from the developmental glue that has given shape to the patient's way of being—and capacity to be—in the world.

Upon first reading, Goldberg's third model (i.e., the functional view) appears closely ties to the foundational view. The distinctive difference is that, in the functional view, religion meets a self-object need and, thus, strengthens the mature or maturing self but, in the foundational view, the self requires religion because of a developmental arrest. Goldberg (1996) follows William James's admonition that clinicians should focus less on pathologies related to religion in the lives of patients and, instead, "proposed that one take a functionalist or pragmatic view" whereby one attended to its "adaptive consequences" (p. 132). In this functional approach to religion, "we are thinking of the self-object functions served by the matrix of religious meaning within which the patient lives" (Goldberg, 1996, p. 132). The self-object functions are those which, in Goldberg's understanding, contribute to the maintenance of a cohesive sense of self. Goldberg acknowledged that this subjective perspective may be a form of countertransference that protects the clinician from having to analyze the patient's actual belief, for example, in "God." The countertransference could be due to the clinician's belief systems or because of the broader cultural stake (and infiltration into the clinical setting) in the separation of church and state.

The most significant distinctive contribution between Goldberg's conceptualization of "foundational" and "functional" approach to religion may lie in the developmental viewpoint. The foundational perspective may be focused on early unmet needs and the functional may focus on how religion is used to alter the state of the self, across a lifespan, to sustain the self-structures that religious experiences are affording the patient. In either case, Goldberg lands firmly within a classical approach to religion, theoretically and clinically, in that it represents psychological needs, evidence of and the site for behavioral pathologies, and the means for attempting to gratify self-object needs. Goldberg does not take up for discussion the "realness" of religion, divinity, or its tenets in her article. Her concern is with the intrapsychic dimension. Goldberg does consider the sociocultural location of religion in her three models and, in this seminal paper, restricted her discussion to the clinical milieu.

Rector completes the circle of those who informed my self-psychological understanding of religion and religious experience in the clinical space. In three important papers, Rector (1996, 2000, 2001) focused on specific self-object functions and their relationship to religious experiences. She first examined the correspondence between early self-object experiences and the God images religious patients present in treatment (Rector, 1996). In that paper, Rector argued that gendered presentations of God develop as responses to unmet early self-object needs and experiences. The article is a pivotal shift in that Rector examines culture and gender, particularly the cultural devaluing of women and its impact on women's development. Rector, relying on feminist theologies' critique of phallocentric psychologies as well as Joan Lang's (1984) early work, contends that Kohut's self psychology left unexamined the blatant devaluing of girls and women in society. Subsequently, self psychology failed to theorize the culturally imposed obstructions (i.e., sexism) that thwart girls' self-development with unforeseen negative clinical implications. Rector argued that these social impediments of the devaluing of women in the broader society have implications for understanding their God representations, the self-object needs expressed in religious engagement, and clinical interventions.

In 2001, Rector next considered mysticism by focusing on idealizing experiences of two of Kohut's patients. Of specific note is her discussion of the development of "the capacity to calm and soothe oneself, to manage anxiety without undue difficulty, to regulate inner tension," arguing that various personality and behavioral difficulties are "evidence, at least in part, of a deficit in the capacity to soothe oneself, and by inference an early" disruption in the idealizing self-object experiences (Rector, 2001, p. 182). Mystical experiences, and the merger experience that characterizes them, are, Rector argued, attempts to resolve or mitigate the absence of an inner sense of strength, values, and "idealism" (p. 191). Rector argued that mysticism need not be understood as an indication of pathology but, depending on the clinical material and transference, may be adaptive to unmet early developmental self-object needs. Mysticism is not, however, limited to early developmental needs but, with maturity, may find sources and expressions less dependent on unmet needs and more responsive to contemporary needs.

For me, these three early self-psychological perspectives established, in large measure, the approach to religion at the CRPC during my tenure there, and the view that I initially adopted. These articles were a part of the research arm of the CRPC with the intention of enhancing clinicians' capacity to engage and theorize patients' religious experience in the clinical milieu, while maintaining Kohut's view of the self, the necessity of developmentally appropriate self-object experiences, and clinical intervention. As such, there was little reconfiguring of Kohut's positing of self-object needs and functions, and religion is understood as, predominately, an individual response to the psychological need to strengthen the cohesiveness of the self. The cultural or group dimensions of religion, as a solution to psychological deficits or as an expression of the need to affiliate, idealize, or to experience religion on its terms were not considered integral aspects of the clinical discussion. This reflects the privileging, in Western cultural milieus, on the individual.

In my clinical work, I found that a functionalist approach had limitations when working from a womanist-informed therapy because, in my view, religion was only understood from its psychological importance for the individual self and, furthermore, could not be theorized as a distinct self-object need, or the way in which religion was very often interconnected to socio-political structures that contributed to the obstacles that Black women faced. One of my colleagues, Celia Brickman (2002), raised important and helpful questions about the uncritical appropriation of the functionalist approaches to religion. She first noted that Freud's views on religion were highly con-tested and were even discredited. Freud equated religious patients with "primitive" peoples and infants—thus equating religious people with what he considered evolutionally and developmentally unformed groups that tended to be based on an embedded racism in his perspective and on his "arm chair anthropology." But Brickman also observed an often-overlooked aspect of Freud's psychology of religion concerned with its sociopolitical and relational dimensions:

> Drawing on the anthropological and social-evolutionary thought current at the turn of the last century, Freud understood primitive peoples as living in subjugation to their patriarchal leaders. He believed that [they] were dominated by external authority in the form of their leaders and gods. Without concurring with his characterizations of primitive peoples, we can nonetheless see that in calling religion primitive, Freud was not only alluding to his belief that . . . religions provide the belief systems that undergird relations of subjugation and domination. (p. 210)

Self psychology had assumed a similar evolutionary perspective. Brickman's reading of the self-psychological functional approach is important and nec-essary because it exposes the social political dimension to psychology of religion. In other words, clinicians need to recognize the ways in which functional explanations reinforce sociocultural–political power relations, and that our responses to religion and religious differences should expose these dynamics and help alleviate patients (and our) internalized acceptance of them. This includes facets of the self and sociocultural context (e.g., gender, race, sexuality, class), and the ways these show up in the clinical room, espe-cially as expressed in the clinical interventions offered by therapists. In my training and beyond, my work to attend to these facets has been crucially informed by womanist theologians.

Womanist Standpoint

As a doctoral student entering the world of self psychology and psycho-analysis, I was also formed by the work of womanist theologians. I was a doctoral student in theology, ethics, and the human sciences and was inspired by Alice Walker's notion of womanist—a perspective, or feminism, that situated Black women's experience of critical inquiry. When speaking of womanism, I first think of it as a method, disposition, epistemological point of reference, as well as a commitment to theorizing that enhances Black women's lives through praxis and critique of society' systemic mistreatment of Black people as well as the cultural misrepresentation of Black women. I found that when we distinguish womanist theology from White feminist perspectives, we highlight Walker's (1983) definition "womanist is to feminist as lavender is to purple" (p. xi) to assert a Black analytical standpoint that involves Black experience, critical social analysis, theo-ethical reflection, and strategic praxis emerging from an acknowledgment of the multiple and inextricably intertwined sites of oppression.

As such, I was committed to bringing an intersectional analysis to my work. That is, keeping in mind the idea of the "simultaneity of oppression" (Smith, 2000, p. xxxiv) *and* what Kimberlé Crenshaw (1989) identified as intersectional analysis. Using the analogy of a car crash at intersecting streets, Crenshaw wrote that intersectional analysis is

> a description of the way multiple oppressions are experienced. A Black woman is harmed because she is in an intersection, her injury could result from sex discrimination or race discrimination. . . . But it is not always easy to reconstruct an accident. (p. 149)

This meant that I entered my clinical practice with a heightened awareness of race, gender, and sexuality as integral to the clinical space, regardless of whether they were acknowledged or analyzed.

As a womanist practical theologian, my research and scholarship are at the intersection of psychoanalysis, culture, and lived religion. Walker (1983) emphasized Black spirituality in a way that much of feminist theology and psychology neglected or ignored. Although her spirituality was informed by Black Southern Christian practices, it was not at this juncture Christian. Walker no longer ascribes to any one religion; she meditates, reads Buddhist teachings on compassion, and finds spiritual meaning in nature. We see the continuing fruits of her definition of womanist as a Black woman "who loves the Spirit" in current research on Black women's lived religion and spirituality, when we read of multireligious belonging, or the incorporation of African religions in the diaspora (see also Coleman, 2011; Hucks, 2001). Womanism is not limited to theology and spirituality, rather it is committed to lived experience of religion. This deep rootedness in "on the ground" understanding of religion and spirituality is one that makes a conversation between the psychological perspective of religion and spirituality and culture ripe for theorizing and clinical innovation.

In using the term "lived religion," I am speaking of how religion and spirituality are lived out in public and in private, internally and relationally, in sustaining practices and ethical decisions and, as a psychoanalyst, how all of these show up in the clinical space. I think the science fiction/fantasy writer and Baptist-raised atheist, Octavia Butler, may have been correct when she said, "Religion is everywhere. There are no human societies without it, whether they acknowledge it as a religion or not" (Goodman & Gonzalez, 2005, 55:20). "Everywhere," I presume, includes the clinical space and, if this is correct, the question that emerges is *how does religion show up in the clinical space?* Furthermore, if religion is showing up everywhere, so is the societal and cultural. How do religion and society show up clinically, possibly tethered, in the psychotherapy space? How do we *think* about religion and spirituality showing up anywhere outside of an explicitly religious setting? How do we respond?

Religion and spirituality are being practiced in the clinical space in explicit and implicit ways. And although we, as clinicians, may have been trained to seek the meaning beyond the religious or spiritual—the intrapsychic meaning of religion in the lives of those who seek psychotherapy with us—our clients, in my experience, often put a hedge around religion. Religion is a given and, often, not subject to the exploratory process of psychotherapy. Obviously, the resistance to engaging religion is not one-sided only on the patient's part. Psychoanalytic theory has a long history of ambivalence directed toward religion and religious patients. Clinicians have often been trained in this ethos of ambivalence, experienced during their own treatment, and carry it into their clinical work.

Clinical Vignette 1: Black Religion and Cultural Self-Objects in the Clinical Space

Early in my career, a senior White male colleague referred one of his patients to me. The patient was a tall Black man, "A," about 40 to 45 years of age, and my colleague made the referral with the notation, "I really think he needs a Black therapist." I could not ascertain from the colleague why "the patient needed a black therapist" or what specifically was not working in his therapy with this Black man. That said, I was a relatively newer therapist, and I wanted more referrals, so I said yes. When I entered the waiting area for our first appointment, I was immediately struck by the huge, black Bible he was hugging close to his chest. Upon sitting in the chair in my office he looked at me hopefully and said, "what Scripture should we use today?" Over a brief 6-week period, we tried to "connect" and could not. All roads led to the Bible and his almost desperate insistence that we open the Bible and find a text to guide our time together. What was clear to me was that the Bible held great importance to him as a spiritual guide for living, but it also was a psychological anchor, such that any work on his "self" had to engage the object representing his "self"—the Bible—that was a primary source for self-confirming experiences. He had memorized large parts of the Bible—it was, as the Bible writes, stamped upon his heart. It was a part of him, affirmed him, and, as I learned, it could restore him from episodes of depression and listlessness.

What I learned, I learned too late. I could not bring myself to actually "practice his religion" in the clinical space. In writing this chapter, I could feel again what I could not name myself at the time and that never emerged in an otherwise very good supervision: I felt dread at the idea of opening the Bible and just letting a scripture guide our work. I imagined some kind of free fall into the lyrical sound of the King James Version. I imagined that the language, the "thou" and "thee," would activate my memories and seduce me into remembering how much as a teenager I loved the Bible and my personal Bible study. This reaction is countertransference because it interfered with the treatment process; unlike countertransference based on a negative affective response, my countertransference was a resistance to positive feelings about the Bible. This can be understood in a variety of ways, but one way is to see it as my overidentification with ambivalence toward religion in the clinical space. As a result, I withdrew from my own affects. By the time I was working with this patient, I had long entered a phase in which I was "religious," but I responded with a "hermeneutic" of doubt. As a result, within about 6 weeks, he decided he needed another Black therapist, one who was a real Christian therapist. This patient, I now think, needed a Black therapist who could see that the continuity of his self-experience was internal and external and was held by the Bible. But he also needed to believe that I was held in a similar manner by the Bible; that I too saw myself in it, and that it was a holding environment for a shared experience between us—patient and analyst. As I facilitated a referral with him, I could not help but wonder what my colleague's fantasy was about *me* that made this seem like an appropriate referral.

Never once in my supervision was countertransference raised as a point of discussion in this case. Given my decline, as it were, of "A's" invitation to join him in integrating his spirituality and religious practice into *his* therapy, his ending of the treatment was inevitable. I did not and could not enter into the play of therapy, that space of liminal possibility, where something both is and isn't—that space where the space becomes clinical because it is co-created. His expectation and request were viewed by me and by my supervisor as an indication of him "not being ready" for psychodynamic therapy. I am not convinced today that this was the case, because I am more convinced that I was not ready to offer him meaningful therapy. Indeed, where I thought he was too concrete and not introspective, I was too concrete. I did not allow my generally operative curiosity or clinical imagination to emerge to wonder what might come of engaging a Bible passage.

Again, there are a number of ways to think about this clinical vignette. Obviously, there were impediments to the treatment, including my countertransference to his affective attachment to the Bible and my disavowal of my attachment to it. I would add, now, that my movement toward a more spiritual practice (i.e., contemplation, mindfully informed ritual, meditation) temporarily made me approach the Bible with ambivalence given its association with Christianity and sometimes a more rigid approach to defining religious experience rather than broader spiritual experience. Second, race and gender seriously may have been silent forces in the construction of the referral, the supervision, and the patient's and my experience. The referring therapist determined that this patient needed a Black therapist and sent him off to me—possibly to take care of a "problem" patient. Possibly this was done to help the therapist ward off his own countertransference to the Bible, the expectation of reading it, or working with a Black man—my curiosity now could lead me to any number of speculations. In any case, the referring therapist seemed to have some sense or fantasies that the patient would fare better with a Black female therapist. I am suggesting that the referring therapist had a fantasy that linked religious behavior and Black people (or Black women), in a way that he did not seem to question. Of course, he knew I was a Christian Catholic and, at this point in my life, a member of a women's Catholic religious community. There was a convergence of ideas about me, such that he imagined that I would be a better "care-taker" of a religious Black man than he. And it is possible, very possible, that although out of my awareness, this contributed to my resistance to engaging my patient. Because I could not speak about or even fully know what I was experiencing, my unconscious reaction to the referring therapist's construction of Black, religious, and gender resulted in me rejecting the referring therapist's ideas by rejection of my patient.

CULTURAL SELF-OBJECTS, RELIGIOUS SELF-OBJECTS: DISTINCT AND OVERLAPPING EXPERIENCES

As a womanist practical theologian and analyst, an intersectional perspective means that I am cognizant in my clinical thinking of how race, gender, sex, class, and sexuality converge with religion in the clinical space.

Womanist and Self Psychology

In privileging experience as a primary source of data for understanding what is happening or what happened in psychotherapy, cultural experience must be considered in terms of the psychological impact for the development of one's self and religious experience.

When we fail to conceptualize the relationship between self and culture (those symbols and practices that glue groups together and create boundaries between groups) and society (those laws, institutions, legal practices that reflect the explicit and implicit values), we are likely to miss important aspects of our patient's religious experience. In this instance, a significant factor in this man's failed treatment was that I saw religion as an external experience rather than one integral to his self-experience and the continuity of how he experienced himself. I have learned in supervising clinicians, both novices and seniors, that relegating religion "out there" is not unusual. The reasons can be summed up as personal and cultural, but regardless, there is always countertransference. Furthermore, psychoanalytic training and treatment centers are reluctant to take culture seriously in clinical work or their institutional life. As a result, training programs are very White, and many clinical practices rarely serve people of color with minimal, if any, training attuned to spirituality and religion. In this sense, countertransference is also a form of cultural hegemony.

At the time, I already was working from a Kohutian self-psychological perspective that emphasized the importance of self-cohesiveness and the need for self-object experiences (i.e., idealizing, mirroring, and twinship) to facilitate the development of self. However, I had not fully taken into consideration Kohut's work on cultural self-objects (Kohut, 1985a, 1985b) as a helpful concept for taking up religion and spirituality in psychotherapy. In brief, the concept of cultural self-object was Kohut's attempt to address the question "How does the social milieu provide stimuli or lack stimuli and . . . and nourish the self or warp the self?" (i.e., idealization and cultural self-objects). How do our interactions and experiences of cultural ideal and social structures shape (and misshape) the psyche—the intersubjective and relational (see also Greene, 2000; Javier & Rendon, 1995; Leary, 1997; Miliora, 2000; Moskowitz, 1995; Roland, 1996; Seeley, 1999)? Let me acknowledge that when Kohut spoke of cultural self-objects, his blind spots included class, race, and sexuality. In my read of his work, he basically meant Western European "high culture"—I would even say "protestant" cultural experience. Kohut recognized that the needs to be affirmed through acceptance and mirroring, and the opportunity to find among one's cultural group figures or values that one can idealize or feel a part, could be satisfied out in the world. Although he did not give significant space to conceptualizing religious experience, he did recognize that it could be an aspect of the cultural self-object context and, as such, contribute to the consolidation of a mature sense of self.

Clinical Vignette 2: In Search of a Contemplative Life

Some years after the first case I mention in Clinical Vignette 1, I was referred another patient for religious reasons. This man was a White, "cisgendered, male" referred to me by a White, cisgendered woman colleague because the patient was suffering anxiety and wanted a therapist who would understand his contemplative life and his desire to live a life as close as possible to that of a Buddhist monk. The referring therapist (my peer in experience) wanted, she said, to work with him and had met with him for an assessment, but thought that given my "meditation practice and religious background," I might be a better therapist. The fact that he could not pay a full fee was never mentioned, but during the course of treatment, he disclosed that she had, in his words, "tried to convince" him that he could pay a higher fee, but given that he was an artist, he could not.

The patient "J" was a Zen Buddhist and lived in a communal house with mostly other Buddhists (although not all his housemates were Zen Buddhists). He had lived in a monastery for 2 years where he studied and had hoped to become ordained. He was highly regarded at the temple and favorably viewed by his teacher. His teacher relied on him to assist during public rituals and retreats.

According to my patient, his status as favorite student made it hard for him to admit to his teacher that he was anxious and depressed. When he finally did tell him, the teacher recommended increased meditation. When his meditation practice did not alleviate his symptoms, he decided on therapy. As he had anticipated, his teacher thought that psychotherapies encouraged one to focus on self (navel gazing) rather than developing "no-self." According to the patient, his teacher was angry.

In telling me about his teacher's reaction, he said, "I heard you are religious and a contemplative. I hope you are stronger than my teacher." In other words, he was afraid that he was in a battle to claim and exert his right to existence. There were sessions where his response to any interpretation or just being in the room would become a teaching on Buddhism, the importance of the relationship between a Buddhist teacher and student, the way one should meditate. The introspection needed for understanding would be sidestepped. Often, I had the thought that, for all his teaching on Buddhism, it was clear he wanted me to see his understanding of Buddhism but did not want to bring it forward for analysis. In this case, I complied for a long time.

What he gradually allowed into the treatment was a fuller picture of his relationship to religious and spiritual practice. The psycho-religious picture that emerged, in brief, was a religious conversion precipitated by a public humiliation involving a loss of status in the art world that resulted in him running to Buddhism, not to hide so much as to be transformed. He had lost control of an institution he had created, because he could not engage in the struggle with a colleague, whom he had trusted with its management while he traveled.

The loss of his status in his art world, he said, "shattered him." Losing his place in the art world left him bereft of his self-object milieu. In other words, his needs for mirroring, twinship, and idealizing were all met in one specific environment and, when he left it, "he ran to Buddhism" to survive, but it was not working.

Initially Buddhism offered him a space to recover and to regain a sense of self. The teacher recognized his artistic gifts could benefit the community, and provided a community for him to attend to the spiritual in a way that being on a public stage had not permitted. Religion then was sought out for its potential for spiritual and psychological healing through a transformation of the self.

However, my patient was not aware of just how enraged he was, and his Buddhist teaching had, because of his interpretation of it, allowed him to disavow it as a focus on the self. This was made most apparent in his art-work, in which violence toward self and others were prevalent themes. As a result, my patient found himself engaging in behavior that was unacceptable to him and, had it been discovered, to his teacher and community. He had begun watching pornography to the point that it became, if you will, almost a ritual practice. He would meditate in the morning, do an afternoon teach-ing, go to his part-time job away from community, and return to community and find pornography on the internet. This came to a crashing halt when a member of the community saw him watching pornography. The person was mortified that he had "intruded" and apologized and, from all accounts had no intention of betraying him. My patient, however, was terrified that he was about to lose his place in the world again. Even after the member of the community left the state, J's terror remained for some time.

J was working at giving up pornography, partly to ensure that he could keep his Buddhist community and, in part, because he was beginning to wonder why he would turn to pornography when it went against his spiritual ideals, his view of how women should be treated, and his understanding of himself. While giving up pornography, his interest in me became more explicit. He wanted to, as he said, learn about me. Months later I learned, in our work, that he had googled me and learned that I was a seminary professor, part of a meditation group, that I had been in a religious community, was a lesbian, and even my partner's first name. He imagined that I had left religious life, so that I could be in a relationship or to become a professor. He imagined me as unambivalently committed to my religious life. I was the contemplative, another teacher for him, and an example.

This idealization was not permanent, of course. And over the course of time, he became angry with me because he discovered my book on psychoanalysis and womanist thought, and he realized I had a life that I had kept from him. I was, he complained, really only interested in Black women and not in his life. His capacity to be with, and express, his feelings of anger was hindered by his views of Buddhism. A shift occurred when his Buddhist teacher suggested that the way to no self was through his anger rather than by denying his anger. The way through included him confronting his colleague who had "taken" his place in the art community and demanding that the former publicly acknowledge, in writing, that my patient was the creative force behind the institution.

This success with "living through his anger" made him trust Buddhism more and its sustaining place in his life. He moved out of the community, retained his "special student status," and was recognized as a teacher of the temple. More importantly, he managed to build what he called "a real life."

I think it is important to note a few subtle, but significant, shifts in my clinical approach as I developed and integrated a womanist perspective. One important aspect of my clinical interventions was to acknowledge his spiritual teacher's religious perspective as valid, such that I would inquire about his anger or pornography from the perspective of the teachings. Second, I recognized that his spiritual teacher was a cofacilitator figure in the clinical space, even though he was not present physically. I welcomed my patient's wrestling with the teachings that he *wanted* to shape his approach to life and how he understood himself and the world. This intervention was in keeping with a womanist understanding of spirituality as infusing all experience. Therefore, while maintaining a clinical interest in how or if the Buddhist teacher or teachings were meeting self-object needs, I did not assume that the patient's desire to bring the teacher's views into the treatment as a form of resistance to me, the transference, or evidence of a regressive pull. There were times when these dynamics seemed operative, and we explored them (e.g., when he wanted to teach about Buddhism in the session rather than be Buddhist in the present).

However, I did think that choosing a Buddhist teacher from an entirely different cultural background was clinically noteworthy, because he also chose me—a Black psychoanalyst. Situating myself in a womanist self-psychological approach meant that we needed to explore what being white meant to him and if choosing two significant persons of color as figures to assist him in his process of change was intentional or even necessary. My approach was to first acknowledge the cultural and racial differences between him and his Buddhist teacher and what this meant for his life. Next, we explored what having a Black lesbian psychoanalyst meant. Although there were some similarities, such as the patient could not become Asian as his teacher was and nor could he become Black, he could grow into the kind of Zen Buddhist his teacher was training him to become. Treating his race (being White), male gender, heterosexuality, culture, and religion as both external and internal realities, and not problems, was important for his treatment.

CONCLUDING REMARKS

The differences in the clinical approaches in these two vignettes are, I think, significant. Specifically, the conscious, but unbiased, admission of religion and spirituality as well as race, gender, and sexuality into the clinical discourse in this latter case was crucial. Second, the acceptance of the Buddhist teacher as a cofacilitator of change in the patient's life, but also in the clinical room through the teachings the patient brought with him, was important because it was a reality for the patient and because it ultimately enhanced his capacity to become consciously selective about what ideologies and values would shape his life during and posttreatment—and this is what I hope for my patients when they leave my care.

REFERENCES

Asante, M. K. (2009, May 17). *Afro-Germans and the problems of cultural location.* http://www.asante.net/articles/17/afro-germans-and-the-problems-of-cultural-location/

Baker, H. S., & Baker, M. N. (1987). Heinz Kohut's self psychology: An overview. *The American Journal of Psychiatry, 144*(1), 1–9. https://doi.org/10.1176/ajp.144.1.1

Bonovitz, C. (2005). Locating culture in the psychic field: Transference and counter-transference as cultural products. *Contemporary Psychoanalysis*, *41*(1), 55–75. https://doi.org/10.1080/00107530.2005.10745848

Brickman, C. (2002). Self and other in the self-psychological approach to religion: A discussion of Pamela Holliman's "Religious Experience as Self-Object Experience." In A. Goldberg (Ed.), *Postmodern self psychology: Progress in self psychology* (Vol. 18, pp. 207–216). The Analytic Press.

Chireau, Y. P. (2003/2006). *Black magic: Religion and the African American conjuring tradition*. University of California Press.

Coleman, M. A. (2011, Spring). The womb circle: A womanist practice of multi-religious belonging. *Practical Matters*, *4*, 1–9. http://practicalmattersjournal.org/wp-content/uploads/2015/08/0600_The_Womb_Circle.pdf

Crenshaw, K. (1989). Demarginalizing the intersection of race and sex: A Black feminist critique of antidiscrimination doctrine, feminist theory and antiracist politics. *University of Chicago Legal Forum*, *1989*(1), 139–167.

Erikson, E. H. (1950). *Childhood and society*. W. W. Norton.

Erikson, E. H. (1958). *Young man Luther: A study in psychoanalysis and history*. W. W. Norton.

Freud, S. (1961). *The future of an illusion* (J. Strachey, Ed. & Trans.). W. W. Norton. (Original work published 1927)

Freud, S. (1962). *Civilization and its discontents* (S. Moyn, Ed.; J. Strachey, Trans.). W. W. Norton. (Original work published 1930)

Freud, S. (1976). Obsessive actions and religious practices. In J. Strachey (Ed. & Trans.), *The standard edition of the complete psychological works of Sigmund Freud* (Vol. 9, pp. 115–128). The Hogarth Press. (Original work published 1907)

Gehrie, M. J. (1980). The self and the group: A tentative exploration in applied self psychology. In A. Goldberg (Ed.), *Advances in self psychology* (pp. 367–382). International Universities Press.

Goldberg, A. (1998). Self psychology since Kohut. *The Psychoanalytic Quarterly*, *67*(2), 240–255. https://doi.org/10.1080/21674086.1998.11927558

Goldberg, C. (1996). The privileged position of religion in the clinical dialogue. *Clinical Social Work Journal*, *24*(2), 125–136. https://doi.org/10.1007/BF02189727

Goldberg, C. (2003). A personal and professional reminiscence of Heinz Kohut. In M. J. Gehrie (Ed.), *Explorations in self psychology: Progress in self psychology* (Vol. 19, pp. 347–358).

Goodman, A., & Gonzalez, J. (2005, November 11). *Science fiction writer Octavia Butler on race, global warming and religion* [video interview]. DemocracyNow.Org. http://www.democracynow.org/2005/11/11/science_fiction_writer_octavia_butler_on

Greene, B. (2000). African American lesbians and bisexual women in feminist-psychodynamic psychotherapies: Surviving and thriving between a rock and a hard place. In L. C. Jackson & B. Greene (Eds.), *Psychotherapy with African American women: Innovations in psychodynamic perspectives and practice* (pp. 82–125). Guilford Press.

Hucks, T. E. (2001). "Burning with a flame in America": African American women in African-derived traditions. *Journal of Feminist Studies in Religion*, *17*(2), 89–106.

Javier, R. A., & Rendon, M. (1995). The ethnic unconscious and its role in transference, resistance, and countertransference: An introduction. *Psychoanalytic Psychology*, *12*(4), 513–520. https://doi.org/10.1037/h0079680

Jung, C. G. (1963). *Memories, dreams, reflections*. Harper Collins.

Jung, C. G. (1973). Religion and psychology: A reply to Martin Buber. In R. F. C. Hall (Trans.), *The symbolic life, Collected works 18* (2nd ed., pp. 663–70). Princeton University Press. (Original work published 1952)

Kohut, H. (1977) *The restoration of the self.* University of Chicago Press.

Kohut, H. (1985a). Idealization and cultural self-objects. In C. B. Strozier (Ed.), *Self psychology and the humanities: Reflections on a new psychoanalytic approach* (pp. 224–231). Norton.

Kohut, H. (1985b). On the continuity of the self and cultural selfobjects. In C. B. Strozier (Ed.), *Self psychology and the humanities: Reflections on a new psychoanalytic approach* (pp. 232–243). Norton.

Lang, J. (1984). Notes toward a psychology of the feminine self. In P. E. Stepansky & A. Goldberg (Eds.), *Kohut's legacy: Contributions to self psychology* (pp. 51–70). Analytic Press.

Leary, K. (1997). Race, self-disclosure, and "forbidden talk": Race and ethnicity in contemporary clinical practice. *The Psychoanalytic Quarterly, 66*(2), 163–189. https://doi.org/10.1080/21674086.1997.11927530

Mason, R. (1980). The psychology of the self: Religion and psychotherapy. In A. Goldberg (Ed.), *Advances in self psychology* (pp. 407–425). International Universities Press.

Meissner, W. W. (1992). Religious thinking as transitional conceptualization. *Psychoanalytic Review, 79*(2), 175–196.

Miliora, M. T. (1997). The cross-culturally disordered self: A self-psychological study and treatment. *Journal of Adult Development, 4*(1), 35–44. https://doi.org/10.1007/BF02511847

Miliora, M. T. (2000). Beyond empathic failures: Cultural racism as narcissistic trauma and disenfranchisement of grandiosity. *Clinical Social Work Journal, 28*(1), 43–54. https://doi.org/10.1023/A:1005159624872

Moskowitz, M. (1995). Ethnicity and the fantasy of ethnicity. *Psychoanalytic Psychology, 12*(4), 547–555. https://doi.org/10.1037/h0079690

Rector, L. J. (1996). The function of early self-object experiences in gendered representations of God. In A. I. Goldberg (Ed.), *Basic ideas reconsidered: Progress in self psychology* (Vol. 12, pp. 269–283). Routledge.

Rector, L. J. (2000). Are we making love yet? The psychology of male domination. In L. Isherwood (Ed.), *The good news of the body: Sexual theology and feminism* (pp. 74–95). Sheffield Academic Press.

Rector, L. J. (2001). Mystical experience as an expression of the idealizing self-object need. In A. Goldberg (Ed.), *The narcissistic patient revisited: Progress in self psychology* (Vol. 17, pp. 179–195). Analytic Press.

Roland, A. (1996). The influence of culture on the self and self-object relationships: An Asian-North American comparison. *Psychoanalytic Dialogues, 6*(4), 461–475. https://doi.org/10.1080/10481889609539131

Seeley, K. M. (1999). *Cultural psychotherapy: Working with culture in the clinical encounter*. Jason Aronson.

Sheppard, P. (1997). *Fleshing the theory: A critical analysis of embodiment in light of African American women's experience* [Unpublished doctoral dissertation]. Chicago Theological Seminary.

Sheppard, P. I. (2017). Womanist-lesbian pastoral ethics: A post-election perspective. *Journal of Pastoral Theology, 26*(30), 152–170.

Smith, B. (Ed.). (2000). *Home girls: A black feminist anthology.* Rutgers University Press.

Strozier, C. B. (1985). Introduction. In C. B. Strozier (Ed.), *Self psychology and the humanities: Reflections on a new psychoanalytic approach* (pp. ix–xvii). Norton.

Walker, A. (1983). *In search of our mothers' gardens: Womanist prose.* Harcourt, Brace, Javonovich.

Winnicott, D. W. (1953). Transitional objects and transitional phenomena; A study of the first not-me possession. *The International Journal of Psycho-Analysis, 34*(2), 89–97.

Winnicott, D. W. (1971). *Playing and reality.* Tavistock Publications.

5

A SUFI MUSLIM MODEL OF SPIRITUALLY INTEGRATIVE PSYCHOTHERAPY

SHAMAILA KHAN

If I am to speak of my psychotherapy work with my clients, I must first speak of who I am as an agent of change in the clinical setting. If I am to speak of integrating spirituality into my psychotherapy work, I need be aware of that aspect of my own identity. So, speaking of my identity—it is multilayered, it is hybrid, it is contextual, it is shifting; it is just complex. Being a woman in this world is complicated, being a person of color is complicated, being Pakistani is complicated, being a young professional is complicated, and you can rest assured that being a Muslim in today's world is complicated. Now, the ways in which all the marginalized aspects of my identity intersect and shift as I transition between different regions in the world is further complicated. In order for me to work with people who enter the therapy room with their own complicated lives, I'd better have my own complicated matters somewhat sorted out or, in the least, be aware of them.

As such, I will begin this chapter by presenting a bit of my personal background, as well as some Sufi Muslim beliefs and values that naturally impact my work. I will locate myself with regard to Islamic traditions, as embedded within my cultural experiences globally that inform utility of my theoretical

https://doi.org/10.1037/0000276-006
Spiritual Diversity in Psychotherapy: Engaging the Sacred in Clinical Practice,
S. J. Sandage and B. D. Strawn (Editors)

frameworks and my overall clinical approach. This will be followed by a demonstration of ways in which this location of the self is expanded upon with three psychotherapeutic and contextualizing theoretical frameworks (i.e., psychodynamic, multicultural, and postcolonial). I then apply this integrative framework in case illustrations.

LOCATING THE TRANSITORY SELF

I was born in Pakistan, and my family immigrated to Libya when I was 3 years old. This was followed by a move back to Pakistan after 11 years in Libya, and then the final move to the United States. Throughout most of my life, these migrations have been the most significant events. Immigrating at a young age, getting accustomed to new cultures and varying ways of life, and learning new languages were all formative experiences. These transitions, with several beginnings and endings, raised questions in my mind about my identity and helped trigger critical reflection. These transitions entailed learning not only about the new culture but also about myself within the new locations—about fitting in and belonging. They altered my definition of the "self" and constructed and reconstructed how I understood and experienced myself to be. This developing curiosity about self and identity, about transitions and changes in people and how they develop, adapt, and come to be based on their histories, naturally led me to be interested in pursuing the field of multicultural psychology, which includes varying intersecting aspects of one's identity. It is only in retrospect that I learned of these as I transitioned between the three continents and learned to converse in multiple languages. Being a Muslim in Pakistan versus being a Muslim in Libya, versus being a Muslim in New York (pre- and post-9/11), and now being a Muslim in Massachusetts are all very different experiences, as each intersected with my ethnic identity. Being a Muslim on various continents—while living in Asia, in Africa, and in North America— expanded my original monolithic sense of what it meant to be a Muslim. These experiences also varied depending on the nations within the continent or the cities within the nations where I lived. The continental and ethnic aspects of my social identity intersected with the religious/spiritual aspect of my identity in nuanced ways.

I also became aware that my experience of being Muslim was different from that of my father and brother, as it was intersecting with the gendered aspect of our identities. Furthermore, there was diversity in how women from different cultures and ethnicities embraced and represented the religious/spiritual aspect of their identity. I encountered Muslim women in varying garbs and upholding their religious identity in such diverse and unique ways, ranging from hijabs to niqabs, to turbans, to head wraps to dupattas and shawls, to none at all. There was such diversity in how faith was reflected outwardly and inwardly, that I found and still find the mainstream stereotypical image of a Muslim woman to be unidimensional, reductive, and monolithic. Contrary to how images define Muslim women, I became interested in figuring out ways of undefining them, and myself in the process.

The experiences of a Muslim woman and a Muslim man are varied, as are the experiences of Muslim men or women from different continents, countries, and cities garbed in multiple ways, and these can further intersect with other aspects of identities (e.g., age, race, sexuality, socioeconomic status, disability). The model of intersectionality (Crenshaw, 1989) within a multicultural framework well captures the complexity of identity. As such, I want to ensure that when I speak to the religious/spiritual aspect of identity, it is understood that it is always intersecting with multiple other aspects of identity and, hence, the experiences are subjective. The multicultural framework within Western psychology is still often neglectful of inclusivity of international and global experiences, and there is a need to further address the oppressive, subjugated, and marginalized aspects of identity that are embedded in sociopolitical histories and ideologies.

SPIRITUAL, EXISTENTIAL, RELIGIOUS, AND THEOLOGICAL (SERT) TRADITIONS

I was born into a Sunni Muslim family and studied about Islam while living in Libya and Pakistan, both of which taught me Islamic perspectives regarding human nature. I learned from a mother who was a practicing Sunni Muslim and a father who was mostly a nonpracticing Sunni Muslim—he chose his practice "a la carte," cherishing individual freedom of belief. Islam was conceptualized and practiced in various ways in my familial home and in the multiple countries where I resided, which allowed me great freedom to employ and embrace it as I saw fit. Although I belong to the religious sect of a Sunni Muslim, my spiritual connection with my divine can veer from traditional forms of practicing to the realm of Sufism.

Islam, like many other faiths, consists of particular beliefs (i.e., the existence of God, judgment day, an afterlife of punishment or reward) and is practiced in the forms of prayer, fasting, and performing the pilgrimage to Mecca, all of which are about an individual's relationship with God. Additionally, Islam is about one's relationship with other human beings; the expression of these relational aspects is demonstrated in certain institutions and laws (e.g., marriage, inheritance, civil/criminal laws) that are faith based. Sufism is the inner mystical dimension of Islam and is referred to as *Tasawwuf* in Arabic. Sufism emphasizes introspection and inner purification, as well as spiritual closeness with the divine. It has been misunderstood as a sect of Islam, but it is actually a broader style of worship that transcends sects, directing its followers' attention inward. Although Sufism is more often followed by the Sunni sect of Muslims, Sufis are adherents of Islam's overall aforementioned beliefs and practices.

Aside from the essential daily prayers, the most central Sufi practice is the recollection of God, referred to as *Dhikr* or *Zikr* (depending on the cultural association) by recitation of the 99 Arabic names of God, as found in the Quran. This internal or external recitation is meant to internalize the Quranic content with the aim of establishing closeness to God. The meditative practices intend to empty the heart of all else aside from God and to begin instituting the qualities of the divine in the person. The function of Tasawwuf, as such, is to perfect the relationship of a person first with God and secondly with fellow human beings. It is about introspection, spirituality transcending religion, and it is apolitical.

In America, I have experienced Islam to be a more private affair, whereas in other settings, it was more communal. Here, I witnessed more syncretism of different faiths—various rituals and beliefs of different faiths are blended, and sometimes faith-based rituals are practiced with detachment from the spiritual base (i.e., meditation, yoga). Personally, I went from being an agnostic, to a monotheist, to a practicing Muslim, to a somewhat practicing Sufi Muslim or Tasawwuf. I landed on it by through the introductory readings of Shahidullah Faridi (1986) and, in particular, his book *The Inner Aspects of Faith*.

Three ideas are central in Sufi Islamic psychology—the *Nafs* (i.e., self, ego, or psyche), the *Qalb* (i.e., heart), and the *Ruh* (i.e., spirit). These terms originated within the Quran, and they have been expanded upon by centuries of commentaries from Sufis. Nafs is considered to be the lowest principle of humanity. Higher than the Nafs is the Qalb and the Ruh (spirit). These notions had a particular appeal for me, and as I delved into studying psychology, I recognized how these notions easily map onto the Freudian notions of id, ego, and superego. Although I am conveying this in a much more simplistic form here, there is great depth and complexity to this Sufi way of thinking, and in many ways it parallels our contemporary theoretical models of psychology. I have found it useful to have an additional language to think of and use in my clinical conceptualizations, particularly when working with some of my Muslim patients, for whom this framework is familiar and easier to grasp. Abu-Raiya (2014) and Ahmad (2010) have looked at these frameworks in some depth and demonstrated their clinical utility. I appreciate when individuals attempt to connect the teachings of faith in light of the knowledge embodied in the modern sciences. Ahmad's work was based on interpreting the Quran in the contemporary idiom. Schacter and colleagues (2010) drew on Ahmad's explanation that the Nafs (akin to the id) is divided into multiple parts. It encompasses how the basic instincts operate on the pleasure principle, which is part of the *Ghaib* or the unconscious.

In particular, *Nafsi Ammar* is the source of harmful inclinations, according to the Holy Quran. It is the primal instinct that, just like the id, is hedonistic and aims to seek pleasure and avoid pain. If human beings allow the Nafs to reign supreme, then they are no better than their lower mammalian counterparts. It is this element of Nafs within the human psyche that Islam seeks to control. In fact, contrary to the popular belief, the highest struggle *(jihad)* in Islam is the struggle against one's Nafs *(Jihad bin Nafs)*. It is this lack of self-control that leads undisciplined men to pick up arms and commit atrocities in the name of faith.

Ruh (partly akin to the superego) is described as a state of super consciousness and is the moral component of the psyche. The concept of Ruh is broader, and it is transcendent, unlike the atranscendent superego. It encompasses *Nafs-e-Mutmainna* (the reassured soul), which results from the *Nafsi lawammah*, prayer and worship. Nafsi lawammah is more akin to how Freud uses superego, where *Lawwam* means to self-incriminate, to self-reproach, or to do *mulamat* (critiquing one's self).

The Qalb (the spiritual heart, which contains spiritual intelligence and wisdom, as well as the ego) is described as reality based, conscious, and in a perpetual state of change. At times, the Qalb is pulled by Nafs on one side and Ruh on the other. The struggle to tilt the Qalb (the present restless state) of a person toward the Ruh is the aim of every Muslim, which will lead to the state of Nafs-e-Mutmainna. Similarly, Abu-Raiya (2014) drew comparisons between the Quranic theory of personality and Freudian and Jungian theories of mind and states:

> Notable similarities were found between the Freudian id, ego, superego and neurosis and the Qura'nic nafs ammarah besoa' (evil-commanding psyche), a'ql (intellect), al-nafs al-lawammah (the reproachful psyche) and al-nafs al-marid'a (the sick psyche), respectively. Noteworthy resemblances were detected also between the Jungian concepts collective unconscious, archetypes, Self and individuation and the Qura'nic constructs ruh (spirit), al-asmaa' (the names), qalb (heart), and al-nafs al-mutmainnah (the serene psyche), respectively. (p. 326)

In his article, Abu-Raiya (2014) discussed the numerous parallels and departure points between the models creating room for new avenues for enriching the dialogue between Western models of the psyche and their Muslim counterparts. Also, within Islam, as explained by Faridi (1986, p. 34), cognition is described as divided in two parts, namely, the Zahir and Ghaib. Zahir is described as the external or conscious, and Ghaib as the internal or unconscious. Believing in the presence of Ghaib is one of the principles of Islam, and it is everything outside of human consciousness. Again, there is a parallel between Freudian notions and Islamic understanding of the differing dynamics within the psyche. Despite these similarities, there are various differences and points of departure between these frameworks. The Quran also enlists other soul structures or dimensions of the Nafs, through which a Sufi may receive, see, or connect with the divine from varying points, depending on the dimension.

There are additional parallels between the Western psychological frameworks and Sufi Islamic frameworks, particularly with regard to treatment of trauma. Calhoun and colleagues (2000) suggested that because trauma involves a loss of existential meaning, there is a significant role for religious beliefs in facilitating personal meaning and purpose of life in the psychological growth that can potentially follow traumatic events. During my disaster relief work, it was notable that people often turned to their faith leaders for the treatment of the psychological problems resulting from natural disasters. Gordon (2006), who treated traumatized individuals in Gaza, noted that Sufi Dhikr was used by people in Muslim regions, and that it is practiced such that the Sufi students arrange themselves into a circle facing the Sufi teacher and chant the name "Allah" or "Hoo," and, while seated or standing, they all make simultaneous light head and body movements as they are chanting. The movement consists of balancing themselves slowly from right to left and from left to right. This type of movement, which can be done with the eyes open or closed, may cause eye movement similar to that used in eye movement desensitization and reprocessing (EMDR). Similarly, Abdul-Hamid and Hughes (2015) proposed that Dhikr fulfills functions similar to the stages of EMDR, where the regular movements of the head from right to left cause a form of eye movements that provide therapeutic effects. They also noted that research trials in Malaysia and Pakistan found that adding aspects of Sufi Islam to the traditional treatment of Muslim patients made the therapy more effective for both depression and anxiety.

KEY SOURCES FOR INTEGRATING SUFI SPIRITUALITY WITH POSTCOLONIAL AND PSYCHODYNAMIC PSYCHOTHERAPY

I have described some of the points of connection between Islam and Western psychology that I have found helpful, and now I want to clarify some of the key theoretical influences that I have found useful for integrating these traditions. First, it is important to recognizing Islam's heterogeneity, with Sufi

Islam being a particular orientation, and my own interpretation of Sufi Islam is primarily influenced by the works of Shahihdullah Faridi (1986), Ibn-Sinha (Avicenna; 2004), Israr Ahmad (2010), and Jalalludin Rumi (2004). I was drawn to Sufism first after learning that my maternal grandmother was a follower of this path. Once I started to explore it, I was further drawn to it when I connected with other followers. I realized it paralleled my innate tendencies, intersected with my cultural identity and with my overall ways of being that are more communal, less orthodox, more diverse, inclusive, and value heterogeneous. I was also attuned to the fact that faith and religion are among the main markers of difference in today's world and have thus created an environment that may breed prejudice, fear, and "othering" of those who are religiously different. This has led to violations of the civil rights of people around the globe. When discussing the incorporation of religious frameworks into our understanding of people and its psychotherapeutic utility, it behooves us to also acknowledge that, at times, contrary to the basics of what each religion essentially promotes, it also can be a detrimental source.

It is also critical to address religion(s) in a nonreductionist framework of being associated solely with rituals and doctrines, and to contextualize it, highlighting how it is embedded within the existing social, economic, and political structures. These contexts are often shifting, which contributes to a variation in ways religion is interpreted and practiced. As such, religions do not dictate what to do, but rather people conduct their actions based on their interpretations of the religion. Given these contextual variations, to speak of *the* Christian, *the* Jewish, *the* Buddhist, *the* Hindu, or *the* Muslim approach to psychotherapy is somewhat of a misnomer. Given the progressively blended and globalized world we live in, the spiritually integrated psychotherapist will need to be spiritually multilingual and a cultural and theoretical polyglot.

Speaking of needing to be a cultural and theoretical polyglot, my psychotherapeutic approach to clinical treatment stems from a particular branch (psychodynamic psychotherapy), although my overall stance and conceptualizations are also often cross- and interdisciplinary, inclusive of not just the SERT traditions above but also of the postcolonial framework inclusive of transgenerational experiences. The spiritual and religious aspects of identity are embedded within this multitude of frameworks for me, and I am guided by the works of Sigmund Freud, Jacques Lacan, Carl Jung, Michel Foucault, Jacques Derrida, Louis Althusser, Gayatri Spivak, Frantz Fanon, Kimberlé Crenshaw, Edward Said, and Homi Bhabha, in addition to the previously mentioned Sufi philosophers. These form the three primary conceptual influences (i.e., psychodynamic, postcolonial, and Sufi) that I seek to integrate into psychotherapy within a multicultural framework.

GROUNDED IN A MULTICULTURAL FRAMEWORK

My beliefs as a Muslim have evolved, ironically, just as America's attitude toward Muslims has devolved. The reality of being a Muslim American today is akin to the reality that people of color, immigrants, the LGBTQ community, women, and others have faced for centuries in this country. As such, my ways of thinking about the religious or spiritual dimension are naturally from within a multicultural framework. Diversity and cultural humility and sensitivity have become core components of the ethical delivery of psychotherapeutic interventions. Multicultural and intersectional aspects of identity are increasingly noted to be crucial components of human psychology, and one is encouraged to examine specific sociocultural groups based on gender, ethnicity, sexual orientation, socioeconomic, and ability status, and yes, religious beliefs.

Mental health professionals are often uncomfortable with issues of religious and spiritual identity, and this may be why these areas have lagged behind other areas of diversity. Being a proponent of diversity, being attuned to all aspects of my identity, I felt that this part of my identity was often marginalized, particularly when it came to psychotherapy, although I considered it to be a very important component of the way I perceived my well-being. Clinicians are encouraged to recognize that individuals are complex beings and are members of multiple groups whose overlapping identities influence their development, social relationships, and worldviews. One's faith is a major component of this identity.

Although psychology is linguistically associated with spirit (psyche), its divide with religion and spirituality has been fraught with many barriers and misunderstandings (Albuquerque et al., 2003). Inquiries about spirituality and religion are often neglected and separated from the treatment process as if it were an esoteric topic that somehow lands outside the bounds of psychotherapy. I have time and again witnessed individuals bring "God," "religion/spirituality," "prophets," and "Satan/Jinn" into the therapy room. There are other clinicians who theoretically understand religion and would like to be more responsive but are ill at ease because they are not able to draw on training experiences to guide them on how to proceed with addressing these aspects. What is ironic is that clinicians happen to address the most private and sensitive of topics, including love, sex, death, jealousy, violence, addictions, and so forth, but are avoidant of this particular aspect. Research data demonstrate that spirituality and religion can constitute important aspects of the person's resilience and ability to cope, particularly during times of distress and trauma (Abdul-Hamid, 2011; Dein, 2006), and they serve as a protective factor against mental health disorders with traumatic bases (Hipolito et al., 2014; Wong et al., 2006). As such, numerous psychotherapeutic movements have attempted to incorporate religion and spirituality into the clinical process (Nizamie et al., 2013; Worthington & Sandage, 2001).

Rising interest in integrating spirituality and religion into therapy is apparent in the establishment of Division 36 (Society for the Psychology of Religion and Spirituality) within the American Psychological Association (Piedmont, 2013). Since its establishment, extensive research has aimed at finding religiously and spiritually based psychotherapies within the larger theoretical and clinical psychological context (Pargament, 2007). Numerous measures assessing religiosity have also been developed, and Abu-Raiya and colleagues' (2008) Psychological Measure of Islamic Religiousness is particularly relevant to my own work. These resources are designed to offer more culturally sensitive approaches to therapy, which include modifications of mainstream frameworks and its accompanying interventions to render them more culturally relevant to the beliefs of varying religious groups, which for me is Sufi Islam. Clinical decisions as to whether this aspect of my identity or conceptualization is implicitly employed or made explicit within the clinical work are dependent on the individual with whom I am working. This is something I am keenly attuned to noticing, if and when it may emerge. Whether religion or spirituality becomes the explicit focus within treatment varies based on the patient.

CONTEXTUALIZED THROUGH A POSTCOLONIAL FRAMEWORK

Additionally, I keep in mind that there are intergenerational experiences that further impact experiences of selfhood as embedded in postcolonial and trauma histories. Therefore, linking the postcolonial and multicultural frameworks is necessary in my view. The postcolonial focus is one of historical legacy based on the impact of the colonial experience on the colonized, as well as on the colonizers. The multicultural focus is concerned with the management of diversity and formulating ways to improve interethnic and intercultural engagements within a particular context. Globalization and international migrations have made this notion of diversity ever more pertinent, reaching global significance. The remote colonial histories within which they are embedded cannot be left out or ignored, as they shape identities. I have found the addition of the postcolonial theoretical framework to my psychodynamic framework to provide a more comprehensive picture of the dilemmas and struggles of my patients, as their experiences are embedded in complex histories and need to be contextualized. Studying the intersection between the aforementioned social categories is not quite as straightforward as it might appear when viewed within context, because each category of oppression has a different ontological basis and the categories themselves have divisions within them. So, treating the categories as homogeneous risks essentializing them.

For instance, as an American Pakistani woman, I belong to not a single diaspora but to several different ones—Asian, Muslim, Pakistani, Punjabi— a complex diaspora with each identity pointing to different experience and expressions and, at times, I keep these identities apart. At other times, I fuse them, most of which is an unconscious process. At different times, I am part of the Pakistani "nation," the Asian "community," the Muslim "congregation," and the Southeast Asian "diaspora." Traversing these varying narratives are the often uncomfortably seated political ideas about the nature of social equality, citizenship, power, morality, and subjugation. Hence, it becomes apparent that being "Pakistani" is far from referring to a fixed or concrete identity and encompasses a historically produced multiplicity shaped by and in response to diasporic and subcontinental movements—of Islam, empire, modernity, and nationalism—that are additionally embedded in spiritual/ religious, regional, and intercultural/linguistic traditions. The identities evoked in the narratives of these varied contexts are at times merged and at times kept strictly separated. These narratives entail imposed silences produced by the mainstream culture's racism and cultural xenophobia, as well as the voluntary silences of submerged identities, highlighted situationally and based on context. Multiculturalism, although often understood somewhat simplistically, is a framework that begins to capture the complexity and counters fragmentation and division while at the same time allowing for the hybrid nature of identities to be sustained situationally. The attempt within a postcolonial framework is to not allow aspects of one's identity to be reified or essentialized but instead to be continually deconstructed so as not to be subjugated (Ashcroft et al., 2006; Spivak, 1999). Multicultural-intersectional and postcolonial frameworks are increasingly important for analyzing how social inequalities are intensified by concurrent membership in a range of stigmatized or devalued categories of gender, race, age, ability, sexuality, and ethnicity. Postcolonialism not only provides a framework for approaching the experiences of the formerly colonized but also can include refugees, exiles, and expatriates (Loomba, 2005; Rushdie, 1991; Said, 1994).

In 1978, with the publication of *Orientalism*, Edward Said outlined a postcolonial theory exhibiting how disproportionate power relations between "The West" and "The East" had dictated the representation of Arabs, Muslims, and others by portraying "The East" as exotic, sensual, feminine, weak, dangerous, eccentric, irrational, and undeveloped. As per Said, this was a reflection of a wider attitude in European thought linked to the experience of imperialism/colonialism and the associated attempt to civilize the individuals from Africa, the Middle East, and Asia, who were seen as inferior by the supposedly superior Europeans. Said was inspired by the writings of Michel Foucault and examined the ways by which "The West" produces knowledge about and, by this means, executes power over "The East." The discourse places "The East" and "The West" into a mutually exclusive and opposing binary relationship where one is better than "The Other" and, hence, has the right to subjugate them. Said (1978) exposed Western stereotypes and distortions of Islam. Additionally, in *Black Skin, White Masks*, Frantz Fanon (1991) was highly critical of racism and colonialism and was a proponent of equality and freedom. The writings of Said and Fanon aimed at freeing the colonized individuals so as to enable them to feel and think independently. The European orientalist tendency was/is the assertion of their supposed authority to describe and define "Others," such as Muslims, while ignoring their own authority to represent themselves. The experience of orientalism impacted ways that colonized individuals identified themselves and, in many instances, Muslims came to accept the orientalist opinion of their societies, such that reform entailed adopting and favoring European ways of being (i.e., becoming Westernized) over their own traditional ways. This parallels the current situation in U.S. society, within which Muslim lives are apparently not as important as lives of other non-Muslim Europeans and Americans, and where Muslims are seen as uncivilized and inherently violent. It is a result of how "The West" is being socialized to believe that Islam is inferior, savage, and an irrational system of beliefs with extremist followers; those stereotypical depictions of Muslims are disseminated and reinforced by the media, further strengthening the existent views and beliefs. According to Said, this reflects the historical influence of ways Westerners needed justification for subordination of "The East," thus depictions of the Orient as inferior, undeveloped, and uncivilized. These inaccurate and Eurocentric cultural representations have persisted and developed into the stereotypes we are very familiar with today.

SPIRITUALLY INTEGRATED CLINICAL PRACTICE

My overall approach to spiritually integrated psychotherapy builds on the theories summarized above and entails understanding people who enter the therapy room and clinical space from a framework that incorporates a blended psychodynamic, multicultural-Sufi Islamic, and postcolonial theoretical orientations. Ironically, the stance of Freud (inclusive of the structural model incorporating the conscious and unconscious, the id, ego, and superego) maps neatly onto the Sufi Islamic notions of Zahir, Ghaib, Nafs, Ruh, and Qalb, although those notions are contrary to Freud's own conceptualization of faith-based ideas,

God, and religion overall as merely being an "illusion." Good (2010) explained how Freud felt that it was important to discourage individuals from seeking assistance for any spiritual concern, and its eradication from one's personal existence would result in the realization of greater psychological well-being. She stated, "Behaviorists also held antireligious points of view, contending that the incorporation of religion into mental health practice invalidated psychology as a science" (p. 8).

However, the field of psychology has recognized the pertinence of multiculturalism and diversity and has become a fervent proponent of these over time. One's faith and one's religion, for me, is a part or an aspect of the multiculturalism, diversity, and social justice orientations, and although psychology has covered ground in terms of speaking of the identity markers of race, ethnicity, gender, sexuality, disability, and socioeconomic status, the aspect of religion has lagged behind and been ignored. Historically, it has not been incorporated into training.

As I conceptualize from within a psychodynamic framework, I expand and build on it from a Sufi Islamic perspective, which for me is embedded in a multicultural framework, and it is understood more specifically from within the intersectionality model of Kimberlé Crenshaw (1989). For Crenshaw, identity is inseparable from lived social relations, and the subcategories of identity (including class, race, gender, sexuality, etc.) are not static but are shifting and mutually constitutive. These different aspects of identity are not comprehensive enough when understood in isolation. Converging the psychodynamic and multicultural frameworks expands my understanding of an individual from a solely intrapsychic to an interpersonal framework. I stretch this framework even a bit further after having learned that peoples' identities are also shaped by colonial and transgenerational histories. I have, therefore, expanded my psychodynamic framework to include the multicultural, international-global, and transgenerational-postcolonial frameworks. So, just as I understand my identity as being hybrid and shifting based on the context, when I am assessing an individual client, I attempt to do so in a multilayered form. This multilayered conceptualization stretches from an intrapsychic to interpersonal, to sociological-political, to an intergenerational-postcolonial space with an overarching multicultural framework inclusive of spirituality/religion in an intersectional format.

Additionally, the psychodynamic notions of transference and countertransference, multicultural notions of conscious and unconscious biases, and Islamic notions of morality (e.g., equality, social justice, compassion) are all embedded and part of the exploratory work in terms of their meanings and how they play out for me in clinical treatment. Composed over time by personal history, each of us brings our own deep-seated assumptions about life to psychotherapy. I recognize I have my assumptions; some I am conscious of, whereas others may be unconscious. The key is to work on being aware and attempting not to impose our personal views on our patients. As stated earlier, my beliefs and values as a Muslim have evolved over time, and there are varying ways in which a Muslim identity and belief system can present itself in a client within your therapy room. Coming from a multicultural and intersectional framework, the key is that of openness, receptivity, humility, sensitivity, being nonjudgmental, curious, and having a check on our own existent or emerging biases.

There are 72 sects within Islam, and the heterogeneity of the religion is apparent in the varied forms of practice and the geographical spread. Furthermore, the ways in which this aspect of identity gets intertwined with one's cultural beliefs and other aspects of one's identity further demonstrate the complexity of an individual's way of operating in the world; hence, any categorical assumptions or stereotypes ought to be deconstructed and challenged. As I stated before, for me, being a Muslim woman in Libya, in Pakistan, in the United States (pre- and post-9/11) are all very different experiences and contributed to my appearing and operating differently in each setting. As such, there is no way of generalizing and categorizing as to what the experience of a Muslim woman would be, as embedded within it is the sect of Sufism, and embedded within each of these are the cultures and ethnicities experienced. Yet people often come to seek treatment with me due to this perceived similarity and sometimes due to the perceived or actual difference. People have conscious and unconscious representations in their minds associated with these aspects of identity that play out in treatment, overlapping and intertwining with their clinical dilemmas and presentations. The sociological and political stances that people have regarding Islam further add to one's way of making sense of themselves and others, and what they bring to treatment and what they leave out. These aspects not only help distinguish whether they seek clinical treatment but also what they bring into the clinical room and what gets left out, what meanings they attribute to their struggles, and how they cope. Hence, I believe in approaching, exploring, and attempting to understand people from a variety of stances (utilizing multiple frameworks), ranging from their intrapsychic representations to their interpersonal ways of relating within families and groups, to how the sociopolitical culture impacts how they are seen and responded to and how history, and even remote colonial histories, shape their sense of self and ways of being.

I conduct therapy in the office and in the field. How one integrates frameworks within a disaster relief setting can look very different from the individual psychotherapy clinical room setting. A great deal of my work since 9/11 has been in the domain of disaster relief and refugee work. I have conducted disaster relief work in Pakistan following the floods in 2010 and the earthquake in 2005, in Haiti in the aftermath of the earthquake in 2010, with the Japanese after the Tsunami in 2011, in the schools in Pakistan after the shootings in Peshawar in 2014, in Boston after the Boston Marathon Bombings in 2013, and in Bangladesh with the Rohingyan refugees in 2018, amongst numerous other local disaster and crisis management situations. Mental health stigma has been apparent in a variety of settings and across a varied demographics of individuals. When people from ethnic minority groups do seek assistance for mental health challenges, they often rely on their faith-based institutions. Many Muslims end up not seeking psychotherapy services because of concerns that typically therapists do not provide treatment within a religious/spiritual context (Amri & Bemak, 2012). When people enter the therapy room, they don't leave their religious and spiritual beliefs behind—they bring them along implicitly or explicitly. We as clinicians need to have an ear out for it when it emerges.

The impact of natural- and human-caused disasters can be far reaching, from the effects on individuals and families to entire communities and nations. Crisis situations often call into question one's basic beliefs. I have seen that suffering may cause religious believers to believe even more strongly in God than they did before, because our minds are designed to seek explanations for the phenomena we see around us that we cannot fully explain. My experience matches Vedantam's (2010) observation:

> Religious believers and non-believers quickly reach diametrically opposing conclusions about the implications of the disaster. For non-believers, natural disasters are evidence that God does not exist—for what kind of benevolent, just or omnipotent figure would cause wanton harm to so many thousands of innocent people? (para. 1)

But believers may experience a reinforcing of their faith. People draw on religious and spiritual methods of coping designed to assist in understanding and dealing with potentially threatening or damaging situations. On the basis of what I have witnessed in disaster settings, religious and spiritual methods of coping are quite varied. The following case examples illustrate these points.

CASE EXAMPLES

Trauma Work With Rohingyan Refugees

On the one hand, religion can bring individuals together in camaraderie and enhance the social fabric of communities. On the other hand, it can also become a source of division and separation within families and neighbors, when it used as an exclusionary tool, especially when religion is blended with ethnicity, race, culture, and other social identities.

In the majority Buddhist state of Burma, aka Myanmar, the predominantly Muslim Rohingya people have long suffered persecution at the hands of the Buddhist community, which denies them citizenship, employment, education, and other basic human rights on the basis of their religion. This ethnic minority is considered "the most persecuted minority in the world" by the United Nations (U.N.; USA for UNHCR, 2021). Their persecution has its roots in Britain's colonization of Burma, and modern-day Myanmar refuses to recognize the existence of a people who have existed for thousands of years. The Rohingya are currently the world's largest stateless ethnic/religious group, and they have been fleeing Myanmar for their lives. The situation and the series of events easily fit the terrifying classification of genocide, as opposed to ethnic cleansing, which is how it is often highlighted.

Although Muslim–Buddhist tensions are historic, they have risen significantly over recent years, and these religious conflicts are now front and center. Local, regional, and international support entities have pursued many different avenues to address these escalating tensions, but the efforts to promote interfaith understanding and tolerance have mostly been futile. The Rohingya have been a state of a major crisis, enduring horrifying atrocities and violations of human rights that have necessitated interventions by the U.N. and the international community. The irony is that the refugee journey is deeply engrained in the teachings and narratives of many religious traditions, and it is an echo of the searing paths that many of our ancestors undertook. The call to welcome the stranger and to support those fleeing conflict, subjugation, and oppression is a fundamental ethical pillar of many faiths. Yet, here faith has precisely been the driving force and the very basis for the persecutory actions.

I traveled to refugee camps in the region on the border of Bangladesh (occupied by around 750,000 people) with the U.N. Refugee Agency and a team of Muslim clinicians, as supported by the Islamic Medical Association of North America, with the aim of providing culturally and religiously attuned trauma services. I was the only woman and the only psychologist on the team (which had its own implications with regard to perceptions of those receiving care from the team, as well as how we operated as a unit). I experienced my time there to be a profound example of bearing witness to the unspeakable trauma that the Rohingya have endured. Sometimes an experience is so profound that there are no words, and we suffer in silence. Yet, the emotional price of remaining silent, without a witness, is costly. The ghosts that they worked hard to keep buried following their arrival were haunting them. I asked myself the question (often at the heart of psychoanalysis) of how I could help them turn their ghosts into ancestors, metaphors as used by Hans Loewald (1960). Although I was pained by these stories, many of the Rohingya did not seem to be. I was feeling what they couldn't feel and was the recipient of their dissociated emotions. They had endured unimaginable atrocities yet were stoic and shared the stories in a factual manner, in a dissociated manner, often without shedding a tear. I worked at a makeshift clinic, where I served Rohingyan women who sought multiple kinds of services, and we provided physical health, supportive, and mental health services. Many of the women were also there for ultrasounds for their pregnancies. I was the sole woman clinician in the setting and, therefore, served in more than one capacity. Most of the pregnant women had become pregnant as a result of rape by militants in Myanmar. I opted to start a psychotherapy group for these women, who had experienced significant trauma and were often dissociating (emotionally/cognitively) as a psychological survival mechanism. They were also dissociated from their physical selves because their bodies were carrying the fetus of their perpetrators. There was a bit of resistance with regard to being a part of the group (even though each one wanted to meet individually), which I interpreted as being shame-related (some had individually shared this sentiment).

I gained a better understanding of the reasons for these emotional dynamics after having connected with a *Hafisa. Hafes* are highly respected individuals who have memorized the Quran and are often descendants of prominent religious figures. They are usually men, but women can also occupy these roles. Female Hafisa are often consulted by other women for their wisdom and guidance on personal matters, and they also give informal religious classes to small groups of girls or women. It was informative and very helpful to have collaborated with the Hafisa, as it not only availed me of information, but it also allowed me to more easily become a part of the group. Apparently, a psychotherapy group had been initiated by the last team on ground, and it was a meditation/mindfulness group. This group had not worked out, and I was just learning the reasons for the failure of that intervention. The group was conducted by clinicians from the United States, where one learns of meditative practices that are often disconnected from the person's spiritual/religious base (i.e., cultural appropriation). The reason for the group's termination was that group members stopped attending. As I explored, I learned that the group members did so because during these mindfulness/meditative exercises, the members were asked to sit still in certain Buddha poses—the group leaders neglected to account for the fact that the perpetrators of the atrocities that were inflicted upon these women were Buddhists. Having recognized this, I thought it would be reparative to engage in meditative practices based in their own faith of Islam, precisely the practice for which they were being persecuted.

As such, we started the group and engaged in *Tasbeehat*, which is a practice within Islam in which one meditates over the *Tasbeeh* (prayer beads). Wernik (2009) explained that typically key phrases such as the divine names and attributes of God are recited during these meditations. This is done in a state of relaxed meditation and focus. When praising or aiming to be in unison with God in Sufi Islam, the precise practice is referred to as Zikr. While in Tasbeehat, one is active in the recitation; it is followed by Muraqaba, when one enters into stillness, silence, and awareness. Faridi (1986) conveyed that on the path of Islamic spirituality, one is continually traveling from self to God. Eventually, one leaves the self behind completely and fully enters the divine presence; and one trains for this ultimate stage of freedom and spiritual awareness. Many of the women within the group had family members who were killed or presumed dead, and often they were not able to retrieve the bodies. When such disasters occur and people are presumed dead because the body is not recovered, it changes everything that traditionally surrounds the natural grieving process. This grieving process as a Muslim typically entails loved ones gathering and reciting Surah Fatiha from the Quran; if this is not done, the Ruh (spirit) is considered to be floating around. Because most of the women had lost someone without ever going through this process, we opted to use the Tasbeeh to recite this Surah Fatiha as a group. This was a pivotal moment in the group. Slowly, over multiple sessions, each woman was able to articulate her story and engage in reciting the surah for the ones they lost, which was very meaningful for each. They articulated initially feeling that they were the only ones who have ever had to go through this anguish, and then how being in the group provided them with a sense of community and shared culture. A culture doesn't have to be characterized solely by a common background, but it is also based on where one feels understood and gets a sense of belonging to help promote resiliency. Once the conversation started flowing, women talked about feeling understood by each other without having to explain too much. At the same time, I provided some psychoeducation about how trauma manifests in its varying forms, noting the varying ways in which people dissociate—emotionally, cognitively, and physically. During this process, the notions of Nafs, Qalb, and Ruh were easily and effectively grasped by the group of women. Framing it in the form of Nafs as part of the Ghaib (or the unconscious) and Nafsi Ammar, as the primal instinct that seeks to avoid pain, and not be in touch with what has happened to them or is happening, it reminded them that one seeks to have self-control using the Qalb, while acknowledging the Ruh pulls one to the other end (a moralistic voice that is hidden within). We discussed the need to keep the Qalb active to continuously attempt to balance off the Nafs and the Ruh, to be in touch with and be able to share both parts of us, to recognize the notion of choice and self-control, and to attempt making decisions that balance the pulls.

This transitioned into discussing their experience of their own bodies and speaking to the unborn children. This was done by thinking through how the Ruh of those deceased stays afloat and not at a resting state until acknowledged, prayed for, and engaged in the burial prayers and rituals. Discussion also entailed focusing on the Nafs (i.e., how it helps meet the basic needs of the body) and using the Qalb to make sense. The group started with four women before expanding to 11, and the group process allowed use of the very religious practices for which they have been persecuted to be acknowledged and utilized for their healing and recovery.

Psychological First Aid Following the Boston Marathon Bombings

I work in the domain of trauma and in disaster response. I provide disaster relief services, as a behavioral health responder, and conduct disaster relief and crisis counseling trainings, locally, nationally, and internationally. My work as a psychologist first responder following the Boston Marathon bombing, in 2013, also revealed to me some of the challenges and possibilities of spiritually integrative intervention. From the moment that the bombing occurred, for me to step in as a first responder, and a Muslim first responder, was a complex state of being. I recall my initial thought in the back of my head, "please don't let the perpetrator be a Muslim," which is a sentiment that many Muslims experience in situations like that. Part of my role that day was helping set up the family assistance center at the hospital and providing psychological first aid to survivors and their friends and family. One of the family members who received devastating news regarding the health status of their son, was immensely distressed. As I provided psychological first aid, and she held my hand, at one point she stated, "How could they do this to us, these Muslims. They need to get out of our country." She stated this under distress, while holding my hand, without knowing that the very hand she was holding was belonged to another Muslim person—that both the perpetrator of the distress and the alleviator of her distress were Muslim. Many inquired as to why I didn't tell her that I was Muslim. For me, in that moment, remembering my role and understanding that my aim was to alleviate this person's distress was important, as it should always be. Knowing our professional aim and role is key, and refraining from being driven to state something biased or reactive in the moment is critical. But for me, personally, this commitment also stems from adherence to the Islamic notions of *Khidmat-e-Khalq* and *Hizmet*. These are ideas embedded in me from my parents and the Islamic teaching reflected in actions of the Prophet Muhammad. Khidmat literally means to help, to assist, and khalq refers to creatures, created by Allah, thus the notion refers to serving humanity. Hizmet is a faith-inspired, civil-society movement that seeks to create a culture of coexistence within universal humanist values; the essence of it is to make a contribution without the expectation of anything in return. I was able to look at all aspects of this person's functioning in that moment— her trauma at this time, what she was engaging in, her projection stemming from the cultural political structure within this country at this time, and her racial privilege and lack of thought or awareness of my possible identity. I could empathize with her loss despite her statement, upon quickly contextualizing it and being clear about my role as a clinician and as a Muslim woman.

Disaster Relief Work With Individuals From Haiti

I have provided trauma and disaster relief services for people identifying as Haitian following the earthquake in Haiti in 2010 (both in Haiti and in the United States). During my time conducting mental health and disaster relief work in Port-au-Prince and Miragoane within Haiti, I experienced assisting people with a variety of belief systems. Haiti is primarily a Catholic country and religious motifs regarding Jesus were everywhere in Port-au-Prince. In addition, the majority of the Haitians practice Voodoo, which is widely accepted but practiced only privately. Voodoo is a mixture of Catholic and African beliefs, and followers believe the world is under the command of *loas* (spirits and deities), who act as arbitrators between people and God. In Voodoo, disasters like the earthquake are not the result of natural forces, but rather discontent of the loas. There is, at the core, the notion that everything you know—people, plants, rocks, everything—has a spirit and a spiritual reality to it that is just as real and as reachable as physical reality. Additionally, Muslims make up 1% of the population of Haiti (Pew Research Center, 2015). While in Miragoane, Mufti Shaheed Mohammed had established a *Darul Uloom* (Islamic seminary) in the area; it caters to Muslims of the entire country (belonging to sects of Sunni and Ahmadi).

With this understanding, faith and spirituality were sometimes in the background and at other times in the forefront within my clinical work in Haiti. There was also an interesting blending of Catholic or Muslim faiths with Voodoo, and determining how each individual blended these and how that contributed to their understanding of suffering and ways of handling of their struggles was a critical part of the work and of alliance building. So, for instance, when an individual walked in speaking of the loas being discontent and being the cause of the disaster and meaning to harm him, as a culturally attuned clinician, one cannot dismiss it. It would be important to inquire as to what would alleviate the discontent, how was this impacting them, and what actions they could take. When the person was Muslim, the option of making a *Dua* (supplication or prayer—to call upon God) for forgiveness was discussed as a possibility. At another time, a person believed in their physical injury being healed by the spirit of the plants, so they covered the injury site where a physician prescribed antibiotics and applied a bandage wrap, followed with a wrap made of leaves. I would listen to the narrative that people ascribed, embedded in their beliefs, and incorporate it respectfully while also sharing additional thoughts about clinical strategies, thus jointly creating spiritually integrative treatment plans, as such.

The notion of stigma regarding mental health was quite prevalent in Haiti and had to be addressed. The notions of Nafs, Qalb, and Ruh were operative in mostly a tacit way with the Muslims. However, I had to be cautious when applying this with the Ahmadi sect of Muslims, as they have been persecuted for their messianic approaches (which have been classified as un-Islamic), particularly in Southeast Asia (including in my homeland of Pakistan). This awareness of my identity as a Sunni Muslim and how it would be perceived was something of which I had to be conscious. Additionally, transgenerational trauma in the country stemming from the political system and the prevalent notion of betrayal from the government needed to be incorporated and understood within a postcolonial framework. There has to be sensitivity to the ways historical dynamics of oppression continue to influence daily life. Haiti was once colonized by France, and those who speak French typically have a higher socioeconomic status than the working-class individuals, who mainly speak Creole. This language distinction also aligns with skin color differences, and these can be the determinants of the resources to get health and mental health needs met.

Working with the Haitian population in the United States also entailed a great deal of collaborative work with faith-based institutions, due to the stigma associated with seeking these mental health services. Haitians are known to be "religious about religion," meaning their faith is known to be deeply important to them. This collaboration was what made for effective provision of services in Massachusetts. I conducted a support group in Boston, and again, it was interesting to see how Haitians who spoke French versus those who spoke Creole perceived each other through the lens of this colonial past in ways that shaped views of socioeconomic status in the present. Therefore, I had to be mindful of possible subgrouping, group cohesiveness, scapegoating, and the way in which existential questions emerged given the diversity of Haitian identities. Here again, the postcolonial framework was immensely effective in helping me get a grasp of the dynamics and the depth of the existing differences in these groups.

CONCLUSION

Although the case examples in this chapter involve disaster field settings, similar experiences play out in individual work in clinical settings. These examples capture the essence of working with people with similar, somewhat similar, and different SERT commitments. I have, on occasion, felt more spiritually related to individuals with different SERT beliefs, due to similar outlooks and values, rather than similar faith-based nomenclature. Not functioning within boundaries and coloring outside the lines are core parts of me, which stem from having traversed multiple settings and boundaries across continents, countries, states, cities, and so on. A part of my way of being is not always fitting in, not fully belonging, and being a hybrid who blends seemingly disparate things with facility. This aspect of my being lends itself easily to blending of multiple theories and integrating them (hence, the appeal for a spiritually integrated theory), and also to naturally being able to engage with different SERT beliefs and variations within the SERT beliefs.

In my individual and group therapy work here in the United States, and in the different disaster and refugee relief field settings nationally and internationally, I have had the opportunity to work with a diverse set of individuals who identified as Muslims while belonging to different nations and ranged on other aspects of identity as well (intersectionality). I have also had the opportunity of working with those who identified with a variety of other religions or with none. Some were atheists, some agnostics, some monotheists, and some polytheists. Clients have identified different aspects of identity-related factors for having sought treatment with me: some due to the religious awareness, some due to religious similarity, some due to cultural awareness or similarity, some due to a linguistic capacity, some due to gender, some due to particular expertise with certain populations, some due to years of experience, and some just due to random assignment. Aspects of faith have been explicit with some and implicit with others. However, at all times, I have had an ear open for the emergence of such narratives.

It fascinates me to witness the beliefs people hold, the tenets to which they adhere, and the ways in which those beliefs and tenets guide their lifestyles. Whether an individual is an atheist, committed to a particular faith, an agnostic, or anywhere in between, there is wisdom to be gained from all the varied beliefs of the world. Each person has their unique relation to their faith, in terms of their beliefs and values, and understanding this relation is an appealing process of the profession.

I have witnessed the ways in which faith is capitalized on as a strength in times of distress and the ways in which it can be used to erase and silence. I have felt the burden of being locked in boxes imposed by myself and society—boxes built with the dust of century-old fallacies decreeing what my faith and beliefs ought to be. Yet, I have learned and relearned from my clinical encounters about the intersectional and pluralistic practices of faiths around the world. I have learned to "discover patients' religion," even if they say that they are not religious, as they have a system of beliefs and values to which they adhere. These clinical encounters have helped me develop a more rigorous and active relationship with my beliefs, often expanding, deconstructing, and reconstructing my relationship with my own SERT traditions, which I truly value.

REFERENCES

Abdul-Hamid, W. K. (2011). The need for a category of "religious and spiritual problems" in *ICD-11*. *International Psychiatry, 8*(3), 60–61. https://doi.org/10.1192/S1749367600002575

Abdul-Hamid, W. K., & Hughes, J. H. (2015). Integration of religion and spirituality into trauma psychotherapy: An example in Sufism? *Journal of EMDR Practice and Research, 9*(3), 150–156. https://doi.org/10.1891/1933-3196.9.3.150

Abu-Raiya, H. (2014). Western psychology and Muslim psychology in dialogue: Comparisons between a Qura'nic theory of personality and Freud's and Jung's ideas. *Journal of Religion and Health, 53*(2), 326–338. https://doi.org/10.1007/s10943-012-9630-9

Abu-Raiya, H., Pargament, K. I., Mahoney, A., & Stein, C. (2008). A psychological measure of Islam religiousness: Development and evidence for reliability and validity. *The International Journal for the Psychology of Religion, 18*(4), 291–315. https://doi.org/10.1080/10508610802229270

Ahmad, I. (2010). *Bayanul Quran* (Vols. 1–7). Tanzeem-e-Islami.

Albuquerque, J., Deshauer, D., & Grof, P. (2003). Descartes' passions of the soul—Seeds of psychiatry? *Journal of Affective Disorders, 76*(1–3), 285–291. https://doi.org/10.1016/S0165-0327(02)00104-0

Amri, S., & Bemak, F. (2012). Mental health help-seeking behaviors of Muslim immigrants in the United States: Overcoming social stigma and cultural mistrust. *Journal of Muslim Mental Health, 7*(1), 43–63. https://doi.org/10.3998/jmmh.10381607.0007.104

Ashcroft, B., Griffiths, G., & Tiffin, H. (Eds.). (2006). *The post-colonial studies reader* (2nd ed.). Routledge.

Calhoun, L. G., Cann, A., Tedeschi, R. G., & McMillan, J. (2000). A correlational test of the relationship between posttraumatic growth, religion, and cognitive processing. *Journal of Traumatic Stress, 13*(3), 521–527. https://doi.org/10.1023/A:1007745627077

Crenshaw, K. (1989). Demarginalizing the intersection of race and sex: A Black feminist critique of antidiscrimination doctrine, feminist theory and antiracist politics. *University of Chicago Legal Forum, 1989*(1), 139–168.

Dein, S. (2006). Religion, spirituality and depression: Implications for research and treatment. *Primary Care & Community Psychiatry, 11*(2), 67–72.

Fanon, F. (1991). *Black skin, White masks*. Grove Press.

Faridi, S. (1986). *Inner aspects of faith* (2nd ed.). Mehfil-e-Zauqia.

Good, J. J. (2010). *Integration of spirituality and cognitive-behavioral therapy for the treatment of depression* [Doctoral dissertation, Philadelphia College of Osteopathic Medicine]. https://digitalcommons.pcom.edu/cgi/viewcontent.cgi?article=1054&context=psychology_dissertations

Gordon, J. (2006). Healing the wounds of war in Gaza and Israel: A mind–body approach. In J. Kuriansky (Ed.), *Terror in the Holy Land: Inside the anguish of the Israeli-Palestinian conflict* (pp. 203–216). Praeger Publishers.

Hipolito, E., Samuels-Dennis, J. A., Shanmuganandapala, B., Maddoux, J., Paulson, R., Saugh, D., & Carnahan, B. (2014). Trauma-informed care: Accounting for the interconnected role of spirituality and empowerment in mental health promotion. *Journal of Spirituality in Mental Health, 16*(3), 193–217. https://doi.org/10.1080/19349637.2014.925368

Ibn-Sinha. (2004). *The metaphysics of the healing: A parallel English-Arabic text al-Ilahiyat min al-Shifa* (M. E. Marmura, Trans.). Brigham Young University Press.

Loewald, H. W. (1960). On the therapeutic action of psycho-analysis. *The International Journal of Psychoanalysis, 41,* 16–33.

Loomba, A. (2005). *Colonialism/postcolonialism* (2nd ed.). Routledge.

Nizamie, S. H., Katshu, M. Z. U. H., & Uvais, N. A. (2013). Sufism and mental health. *Indian Journal of Psychiatry, 55*(6), 215–223. https://doi.org/10.4103/0019-5545.105535

Pargament, K. I. (2007). *Spiritually integrated psychotherapy: Understanding and addressing the sacred*. Guilford Press.

Pew Research Center. (2015, April 2). *The future of world religions: Population growth projections, 2010–2050.* http://www.globalreligiousfutures.org/countries/haiti#/?affiliations_religion_id=0&affiliations_year=2010&region_name=All%20Countries&restrictions_year=2016

Piedmont, R. L. (2013). A short history of the psychology of religion and spirituality: Providing growth and meaning for Division 36. *Psychology of Religion and Spirituality, 5*(1), 1–4. https://doi.org/10.1037/a0030878

Rumi, J. (2004). *The essential Rumi* (C. Barks, Trans., New ed.). Harper One.

Rushdie, S. (1991). *Imaginary homelands: Essays and criticism*. Granta Books.

Said, E. W. (1978). *Orientalism*. Random House.

Said, E. W. (1994). *Culture and imperialism*. Vintage Books.

Schacter, D. L., Gilbert, D. T., & Wegner, D. M. (2010). *Psychology* (2nd ed.). Worth Publishers.

Spivak, G. C. (1999). *A critique of postcolonial reason: Toward a history of the vanishing present*. Harvard University Press. https://doi.org/10.2307/j.ctvjsf541

USA for UNHCR. (2021). *Rohingya refugee crisis.* https://www.unrefugees.org/emergencies/rohingya/

Vedantam, S. (2010, January 20). Haiti: Natural disasters and religious belief: What happens to religious faith after a disaster? *Psychology Today.* https://www.psychologytoday.com/gb/blog/the-hidden-brain/201001/haiti-natural-disasters-and-religious-belief

Wernik, U. (2009). The use of prayer beads in psychotherapy. *Mental Health, Religion & Culture, 12*(4), 359–368. https://doi.org/10.1080/13674670902732781

Wong, Y. J., Rew, L., & Slaikeu, K. D. (2006). A systematic review of recent research on adolescent religiosity/spirituality and mental health. *Issues in Mental Health Nursing, 27*(2), 161–183. https://doi.org/10.1080/01612840500436941

Worthington, E. L., Jr., & Sandage, S. J. (2001). Religion and spirituality. *Psychotherapy: Theory, Research, Practice, and Training, 38*(4), 473–478. https://doi.org/10.1037/0033-3204.38.4.473

6

CHRISTIAN SPIRITUALLY INTEGRATED PSYCHOTHERAPY

A Wesleyan Model

BRAD D. STRAWN

While most practitioners are aware that psychology and psychotherapy have a long history of antagonism with spirituality and religion (SR), many are unaware that there is an equally long history of intellectual inquiry between the two (Hoffman, M. T., 2011; Vande Kemp, 1984). In fact, for many psychologists, SR has never really been a problem but something to understand. In conservative Christian circles, however, this has not always been the case. In these settings, psychology was often equated with secular humanism, undercutting religious explanations and authority as well as personal responsibility (Vitz, 1977). A rapprochement between Christian faith and psychology began in the mid-1960s with the advent of several American Psychological Association (APA)–accredited doctoral programs in clinical psychology specializing in SR (e.g., Fuller Graduate School of Psychology, Rosemead School of Psychology, George Fox Graduate School of Psychology, Wheaton Graduate School of Psychology) and the development of journals (e.g., *Journal of Psychology and Christianity*, the *Journal of Psychology and Theology*) and organizations (e.g., The Christian Association for Psychological Studies) specializing

https://doi.org/10.1037/0000276-007
Spiritual Diversity in Psychotherapy: Engaging the Sacred in Clinical Practice,
S. J. Sandage and B. D. Strawn (Editors)

in the dialogue. *Integration* (i.e., the interdisciplinary conversation between psychology and Christian theology) was the term coined in Christian evangelical settings to describe this dialogue (Vande Kemp, 1984).

Outside specifically Christian settings, the dialogue between psychology and SR has also been growing (see the Introduction to this volume). The APA has supported the idea that a client's SR is a central aspect of their culture, expecting clinicians to develop competence in the same manner as culture. In the APA (2002) *Guidelines on Multicultural Education, Training, Research and Practice and Organizational Change for Psychologists*, *culture* is defined as

> the belief systems and value orientations that influence customs, norms, practices, and social institutions, including psychological processes (language, care taking practices, media, educational systems) and organizations (media, educational systems; Fiske, Kitayama, Markus, & Nisbett, 1998). Inherent in this definition is the acknowledgement that all individuals are cultural beings and have a cultural, ethnic, and racial heritage. Culture has been described as the embodiment of a worldview through learned and transmitted beliefs, values, and practices, *including religious and spiritual traditions* [emphasis added]. It also encompasses a way of living informed by the historical, economic, ecological, and political forces on a group. These definitions suggest that culture is fluid and dynamic, and that there are both cultural universal phenomena as well as culturally specific or relative constructs. (p. 8)

The term "spiritually integrated psychotherapy" (Pargament, 2007) emerged from a nonreligious setting to describe a manner in which therapists might work in SR-competent ways. Unfortunately, research demonstrates that students trained at nonreligious doctoral programs obtain very little training in SR (Pargament, 2007). Most young professionals leave graduate school unprepared to address the SR issues that they will face in their work. This state of affairs is a reflection of the deeply seated assumption within the mental health field that spirituality is, at most, a side issue in psychotherapy, one that can be either sidestepped or resolved through an education to reality (Pargament, 2007, p. 9).

This reality makes a volume like the present one vitally important. The present chapter will attempt to demonstrate the importance of SR competence in spiritually integrated therapy from a particularly Christian perspective.

For the sake of this book and chapter we refer to one's spiritual, existential, religious, and/or theological (SERT) tradition (Rupert et al., 2019). This implies that therapists and/or patients may have spiritual, existential, religious, and theological leanings, conscious and unconscious, that are an important aspect of their sense of self and the way in which they make sense of their world. While there are important differences between spirituality and religion, the term SERT helps cover a variety of ways in which individuals may organize their reality through interaction with something sacred and transcendent. SERT is used in this chapter as inclusively as possible.

When discussing spiritually integrated psychotherapy, it is essential to clarify *whose* spirituality is being referred to. While spirituality is often used in vague transcendent ways, spirituality is ultimately defined by the adjective that proceeds it (Clapp, 2004); thus, this chapter describes a *Christian* spiritually integrated therapy and its implications for working with religious clients. With hundreds of different groups all claiming to be Christian, it is equally important to resist a monolithic generalization of Christianity but rather to contextualize the particular Christian tradition of therapist and client as this will have important bearing on the work (Strawn et al., 2014; Wright et al., 2014). Therefore, due to the author's specific SERT tradition, the focus of this chapter is on a Christian *Wesleyan* model of spirituality and its implication for psychotherapy.

A BRIEF HISTORY OF WESLEYANISM

John Wesley, the theological father of Methodism, was a 19th-century cleric in the Church of England, who attempted to ignite a renewal movement within the Church of England (Maddox, 1994). Wesley was concerned that the Church of England had lost its way. He specifically feared that the church had forgotten its mission and calling. This was particularly evident in developing socio-economic disparities between the laity within the churches and a neglect of the poor.

Wesley was not primarily a parish priest. Rather, he was an itinerant preacher, traveling and preaching to those who no longer felt welcomed or comfortable in the church. His mission included traveling, preaching, and then setting up discipleship groups for those interested in ongoing spiritual formation. These groups followed a strict set of criteria (e.g., methods) for formation, including regular confession to one another as well as financial giving and ministry to the poor. Wesley's small groups were a powerful means of spiritual formation and have been credited with influencing the church small group movement, Alcoholics Anonymous and even group therapy (Malony, 2010). Wesleyan theology emerged primarily from the preaching, teaching, writing, and practices of Wesley. He was a praxis theologian, rather than a systematic one, and therefore he never wrote a doctrinal opus. His focus was not on the intellectual tenants of doctrine but rather on the daily lived-out practices of faith whose goal was personal transformation. Therefore, his theology is mostly gleaned from published sermons and a small number of short books and tracts (Maddox, 1994).

WESLEYAN THEOLOGY TODAY

Wesleyanism today is part of the Protestant movement in Christianity and is most widely associated in the United States with the mainline United Methodist denomination.[1] Some Wesleyan traditions would consider themselves evangelical, whereas others would eschew the concept. Wesleyanism ascribes to the central tenets of Orthodox Christian faith. In summary, these include the Trinitarian God—one God in three persons (Father, Son, and Holy Spirit)—who created the world, sent his son, Jesus Christ, to show humanity how to live, suffered, died and was resurrected reconciling all people to God. Wesleyans believe that the Holy Spirit is the source of ongoing life and is the teacher and comforter in Christ's physical absence. Wesleyans believe that the ongoing work of God through the Spirit is not limited to those who claim a relationship with God but is the source of life and transformation, constantly wooing humanity to God's self and into a life of peace, shalom (wholeness of mind and body), and love. For this reason, many Wesleyans are pluralistically open when it comes to other faith traditions (Stone & Oord, 2001). Finally, Christ will return to usher in God's eternal Kingdom where those who choose life with God will live forever.

Importantly, Wesleyans are not biblical literalists or inerrantists and therefore not fundamentalists. They view the Bible (the 66 books of the Old and New Testaments) as a divinely inspired text, written by human individuals, in particular social locations, to particular people, attempting to make particular points. So, it is while an inspired text, it contains human fingerprints. Furthermore, the Bible consists of numerous genres, such as poetry, liturgy, narrative, letters, and so forth. Therefore, the Bible is not considered a book of history or science but must be read in light of genre and interpreted through the lens of tradition, reason, and experience (Gunter et al., 1997). While not an inerrant book, the Bible does teach a way of morality as demonstrated through the life and death of Jesus Christ (see especially the Sermon on the Mount found in Matthew 5, 6, and 7). This biblical openness has allowed some of the more mainline branches of Wesleyanism (including some United Methodists)

---

[1]There are a number of other denominations that are theologically Wesleyan, including but not limited to: The Wesleyan Church, Free Methodist, Nazarene, and African Methodist Episcopal (AME).

to openly affirm the LGBTQI2 community. It has also allowed Wesleyans to embrace sources of truth outside of the Bible, including but not limited to, the science and practice of psychotherapy.[2]

Wesley emphasized human freedom more than Calvinist theology, which stresses God's sovereignty. Calvin's belief in God's all-controlling sovereignty (e.g., nothing happens outside of God's will) led him to the doctrine of predestination—God preordains which persons will obtain heaven or hell (Wynkoop, 1972). Wesley emphasized human freedom, which he conceptualized as emanating from God's essential nature of love (Stone & Oord, 2001). Because God could not act contrary to God's nature, God loves humans with an *uncontrolling love* (Oord, 2019). God cannot intercede in persons' lives in any way that violates their freedom; otherwise, God is controlling and no longer love. Therefore, to preordain persons to heaven or hell would be contrary to God's nature. This means that humans are free to accept or reject God's saving love. This also means that God is not the source of creation's suffering; neither does God allow it. God grieves with creation's suffering and is at work to do all God can to bring about restoration. But again, because of God's uncontrolling love, God cannot singlehandedly stop creation's suffering. Therefore, there is room for the important collaborating activity of humans with God, such as that seen in the practice of medicine, psychological science, and psychotherapy.

Wesley did not endorse the deist position, which asserted that God created the world and since then no longer interacted with it. Wesley believed that the uncontrolling love of God naturally led to a cooperative relationship between God and humans. God could not overpower a person's freedom, nor singlehandedly stop suffering, but that didn't mean that God wasn't still at work for the good of the person.[3] Humans who remained open to God's uncontrolling influence could make decisions in light of that influence. To remain open to God's leading is facilitated by engaging in spiritual practices, or *means of grace* (e.g., physical and tangible elements and acts such as reading scripture, receiving the eucharist, prayer, worship, acts of mercy toward others), which not only allow God to speak to the person (e.g., through the Holy Spirit) but also shape human character to grow in embodiment toward the image and likeness of God—best captured in a life of love, participating with God to usher in God's reign of peace and shalom. The Wesleyan concept of uncontrolling love, free will, and Divine-Human cooperation suggests that

---

[2]Wesley was deeply interested in science, medicine, and electricity. Malony (2010) has referred to him as an 18th-century health psychologist.
[3]This perspective has been most closely aligned with what has been described as Open Theism or Process Theology.

psychotherapy may be considered an aspect of God's ongoing work in concert with humans to bring about restoration and healing to individuals, communities, and the world.

Theologically Wesley read widely in the Christian tradition, integrating ideas from both Western (Protestant) and Eastern (Orthodox) branches of Christianity in his sermons and writings. From the West he incorporated *saving* grace or justification by faith. This doctrine emphasizes God's unmerited grace through the life, death, and resurrection of Jesus Christ forgiving humans from sin and reconciling them to God's self. Justification by faith implies that there is nothing persons can do to earn God's love and forgiveness; it is offered freely to those who accept it. From the East he incorporated the concept of *sanctifying* grace, which emphasizes the transforming power of God via the Holy Spirit to form persons into the image and likeness of God. Being formed into Christ-likeness means that persons would develop to live and love as Christ had. Saving grace has been compared to God's *juridical* activity and sanctifying grace to God's *therapeutic* activity (Maddox, 1994).

This therapeutic activity (i.e., sanctifying grace) is the cooperative work of God and persons, via spiritual practices, empowered by the Holy Spirit, to transform persons from self-centered preoccupation to a life of holiness or sanctification—to love as Christ loved. Wesley referred to these transformative practices as means of grace in which a tangible physical article (e.g., the Eucharist) or event (e.g., small group meeting) became the mediation of God's grace (Maddox, 1994). While there are a variety of interpretations of holiness and sanctification within the Wesleyan tradition, the most psychologically minded emphasizes persons moving from a self-centered preoccupation to an *other* orientation—living out a virtue of love for God and neighbor. Although certain branches of Wesleyan interpretations of holiness unfortunately led to an emphasis on "works righteousness" culminating in legalism, a more accurate understanding of sanctification is the development of the virtue of love within persons and their communities (i.e., the church) for the sake of the world. Therefore, Wesleyanism is equally interested in the transformation of persons into the virtue and character of love as salvation from sin (Maddox, 1994, 2004; Wynkoop, 2015). For a Wesleyan, transformational activities such as psychotherapy, can be understood as religious, spiritual, or sacred in nature, means of grace, even if they are not connected to a person's eternal salvation.

A final theological concept that has import for Christian Wesleyan spirituality is what has been referred to as *immanental cosmology* (Lodahl, 2003). A Wesleyan theology espouses that God is both transcendent (i.e., a wholly other being who is free to move and act in God's creation as consistent with God's nature) and immanent (i.e., through the power of the Holy Spirit—third of the Trinity—God is at work in the very nature of creation, sustaining all of creation and attempting to woo all toward growth, and love). For this reason, a Wesleyan can conceptualize God as working in many spheres of life, including other religious traditions. This has sometimes been referred to as *big tent theology*, meaning that one can claim both clear theological doctrine practices and ethics for the life of faith, while remaining open, welcoming, and hospitable to seekers of other traditions as well.

In summary, a nonliteralist, nonfundamental view of scripture allows a Wesleyan to incorporate other sources of knowledge regarding life, including the science and theory of psychotherapy. A Wesleyan will eschew the dichotomy of sacred (e.g., religion) and secular (e.g., science) as God's activity in the world is seen in the work of the Spirit. This means that God is at work in various means of grace including psychotherapy, where the aim may be conceptualized as the restoration of human love. Furthermore, Wesleyans are not solely interested in salvation—getting one's ticket stamped for heaven—but in the ongoing transformational work of the Spirit moving persons from self-centeredness to other—love centered.

This chapter attempts to illustrate how one might conduct psychotherapy with a Christian Wesleyan spirituality. It will keep in mind (a) convergences and divergences, (b) the impact of both the therapist's and client's SERT traditions on the work, and (c) illustrate the challenges through case material.

PERSONAL SERT TRADITION

What is now referred to as *spiritually integrated psychotherapy* might be referred to as *clinical integrative practice* in evangelical Christian circles (Strawn, 2020). However, it is important to recognize that while there are "Christianities," there are also various types of evangelicals. Splits and divisions have occurred within evangelicalism. While these splits have been happening for some time, they recently and dramatically reoccurred during the presidential election of 2016. Depending on which source you read, the vast majority of self-proclaimed evangelicals supported the Republican candidate, while an alternative group, best described as neo-evangelicals (Labberton, 2018; Scalise, 2015), did not.

My religious background is replete with scraps of fundamentalism, having grown up in an evangelical church that emphasized personal holiness often leading to legalism, purity culture, and othering (e.g., forming ingroups and outgroups based on religious membership). We focused on sin management, rule-following, and getting our tickets stamped for heaven in the next life. Doing right also meant staying away from all those places and people that didn't and led to othering. My psychological training must certainly be credited with the expansion of my narrow, fundamentalist, literal, and legalistic Christian worldview. Conducting therapy with individuals who were very different from myself facilitated my seeing clients not as categories or labels but as persons with names, histories, loves, pains, similarities, and differences who exhibited both challenges and strengths. The black-and-white thinking of my particular evangelicalism became nuanced, open, and most importantly, loving toward all of God's creation.

But my theological training also deserves recognition. During my doctoral psychology training I also studied theology proper in a seminary setting. Scriptural issues of justice, reconciliation, and liberation of the oppressed came to the foreground. My religious focus shifted from self-monitoring sin management, in order to get to heaven, to participating with God in bringing God's peace, or shalom, to *all* persons. I describe this as a movement out of a kind of fundamentalistic evangelicalism into a Wesleyan neo-evangelicalism. One of the huge aspects of this was that it meant that knowledge or truth might be obtained through multiple sources in addition to the Bible, such as science, history, philosophy, logic, anthropology, and so on. Even more radically, I came to understand that biblical knowledge is in part human interpretation (i.e., hermeneutics) and therefore could be aided and enhanced through the use of these other sources.

Finally, these psychological and theological changes led me to recognize and respect issues related to race, culture, ethnicity, gender, and sexual orientation, as well as to critique traditions of the Christian Church that have contributed to issues such as White supremacy and colonialism. As a White, heterosexual, cisgendered male, I attempt to remain mindful of my position of great privilege, knowing it impacts my work in unrecognized ways. It is also true that my social location within neo-evangelicalism also marks me as a "safe psychologist" to *some* clients who see me as sharing their religious worldview.

SPIRITUALLY INTEGRATED PSYCHOTHERAPY–A WESLEYAN CHRISTIAN PSYCHOANALYTIC PERSPECTIVE

I practice from a pluralistic relational psychoanalytic orientation. I concur with Nancy McWilliams (2004) that while psychoanalytic pluralism does not always make sense theoretically, it often does phenomenologically. Different cases and patients may best be conceptualized through a variety of psychoanalytic perspectives. I also hold respect for nonanalytic therapies. So, while conceptualizing a client psychodynamically, I remain open to interventions from other theoretical orientations when they enhance the treatment. Being psychoanalytically informed, I explore and emphasize a client's history, their physical and biological realities, as well as their social location (e.g., race, culture, ethnicity, sexual orientation). I make use of such psychoanalytic concepts as the unconscious, transference–countertransference enactments, defenses, dissociation, multiple self-states, rupture and repair, mutual recognition, and the Third (i.e., therapist and patient hold the tension of recognizing one another as separate minds that can at times be shared; Benjamin, 2018; Bromberg, 2001; McWilliams, 2004; Safran & Muran, 2000).

One of the hallmarks of a relational psychoanalytic approach is the centrality of the therapist's contribution to the therapy (Aron, 1991; Hoffman, I. Z., 1983; Renik, 1993). This contribution goes well beyond countertransference as the therapist's unresolved issues or as projection from the client onto the therapist who then identifies with and experiences the projections as their own feelings (i.e., projective identification), to include the real qualities and history of the therapist and the way he or she unconsciously brings these to the work. The therapeutic relationship is genuinely mutual although asymmetrical (Aron, 1996). Relational therapy is egalitarian, democratic, narrative, hermeneutical, and constructivist (Sorenson, 2004). Therapy consists of ongoing and unavoidable transference–countertransference enactments in which patient and therapist become intertwined in one another's stories. These enactments can have a pathological repetitive dimension as well as a forward-moving, generative dimension and therefore are essential to growth (Atlas & Aron, 2018). From this relational perspective, the focus of therapeutic change is not solely interpretation or intervention, both of which attempt to change one's cognitions, but a kind of "dramatic dialogue" (Atlas & Aron, 2018) in which issues are worked through (sometimes without narration) by the sheer act of performing the enactments together. Through these processes, developmental deficits may be filled, dissociated self-states and their accompanying affects may be reintegrated, and unconscious defenses may be relinquished. As Atlas and Aron (2018) stated:

> Our conceptualization of contemporary clinical practice featuring dramatic dialogue makes use of this common theme: the analyst's facilitating the emergence of multiple selves, characters, internal objects onto the analytic stage where in scene after scene they are lived, articulated, developed, processed, and transformed. Generative enactment thus becomes not just an occasional mishap, but the *modus operandi* of psychoanalysis. (p. 118, italics in original)

Of course, one's anthropology is central to psychotherapy. What is a human, how do humans develop, and how do they become wounded and healed? As a spiritually integrated psychotherapist, I also (consciously and unconsciously) integrate my understanding of theological anthropology into my psychological conceptualization. John Wesley, operating from within 18th-century British empiricism, believed that affects—transient emotions—could become habituated (i.e., tempers), via ongoing relational experiences and behavior, culminating in the motivational dispositions of a person. John Wesley believed these habituated tempers could be either sinful and selfish or holy and loving. His "methods" of spiritual formation were God's spirit working through the means of grace (e.g., prayer, Bible study, group meetings, sharing in the eucharist) aimed at reforming malformed tempers. The central goal of religion was the restoration of moral affections of heart (Maddox, 2004; Strawn, 2004) transforming persons into the image and likeness of Christ. This meant that "love" would become the central virtue, ruling in a person's life and lived out toward God, self, and other (Maddox, 1994).

This Wesleyan moral affectional psychology (Maddox, 2004) has deep resonance with contemporary psychoanalytic theory and cognitive neuroscience, which both suggest that human affect, cognition and behavior are deeply influenced by experiences (developmental and traumatic) that operate outside of conscious awareness (Cozolino, 2002; Damasio, 2005; Schore, 2015; Wilson, 2002). These developmental or traumatic experiences may lead to behaviors whose ultimate design is to protect persons from unconscious fears of retraumatization; however, they often tend to become enacted in problematic interpersonal behaviors. A Christian Wesleyan spiritually integrated psychoanalytic psychotherapy will focus on working through (i.e., empowered by the Spirit's immanental presence) these early experiences, restoring a person's capacity to self-awareness, mentalization, spontaneity and love in virtuous ways. This may mean working overtly within the client's SERT tradition, including use of resources and practices from their tradition. For example, some clients may desire the use of spiritual practices such as prayer or sacred texts or even engagement with religious authorities from their tradition to be a necessary aspect of therapy. This will demonstrate that therapy respects the client's SERT tradition and ensure that the therapist's tradition doesn't set the clinical agenda. While other religious or spiritual clients will have no desire to utilize elements of their tradition in the therapy, either way it can be good spiritually integrated therapy. Good spiritually integrated therapy is first of all, good therapy.

SERT TRADITIONS WITHIN PSYCHOTHERAPY

A clinician's SERT tradition is as likely to influence one's therapeutic work as their social location (e.g., culture, race, ethnicity, sexual orientation). Students are often trained that the first step in becoming interculturally competent is to begin by understanding one's own culture. The same is true for SERT traditions. This must be done not only when the therapist has an active SERT tradition but even if they have eschewed a previous tradition. For example, a nonreligious therapist growing up with no awareness of a SERT tradition may have still internalized Judeo–Christian values of the surrounding culture or may unconsciously maintain remnants of previous generational religious traditions. One may physically leave home and history, but these never fully leave us. To be SERT competent, we must respect and understand our clients' SERT traditions, and we must understand how those interact with our own (Crabtree et al., 2020; Morgan & Sandage, 2016; Strawn et al., 2014; Wright et al., 2014).

Equally important is to understand how one's *psychotherapeutic orientation* and theory contain elements of SERT traditions. Numerous writers have noted that embedded within seemingly neutral psychotherapy theories are assumptions about normality, morality, and images of the good life. These concepts fall within the philosophical category of ethics, which historically fall under the academic category of theology. Therefore, embedded within our very psychotherapy theories are implicit cultures that possess religio-ethical systems or moral philosophies (Browning & Cooper, 2004). For example, Freudian theory espouses a culture of detachment, whereas humanistic theories offer a culture of joy. Each of these cultures offers deep metaphors suggestive of human capacities and expectations. Where the culture of detachment suggests that the world is basically hostile and humans are self-absorbed, the culture of joy suggests the world is basically harmonious and human wants and needs are basically harmonious (Browning & Cooper, 2004, p. 5). These theories then implicitly prescribe how humans are to live and how to envisage the good life.

That psychotherapy theories contain these deep cultural metaphors and corresponding moral philosophies is understandable because they are products of particular theorists in particular times and settings, responding to current cultural problems. As Cushman (1995) and others have noted, our theories can't help but incorporate some of the values and ethics of the culture in which they were developed. Again, this is not necessarily a problem, but it may become problematic if these ethically laden theories present themselves as value-neutral. Rather than morally neutral, psychotherapy is a moral discourse (Cushman, 1993) consisting of at least three conversation partners: the client, the therapist, and the therapist's theory. One may speak of the four moral strands of relational psychotherapy always at play (Barsness & Strawn, 2019): professional (ethics of the professional guild), personal (ethics learned from one's personal social location), theoretical (ethics embodied both within the theory itself as well as the theories stated or unstated telos), and communal (a potential ethic in which a therapist may ground their work in a thick SERT tradition which offers more than a kind of individual ethic based on emotion, which implies if it feels good to me it is ethical). Clients and therapists both have explicit and implicit personal ethics. These work together with our psychotherapeutic orientations serving as implicit moral philosophies for how one should live. Therefore, it is imperative that therapists recognize that there are at least *three* SERT traditions at work in any *one* therapy: the therapist's, the client's, and the theory's.[4]

CASE EXAMPLE: JOSHUA

I now turn to a clinical vignette illustrating the vital importance of being cognizant of the multiple SERT traditions (and their unacknowledged ethics) in therapy. Identifying information has been changed to maintain client confidentiality.

Whose SERT Is It?

A White, heterosexual, cisgendered man in his late 50s came to therapy because he was indecisive about divorcing his wife of some 30 years. He didn't choose me as a therapist because I was religious, although he knew I was from the referral source. His marriage had been difficult from the beginning, with constant vitriolic fighting resulting in deep shame being inflicted on one another. He reported that all his life he had been indecisive about most decisions and married his wife only because he felt he had little choice. He was not raised in a practicing religious context but internalized some of the ethics from the larger Christian context of his extended family (i.e., Christian Science).

In an early session he spent considerable time describing his wife, what he believed she wanted and needed from him. He was conflicted about leaving her but certain that she still wanted to make the marriage work. He spoke at length about the negative impact a brief separation had on her years ago and how poorly she would take a divorce. As he droned on and on about her, I found myself feeling frustrated. He came to therapy due to indecision, and here he was again, unable to even make the decision to focus on his own experience but instead spending his time privileging his wife's. Finally, I interjected and noted, "It's clear to me that you have a lot of thoughts about

---

[4]Further ethical contributors are the often disguised, systemic, and conflicting traditions found in the larger sociopolitical context which the therapist and client inhabit. Examples may include White supremacy, classism, sexism, and so on.

what your wife wants and needs and how a divorce might negatively impact her, yet you are not telling me anything about what *you* want or need." Without missing a beat, the client responded, "Well, that's the difference between psychology and religion, isn't it? Psychology is all about the self and religion is all about the other?"

While my client's understanding and exposition of psychology and religion could be questioned or at least nuanced, he *was* on to something. It might be tempting to reduce his comments to defense or resistance, but even if they were, that doesn't mean he is wrong. The client rightly noted an implicit religio-ethical system, or practical moral philosophy within much of psychotherapy theory, that favors individualism and self-interest (Browning & Cooper, 2004; Vitz, 1977). And even though my personal SERT tradition would not endorse an individual or self-focused ethic, clearly there was a way in which my theory did. Not being fully aware in the moment of the complicated, and potentially conflicting, SERT traditions in the room, I intervened in a way that was in conflict with my own values and perhaps the client's as well. It bears pointing out that Christianity does in fact value love and care for the self, but this has often been overlooked, and therefore a more humanistic psychology has been an important correction (Browning & Cooper, 2004). From my personal SERT tradition, love of self and neighbor is not just a balance but an inextricable connection that is reciprocal and mutual. But in that moment with my client, I felt "caught," leaning too far away from the client's (and my own) SERT tradition and subsequently missing him.

My intervention could be understood in a number of ways. Was I being unconsciously invited into a dramatic dialogue in which I played the impatient parent who was pushing my patient to "hurry up and make a decision already," becoming frustrated when he took his time, perhaps like his "unhappy wife"? Did I have my own issues with procrastination and indecision and projected those on my patient? Or could it be that we two were somehow grappling with the way that self, other, and relational ethics had always been a part of his struggles growing up, even part of the human dilemma? Probably all of this is true and more. The good news is that all of this could be processed and worked through. The truth, however, is that in that moment I was not cognizant of my client's tradition and was only vaguely aware of the conflict between my own and that of my theory. If I had been aware, I might have said something more like, "Given your concerns for your wife, I wonder what kind of opposing desires you have and what that is like for you?" or "Given your values, what are your thoughts about acting on your wish to leave?" or "You seem deeply concerned and responsible for your wife regarding the possible decision to leave the marriage. Can you say more?" Of course, there are multiple ways to intervene that would acknowledge and make space for all the traditions in the room, but the central point is that if clinicians are not working toward SERT competence, they may do similar damage to a patient as is done when a clinician is not aware of the various cultures in the room (i.e., client's, therapist's, and theory).

I now turn to an example of my Christian Wesleyan spiritually integrated psychoanalytic therapy in which the clinician and client are from different Christian traditions.

How Orthodox and Armenian Am I?

Joshua (Josh) was a single Armenian American, cisgendered man in his 30s who identified as heterosexual. He came to therapy to work on relationship issues and frequently suffered from both mild depression and anxiety. Josh's parents separated and divorced shortly after his birth leaving him to never know his European American father. He was raised primarily by his Armenian grandparents and infrequently by his Armenian mother, who dated a series of men but never settled down with any.

Josh was raised in a very Armenian household, but physically resembled his non-Armenian father with blond hair and blue eyes. His Armenian side of the family tended to be darker skinned, with dark hair and eyes. His family was deeply Orthodox, but for some unknown reason Josh's mother sent him to a very conservative private evangelical school. Josh always felt like a "man without a country." He was Armenian but didn't look it, and he was Orthodox but was steeped in evangelicalism with all of its religious exclusion (including rejection of Orthodoxy) and scare tactics. While Josh was still in elementary school, his mother adopted her nephew, who had been essentially abandoned by his mother (the father had died), and raised him as her son. Their relationship was very close, and Josh felt replaced by his cousin. Josh had no place in which to discuss this sense of displacement and "not belonging." He was Armenian, but not Armenian enough. He was Orthodox, but not Orthodox enough. He was evangelical, but not evangelical enough. He was a son, but not son enough to be chosen by his own mother, or to be known by his father.

Over time, we came to understand that Josh in fact didn't feel that he was ever wanted—left by his biological father, rejected by his mother, and treated with ambivalence by his extended family. His evangelicalism caused him to live in fear of doing something sinful and ending up in hell, while at other times he wondered if all this religious stuff was made up, a thought that deeply disturbed him. Josh was a highly educated person (he was very intelligent and had obtained a post-baccalaureate degree) and had some ideological problems with some of the Orthodox church's beliefs further adding confusion to his Orthodox identity.

Josh knew that I was an evangelical and an ordained minister. This often affected our work. Was I like a priest in the Orthodox Church (Josh loved his priest, but he couldn't imagine telling him some of the things he told me) or like an evangelical pastor at his school (with whom he didn't feel safe)? Because so many others had left him and/or passively put up with him, I sensed that it was important for Josh to know that I welcomed him and chose to be with him. I enjoyed working with Josh and found him thoughtful, intelligent, and funny, but also in deep pain. Trusting me was an issue, as was his self-disclosure. I suggested that we move to twice-weekly therapy, and after some ambivalence regarding fears of dependency, being "too much," or "not enough," Josh agreed.

As a neo-evangelical, I could deeply identify with Josh's fears and concerns about evangelicalism. As a Wesleyan, I resonated with many of the Orthodox doctrines (e.g., theosis as akin to sanctification) and their spiritual practices (e.g., means of grace). The uncertainty Josh had regarding his self-states mingled nicely with my own self-states. I began to suspect that the dramatic dialogue that Josh and I would engage in would be related to these central issues, particularly as they related to Josh's sense of self. Who was he and who wanted him? Who was I and what did I want from him, and would he be able to deliver? Would Josh be enough for us, or would he be too much? Would I be enough or too much? Either way, he might lose.

Not surprisingly, many of Josh's most troubling issues revolved around relationships. His fear of not being relationally wanted, accepted, or welcomed created in him an accommodating personality (Brandchaft, 2010). If there was any hope of being cared for or even important to the other, Josh had learned to silence his voice, deny his needs, and acquiesce to the other. Interpersonally, Josh was quickly liked by others who often felt more intimate with him than he did with them. And certain types of individuals were prone to take advantage of Josh, including making him the recipient of their projections and even blame.

Understandably, Josh went through some terrible relational work situations with supervisors, and I was the only person he could confide in about these. He was full of doubt about his perceptions of the situations. Supervisors would make Josh "special" only to pit him against others, project things upon him, and blame him when things didn't go well. He experienced much of his psychological distress somatically, and his immediate family had grown weary of hearing about his very real physical problems, which had no identifiable causes or cure. Together we explored these relational conflicts, with me supporting and confirming Josh's experience. When he was somatic and feared something awful was happening to him, we attempted to understand together what his body might be saying and tried to find ways to soothe his anxiety primarily by letting him know that all of his thoughts and feelings were welcome. It wasn't hard to be the "good object" that Josh needed. During this time, I often wondered, sometimes aloud, if or how Josh's SERT tradition did or didn't assist him in times of distress. My own SERT tradition, having expanded from my early fundamentalist years to the "big tent" theology of Wesleyanism, made it easy for me to hold Josh's different psychological, cultural, and theological perspectives. Nevertheless, Josh seemed somewhat hesitant to talk of religion and when he did, the conversation inevitably returned to his terrible evangelical experience or his fear of religion "not being true." Again, would I be a new kind of priest he could open up to or a condemning evangelical pastor like he experienced in school?

Greenberg (1986) wrote, "If the analyst cannot be experienced as a new object, analysis never gets under way; if he cannot be experienced as an old one, it never ends" (p. 98). It was inevitable, therefore, that we would have a rupture in which I would become an old bad object from Josh's past. In our dramatic dialogue, or enactment, in which Josh's unconscious history and mine intertwined, two main issues emerged for me. First, for the longest time, Josh had a hard time sharing with me his deep personal feelings—especially as they pertained to me. It seemed that he did in fact have thoughts (and even dreams) about me, but he just couldn't bring himself to say them aloud. While this was understandable, I felt it slowed the pace of the therapy. Josh knew this and I believe that even though I told Josh we were not in a hurry, I think my personal need to feel helpful unconsciously communicated to Josh that I was impatient. Secondly, Josh seemed to continually get stuck between two supervisors who both demanded loyalty, and both had power to make his life miserable. I believed that because Josh never felt like he had a home or was truly wanted, these situations set up terrible conundrums for him. He felt powerless in these situations, wanting to be chosen and liked by all but equally afraid of being exposed as either "too much," or "not enough." I was being unconsciously invited to play a role in Josh's script in which I would become the rejecting parent (or pastor), frustrated with Josh for not moving things along, or as the dismissive and abandoning parent who would give up on Josh because he was "too much" (i.e., too dependent) or "not enough" (e.g., not sharing enough in the session). As is inevitable in these kinds of enactments, things were destined to come to a head, to be felt in real time, in order for working through to occur.

On the day in question, Josh was telling me yet again about another supervisor who seemed to be bullying and manipulating him. He explained how he felt powerless and at the complete whim of the supervisor. While I was conscious of wanting to help Josh not feel powerless, I was not fully aware of other factors at work in me and between us. I suddenly blurted out, "You could have just walked out of the meeting, right?" Instantly Josh became both tearful and angry, saying, "How am I supposed to just do that?" I immediately realized we had experienced an empathic rupture but also sensed that it was inevitable and important.

In a moment I had gone from the one safe person who saw him, chose him, and understood him, communicating to him that he was neither "too much," or "not enough," to one of the many who eventually became frustrated with him, possibly leaving and punishing him. Benjamin (2018) described this as a "doer-done-to" complementarity in which I stopped empathizing with Josh, leaving him to experience me as doing (i.e., the doer) something painful to him (i.e., forcing my perspective and expectations on him) making him the "done to." In his angry response to me, we could quickly switch positions, with me slipping into the "done to" position, experiencing Josh as overreacting and not giving me credit for the years of support I had offered him in the past (Josh became the doer). Regaining my emotional footing and empathy for Josh, I acknowledged his understandable anger and owned that I had spoken poorly. Of course, it was easy for *me* to imagine walking out of the meeting with the supervisor, but not for Josh, both because of his history and because of the actual power differential in the room. And in responding as I had, I inadvertently sent the message to Josh that once again he was "too much," too needy, too dependent, too sad, or "not enough," not assertive enough, not strong enough, not enough to keep people near, and so on. By acknowledging how I had been unempathic to Josh, we were able to move toward mutual recognition, repairing the rupture and entering the Third (Benjamin, 2018) where understanding, connection, and support returned. This exchange was an enactment, a dramatic dialogue in which both Josh and I played roles that represented his core challenges (and mine) and asked the questions *Who am I?* and *Am I too much or not enough?*

Over time, these themes of who he was and how he could be with others continued to show up in various ways. He was in fact starting slowly but surely to lean into who he might be. In our sessions, Josh also struggled with his Orthodox beliefs. He loved the worship, the doctrine, and the practices but, as mentioned earlier, he had some problems with some of the orthodox beliefs around gender and sexuality. One day I casually remarked, "Sounds like you are exploring what it means for *you* to be Orthodox." Josh smirked at me and replied, "We don't do that in the Orthodox Church." I recognized, that while that kind of spiritual exploring might be okay for a neo-evangelical (my SERT tradition and the individualism inherent in my psychotherapy theory), it was not okay for someone from the Orthodox tradition, which has a much more collectivist ecclesiology. Although this was a kind of therapeutic mistake, it also solidified for me a central question of Josh's that I wasn't fully cognizant of at the time: Was Josh Orthodox enough?

In a subsequent session, Josh took a big step by bringing in a prayer book. He wanted my opinion on the prayers, and at first I wasn't sure why. I came to understand that Josh valued the prayers highly but worried that they were not psychologically healthy because of their self-negating language.[5] Once again there was a possible impediment to his accepting his Orthodox self-state. This time maybe the faith was "too much," or maybe he couldn't accept the prayers and subsequently he would not "be enough" of a good Orthodox person. Once again, my SERT tradition (and my theory's) and my own self-states were interacting with Josh's. How would this neo-evangelical therapist/pastor respond to Josh's Orthodox self-state? I was reminded of when Josh asked me to watch a YouTube video of an Armenian fundamentalist evangelical viciously attacking the Orthodox faith. This had made him highly anxious. Was this Armenian evangelical right or was Armenian Orthodoxy right? And who might I be in the drama? Was I the evangelical or would I side with Josh's Orthodox self? I read the prayers and noted how the writer did in fact use powerful language to describe human status as lowly in comparison to the greatness of God. From my SERT tradition the language did feel a bit strong and even self-negating, but then I remembered Ghent's (1990) work on surrender. Ghent argued that there is a significant difference between a pathological masochistic submission to a powerful other and a more universal and healthy surrender to something outside one's self that can be trusted. In the context of the Orthodox tradition, the prayers didn't feel like self-degradation, or masochism, but rather surrender to the infinite, all-powerful, ineffable God. I told Josh that I thought the prayers were beautiful and that to me the strong self-negation language of the prayers was about holding God in high esteem and surrendering to that as an act of faith and trust, rather than a devaluation of the self. Josh resonated deeply with this. My ability to know and hold my own SERT tradition, while attempting to understand Josh's, made this exchange possible.

In that moment I remembered that I had a book on Orthodox therapy on my shelf, literally within my reach (Metropolitan Hierotheos of Nafpaktos, 2005). I said, "I have this book on Orthodox therapy and wonder if you would like to borrow it for a while?" Josh excitedly said yes and that he

---

[5]Here is also an example where Josh may have internalized consciously or unconsciously the ethic embedded in the therapy we were doing that favored self-esteem, worth, and value over humility.

would bring it back next time. He returned the very next session having read a great deal, and he had even copied some of the pages. As he handed it back to me, he smiled and said, "I am more Orthodox than I knew!" This was an important moment of incorporating a self-state that Josh had not felt fully comfortable incorporating, and in so doing it helped solidify his sense of self.

In a similar way and deeply connected to his SERT tradition, Josh's Armenian self-state was also, at times, difficult to own. In a session in which he was struggling with being Armenian enough, I said, "Josh, I think you sometimes worry that you are not Armenian enough, but I think you are very Armenian," and I pointed out ways that I knew this to be true. He smiled broadly and agreed. These multiple events, among others, can be conceptualized as dramatic dialogues in which our histories and self-states mingled and interacted together allowing us to work through issues in affective and even unformulated ways rather than intellectually figuring something out.

It was the dance of both Josh's Armenian/American, Orthodox/Evangelical self-states and my neo-evangelical/Wesleyan, pastor/therapist self-states that helped Josh begin the process of incorporating his own. Perhaps it was our dialect of difference (Bollas, 2018) that made this even more possible than if I had been an Orthodox therapist, or a conservative evangelical.

From my Christian Wesleyan spiritually integrated psychoanalytic psychotherapy approach I assert that we have been unraveling Josh's internal conflicts, dissociated self-states, and affects in and through the enactments of our dramatic dialogue. Whereas Josh was trained from an early age to accommodate those around him, fearing that he was "not enough of something" or "too much of something else," our relationship not only negated those feelings but also began to help him move confidently into owning those dissociated parts of himself of which he had felt uncertain (i.e., Orthodox and Armenian).

In the language of my SERT tradition, although kind and considerate, Josh's moral affections had not had the chance to be formed into true love of self or others. Pathological accommodation (Brandchaft, 2010) is not genuine other-love, but rather self-preservation as a function of caring for the other. Josh certainly did not love himself, and his accommodation was not a generative kind of other-love but a learned and necessary survival mechanism. He learned to tell people what they wanted to hear and behaved in ways that meet their narcissistic needs. Our psychotherapy, through the immanental work of the Spirit, has become a "means of grace" in which God works to restore Josh's malformed moral affections of self-preservation and accommodation to authentic love of self, other and even God. This "therapeutic aspect" of grace is the sanctifying work of psychotherapy (Strawn, 2004). In the language of Josh's tradition, the therapy is in service of the theological task of theosis—transforming Josh into the image of God. Being aware of my own SERT tradition, Josh's, and those underlying my psychoanalytic theory enabled us to acknowledge, respect, and incorporate Josh's into our work.

While therapy is ongoing, Josh is definitely using his voice more in therapy, with peers, family, and superiors and he seems less apologetic for the "space" he takes in the world. He stands up for himself better, extricates himself from unhealthy relationships faster, and feels more "enough" and less "not enough." This is in part because he is owning his once dissociated self-states, leaning into his Armenian heritage without eschewing his American roots, embracing Orthodoxy while accepting the evangelical influence. It's not always clear to me how much of a source of psychological support his Orthodox faith is, but I do believe his evangelical roots have become less of a hindrance. Anxiety and somatization are still challenging for Josh, but we are attempting to develop a different relationship to these by accepting them, listening to them, and welcoming them as another kind of self-state, there to help us both as we continue this sanctifying work together.

CONCLUSION

This chapter has demonstrated how a spiritually integrated psychotherapy from a Christian Wesleyan perspective might be conceptualized and practiced. I have emphasized the value of the therapist's knowing one's own, the patient's, and even the theory's SERT traditions. My SERT tradition finds great resonance with a contemporary relational psychoanalytic approach which emphasizes the unconscious, transference-countertransference enactments, dramatic dialogue, rupture-repair and mutual recognition, and thirdness. Because of the openness of the Wesleyan perspective, this approach can be used with those from other religious traditions or those with no tradition. By accepting their traditions and being aware of my own, I am better equipped to recognize when my own tradition is influencing my experience and reactions. My SERT tradition not only helps illuminate what is happening theologically in psychotherapy, but is the impetus for what I do. As a follower of Jesus Christ, I understand my therapeutic work as participation with the Spirit in the restoration, reconciliation, and liberation of all of creation, and the establishment of God's peace, or shalom, on earth as it is in heaven.

REFERENCES

American Psychological Association. (2002). *Guidelines on multicultural education, training, research, practice, and organizational change for psychologists.* https://www.apa.org/about/policy/multicultural-guidelines-archived.pdf

Aron, L. (1991). The patient's experience of the analyst's subjectivity. *Psychoanalytic Dialogues, 1*(1), 29–51. https://doi.org/10.1080/10481889109538884

Aron, L. (1996). *A meeting of the minds: Mutuality in psychoanalysis.* Analytic Press.

Atlas, G., & Aron, L. (2018). *Dramatic dialogue: Contemporary clinical practice.* Routledge.

Barsness, R. E., & Strawn, B. D. (2019). Relational psychoanalytic ethics: Professional, personal, theoretical and communal. In R. E. Barsness (Ed.), *Core competencies of relational psychoanalysis: A guide to practice, study and research* (pp. 179–200). Routledge.

Benjamin, J. (2018). *Beyond doer and done to: Recognition theory, intersubjectivity and the third.* Routledge.

Bollas, C. (2018). *Forces of destiny: Psychoanalysis and human idiom.* Routledge. https://doi.org/10.4324/9781315533414

Brandchaft, B. (2010). *Toward an emancipatory psychoanalysis: Brandchaft's intersubjective vision.* Routledge.

Bromberg, P. M. (2001). *Standing in the spaces: Essays on clinical processes trauma and dissociation.* Routledge.

Browning, D. S., & Cooper, T. D. (2004). *Religious thought and the modern psychologies* (2nd ed.). Fortress Press.

Clapp, R. (2004). *Tortured wonders: Christian spirituality for people, not angels.* Brazos Press.

Cozolino, L. (2002). *The neuroscience of psychotherapy: Building and rebuilding the human brain.* Norton.

Crabtree, S. A., Bell, C. A., Rupert, D. A., Sandage, S. J., Devor, N. G., & Stavros, G. (2020). Humility, differentiation of self and clinical training in spiritual and religious competence. *Journal of Spirituality in Mental Health.* https://doi.org/10.1080/19349637.2020.1737627

Cushman, P. (1993). Psychotherapy as moral discourse. *Journal of Theoretical and Philosophical Psychology, 13*(2), 103–113. https://doi.org/10.1037/h0091120

Cushman, P. (1995). *Constructing the self, constructing America: A cultural history of psychotherapy.* Addison Wesley.

Damasio, A. (2005). *Descartes' error: Emotion, reason, and the human brain.* Penguin.

Fiske, A. P., Kitayama, S., Markus, H. R., & Nisbett, R. E. (1998). The cultural matrix of social psychology. In D. T. Gilbert, S. T. Fiske, & G. Lindzey (Eds.), *The handbook of social psychology* (4th ed., Vol. 2, pp. 915–981). McGraw-Hill Co.

Ghent, E. (1990). Masochism, submission, surrender: Masochism as a perversion of surrender. *Contemporary Psychoanalysis, 26*(1), 108–136.

Greenberg, J. R. (1986). Theoretical models and the analyst's neutrality. *Contemporary Psychoanalysis, 22*(1), 87–106. https://doi.org/10.1080/00107530.1986.10746117

Gunter, W. S., Jones, S. J., Campbell, T. A., Miles, R. L., & Maddox, R. L. (1997). *Wesley and the quadrilateral: Renewing the conversation.* Abingdon.

Hoffman, I. Z. (1983). The patient as interpreter of the analyst's experience. *Contemporary Psychoanalysis, 19*(3), 389–422. https://doi.org/10.1080/00107530.1983.10746615

Hoffman, M. T. (2011). *Toward mutual recognition: Relational psychoanalysis and the Christian narrative.* Routledge. https://doi.org/10.4324/9780203881279

Labberton, M. (2018). Introduction: Still evangelical? In M. Labberton (Ed.), *Still evangelical? Insiders reconsider political, social and theological meaning.* InterVarsity Press.

Lodahl, M. (2003). *God of nature and grace: Reading the world in a Wesleyan way.* Kingswood Books.

Maddox, R. L. (1994). *Responsible grace: John Wesley's practical theology*. Kingswood Press.

Maddox, R. L. (2004). Psychology and Wesleyan theology: Precedents and prospects for a renewed engagement. *Journal of Psychology and Christianity, 23*(2), 101–109.

Malony, H. N. (2010). John Wesley, John Calvin, and Martin Luther: An unholy triumvirate of import for psychology. In L. Hoffman (Ed.), *Toward a Christian clinical psychology: The contributions of H. Newton Malony* (pp. 92–103). Fuller Seminary Press.

McWilliams, N. (2004). *Psychoanalytic psychotherapy: A practitioner's guide*. Guilford Press.

Metropolitan Hierotheos of Nafpaktos. (2005). *Orthodox psychotherapy: The science of the fathers*. Birth of the Theotokos Seminary.

Morgan, J., & Sandage, S. J. (2016). A developmental model of interreligious competence: A conceptual framework. *Archive for the Psychology of Religion, 38*(2), 129–158. https://doi.org/10.1163/15736121-12341325

Oord, T. J. (2019). *God can't: How to believe in God and love after tragedy, abuse, or other evils*. SacraSage Press.

Pargament, K. I. (2007). *Spiritually integrated psychotherapy: Understanding and addressing the sacred*. Guilford Press.

Renik, O. (1993). Analytic interaction: Conceptualizing technique in light of the analyst's irreducible subjectivity. *The Psychoanalytic Quarterly, 62*(4), 553–571. https://doi.org/10.1080/21674086.1993.11927393

Rupert, D., Moon, S. H., & Sandage, S. J. (2019). Clinical training groups for spirituality and religion in psychotherapy. *Journal of Spirituality in Mental Health, 21*(3), 163–177. https://doi.org/10.1080/19349637.2018.1465879

Safran, J. D., & Muran, J. C. (2000). *Negotiating the therapeutic alliance: A relational treatment guide*. Guilford Press.

Scalise, C. J. (2015). What does Fuller mean by "Evangelical"? *Fuller, 2015*(2), 44–47. https://fullerstudio.fuller.edu/fuller-mean-evangelical/

Schore, A. N. (2015). *Affect regulation and the origin of the self*. Routledge. https://doi.org/10.4324/9781315680019

Sorenson, R. L. (2004). *Minding spirituality*. Analytic Press.

Stone, B. P., & Oord, T. J. (2001). *Thy nature and they name is love: Wesleyan and process theologies in dialogue*. Kingswood Books.

Strawn, B. D. (2004). Restoring moral affections of heart: How does psychotherapy heal? *Journal of Psychology and Christianity, 23*(2), 140–148.

Strawn, B. D. (2020). Clinical integrative practice (CIP). *Journal of Psychology and Theology, 48*(4), 237–238. https://doi.org/10.1177/0091647120956964

Strawn, B. D., Wright, R. W., & Jones, P. (2014). Tradition-based integration: Illuminating the stories and practices that shape our integrative imaginations. *Journal of Psychology and Christianity, 33*(4), 300–310.

Vande Kemp, H. (1984). *Psychology and theology in Western thought, 1672–1965: A historical and annotated bibliography*. Kraus International Publications.

Vitz, P. C. (1977). *Psychology as religion: The cult of self-worship*. Eerdmans.

Wilson, T. D. (2002). *Strangers to ourselves: Discovering the adaptive unconscious*. Belknap Harvard.

Wright, R., Jones, P., & Strawn, B. D. (2014). Tradition-based integration. In E. D. Bland & B. D. Strawn (Eds.), *Christianity & psychoanalysis: A new conversation*. InterVarsity Press.

Wynkoop, M. B. (1972). *Foundations of Wesleyan-Arminian theology*. Beacon Hill Press.

Wynkoop, M. B. (2015). *A theology of love: The dynamic of Wesleyanism* (2nd ed.). Beacon Hill Press.

7

RAISING THE SPARKS

Psychotherapeutic Process as Tikkun Olam

KAREN E. STARR

The subject matter of this chapter combines two of my deep interests: Judaism, in particular, the Jewish mystical tradition, or *Kabbalah*, and psychoanalysis, in particular, the relational tradition. Although on the surface these two disciplines seem very different, both have in common a concern with personal transformation. Each places great value on the individual's effort to know the self more deeply. In this chapter, I offer a perspective on psychoanalysis and psychotherapy (I use these terms interchangeably) as seen through a kabbalistic lens. Viewed from the standpoint of modern psychology, kabbalistic formulations may be understood as an attempt to express psychological concepts that did not yet exist. But by embedding the search for the self in the larger context of the individual's relationship to the universal, the kabbalists gave expression to a spiritual and moral basis for an endeavor that in modern times, in the form of psychoanalysis, has been criticized for its focus on the individual to the exclusion of their relation to the larger whole.

Some of the material in this chapter has been adapted from my book, *Repair of the Soul: Metaphors of Transformation in Jewish Mysticism and Psychoanalysis* (Starr, 2008b).

https://doi.org/10.1037/0000276-008
Spiritual Diversity in Psychotherapy: Engaging the Sacred in Clinical Practice,
S. J. Sandage and B. D. Strawn (Editors)

The kabbalistic goal of *tikkun olam*, repair of the world, has been taken on by many Jewish organizations as a challenge to effect social change by adding a spiritual dimension to movements such as the environmental movement and the movement for social, economic, and political justice. Here, I propose that the notion of tikkun applies as well to the psychotherapeutic endeavor—that the therapist's aim of healing the individual is inexorably linked with the desire to make the world a better place by doing so.

In offering this spiritually inflected framework for thinking about psychotherapy process, I want to emphasize that I hold these metaphors lightly. In other words, while the spiritual dimension of the work I do with patients is meaningful to me personally and, at times, informs how I conceptualize my own engagement with the psychoanalytic task, it operates in the background rather than in the foreground of my clinical work. It is very rare that I draw upon any of these metaphors explicitly with patients, whether they are Jewish or not. But, especially with patients who are suffering a spiritual or moral crisis or a crisis of identity, whether they adhere to a particular religious belief or to none at all, I have found these metaphors useful as I think about what we are both trying to do together. At the end of this chapter, I offer a clinical vignette of my treatment with a patient who was raised Catholic and who identified as atheist, but whose struggles to find meaning and purpose in his life, I believe, are relevant to the spiritual dimension of the psychotherapeutic endeavor that I am attempting to articulate here.

In my approach to a spiritually inclusive psychoanalysis, I do not propose that psychoanalytic formulations be discarded in favor of spiritual metaphors, nor do I wish to explain away spiritual experience in psychoanalytic terms. Rather, I suggest that in playing with the possibilities created by opening a dialogue between them, we can gain a more expansive perspective of the therapeutic undertaking. Hasidic master Rabbi Nachman of Bratzlav said, "In working with people to bring them to themselves, one must work at great depth, a depth scarcely imaginable" (Schachter & Hoffman, 1983, p. 13). I believe these are apt words to describe both the kabbalistic and psychoanalytic endeavors.

> I begin by offering a brief overview of some of the psychoanalytic theorists who have influenced my thinking in this area. I provide some historical background on Kabbalah, and then explain in detail some of the kabbalistic metaphors, tying them in with psychoanalytic concepts. I offer brief vignettes drawn from the Torah, kabbalistic commentary, and my own clinical practice. The ideas presented in this chapter are just a brief overview of a complex body of scholarship in Jewish studies and psychoanalysis. These concepts are elaborated in greater depth in my book, *Repair of the Soul: Metaphors of Transformation in Jewish Mysticism and Psychoanalysis* (Starr, 2008b).

THEORETICAL ORIENTATION

While I have been trained in both cognitive behavioral and psychoanalytic approaches, my preferred orientation is psychoanalytic. Psychoanalysis provides me with an exquisitely rich and nuanced framework with which to consider the myriad of factors that shape human experience. I believe in the power of the unconscious, or that which is outside our awareness, and that it needs to be taken into account in attempting to both understand and to change human behavior. In particular, I am drawn to the relational psychoanalytic paradigm as the framework with which to conceptualize experience. The relational umbrella is a wide one—it includes ideas from self-psychology, interpersonal theory, and object relations, all of which presume that human beings develop in a matrix of relationships that shape our experience of ourselves and the world we live in.

The paradigm shift in contemporary psychoanalysis from a one-person to a two-person psychology has been accompanied by a greater emphasis on the mutative role of the analytic relationship as a facilitator of psychic change. In this two-person paradigm, one of the important goals of analysis is the creation of an environment of emotional intimacy that potentiates the emergence of a deeply personal sense of authenticity. Rather than viewing the analyst as objective observer, blank slate, or reflecting mirror (a one-person psychology), the relational paradigm (a two-person psychology) acknowledges that the analytic process affects both participants in the dyad, the analyst as well as the patient. It views the relationship between analyst and analysand as mutual, yet asymmetrical (Aron, 1996).

One aspect of the contemporary relational psychoanalytic paradigm that appeals to me is that it has promoted healthy debate within psychoanalysis about theory and technique. I have written elsewhere about the suitability of relational psychoanalysis for integration with other forms of psychotherapy that have traditionally been considered "nonanalytic" (Bresler & Starr, 2015). The contemporary relational framework, with its interest in attachment theory, infant research, embodied experience, dynamic systems theory, cognitive science, and neuroscience, makes possible a more open dialogue with therapeutic approaches that have traditionally remained outside the psychoanalytic sphere than was feasible within the more inward-focused classical psychoanalytic framework. Further, and relevant to theme of this book, because it has reenvisioned fantasy and illusion as essential to living a life of creativity, vitality, and meaning, I believe relational psychoanalysis is also particularly well suited for a conversation with religion and spirituality.

While Freud (1927/1968) famously referred to religion as a "mass delusion" (p. 85), contemporary psychoanalytic scholarship has been more attuned to humanity's spiritual and aesthetic yearnings. (For a thorough investigation of Freud's relationship to Judaism, his own Jewish identity, and its impact on the development of psychoanalysis, see Aron & Starr, 2013.) This shift can be traced to Winnicott's (1967) ideas about transitional space and transitional experiencing, in which Winnicott reframed illusion as a way for human beings to *relate* to reality, rather than as an evasion of reality that should be avoided. For Winnicott, artistic creativity and religious feeling were both manifestations of transitional experiencing, characterized by the growth-enhancing ability to enter into shared illusions, to relate inner and outer reality. He viewed the capacity for illusion as a necessary step toward emotional maturity and relationship with others, and as a potential source of truth linked with creativity and insight. Winnicott extended the idea of transitional space to include the analytic situation, in which the analytic hour is used as a potential space for entering into collaborative exchange.

Following Winnicott, psychoanalyst Emmanuel Ghent (1990) linked the transformative possibilities of religion and psychoanalysis, referring to a "longing for surrender" of what Winnicott called the false self for the sake of authenticity, "the discovery of one's identity, one's sense of self, one's sense of wholeness, even one's sense of unity with other living beings" (p. 111). In Ghent's (1990) view, the sense of unity is an emotional achievement, recognition of what we have in common as human beings. Transformative rather than informational, *being* rather than *knowing*, surrender results in a feeling of spontaneity and aliveness, openness to experience, and the enhanced ability to relate to others from a position of authenticity.

Hans Loewald considered himself an interpreter of Freudian theory, but his exegesis can be considered a radical one, mystical in its implications, even while cloaked in orthodoxy. Loewald (1978) translated Freud's "Wo Es war, soll Ich werden," as "where id was," there shall "ego *come into being*" [emphasis added] (p. 497), contending that psychic transformation is a matter of the ego's renewal by the dynamic unconscious. Loewald believed that the interplay between the dynamic unconscious and the ego, a reciprocal shaping of different levels of mentation, is what makes human life human. Irrational forces have the potential to enrich and transform the rational. Loewald (1988) used the term *conscire* (p. 49), knowing together, to describe the intersection of unconscious with conscious knowing, explicitly connecting this form of knowing with mysticism. Loewald's (1980) vision of a rich human life, and by extension, a successful analytic outcome, is like Winnicott's—a sense of aliveness and openness to experience without which the human condition would be desolate.

Psychoanalyst Wilfred Bion (1977a, 1977b) steeped himself in the Eastern mystical traditions. Aware that his views would disturb the psychoanalytic establishment, he questioned the notion that science is limited to objective discovery. Bion insisted that psychoanalysis, mysticism, and scientific discovery all had in common the seeker's "at-one-ment" with ultimate reality or absolute truth, the truth of an object that could never be known but whose presence could be intuited.

For Bion, at the heart of the question of what is transformative in psychoanalytic process is the enigma of how the patient moves from insight to change, from intellectual understanding to a newly felt way of being. Bion (1977b) phrased the problem as "how to pass from 'knowing' 'phenomena' to 'being' that which is 'real'" (p. 148). He conceived of the sign "O" to designate absolute truth and ultimate reality, encompassing both good and evil—from a mathematical vertex, the infinite, and from a religious vertex, the Godhead. For Bion, transformation involves "being" rather than "knowing" and entails "being in O," at one with the truth of the psychoanalytic session. In Bion's framework, ridding oneself of memory and desire makes possible the awareness of phenomena that are evolutions of O. Bion offered no rules for interpretation, only rules for the analyst to help him "achieve the frame of mind in which he is receptive to O of the analytic experience." (Bion, 1977a, p. 32) For Bion, being receptive to O requires an act of faith.

In the beginning, Freud championed positivism, rationality, and objective discovery as the foundations of psychoanalytic knowledge. Later theorists felt it necessary to find a place for the nonrational in formulations that attempted to explain the mystery of psychic enlargement and renewal. The creation of a space within psychoanalytic theory for an appreciation of the transformative possibilities of aesthetic and creative experiencing, and for intuition as a source of truth, makes the boundary between religion and psychoanalysis a more permeable one, allowing for a potentially fruitful collaborative exchange.

Stephen Mitchell (2000), a founder of relational psychoanalysis, highlighted the significance of Loewald's theoretical contributions in radically transforming the basic values that guide the psychoanalytic undertaking. Meaning, imagination, and aliveness are now at the heart of the psychoanalytic enterprise. Rather than the triumph of the rational over the irrational, the goal of the analytic project becomes the ability to move fluidly from one realm of experience to the other.

Drawing upon Loewald's vision of mind as embedded, from the beginning, in an interactive field with other minds, and further developing from these interactions, Mitchell (2000) proposed a system of mutual influence between the individual and the larger relational matrix, in which each, the microcosm and the macrocosm, shape and transform one another:

> In the beginning . . . is the relational . . . matrix in which we discover ourselves. . . . Within that matrix are formed . . . individual psyches with subjectively experienced interior spaces. Those subjective spaces begin as microcosms of the relational field, in which macrocosmic interpersonal relationships are internalized and transformed into a distinctly personal experience; and those personal experiences are, in turn, regulated and transformed, generating newly emergent properties, which in turn create new interpersonal forms that alter macrocosmic patterns of interaction. (p. 57)

I believe that Mitchell (2000) is expressing here in psychological terms what the kabbalists articulated on the spiritual plane, projecting their vision further outward into the cosmos: namely, that there exists a relationship of reciprocal influence between the microcosm and the macrocosm, between the individual and the larger whole of which she is an inextricable part. Further, as Mitchell suggested, and as the kabbalists intuited in their development of their theosophical and sefirotic (attributes/emanations of the manifestation of God) systems, there exist modes of organization that vary according to degrees of articulation of spatial, temporal, and perceptual boundaries. The specific world of reality that we perceive in our everyday lives is the result of an infinitely complex interaction, back and forth among these different dimensions of being. Although one may feature more prominently in the foreground of conscious awareness at any given time, they each exist, and continue to operate, in dialectical and dynamic relationship to one another. In both psychoanalytic and kabbalistic formulations of transformation, living a life of vitality and meaning requires moving fluidly among these varying domains of experience, cultivating the life-sustaining channels of mutual influence between the primal dense unity of being and the demarcated boundaries of individual existence.

SPIRITUAL TRADITION

My father came from a secular Jewish family, my mother from an Orthodox Jewish one. Although we were not strictly observant, we kept a kosher home, my mother lit Shabbat candles every Friday night, and we celebrated the Jewish holidays. As a child, I attended an Orthodox Jewish day school where I spent half my school day studying Jewish texts and the commentaries on those texts. I became absorbed in the Hebrew language, fascinated by the shape of its letters and the roots and meanings of its words. I was intrigued by the rabbinic method of interpretation—the use of association and word play to expand upon the simple, more obvious explanations of the text, and to find deeper meanings. Even then, I was awed by the multiplicity of meanings made possible through interpretation. Later, I experienced this same sense of awe studying literary criticism at Barnard, learning how to take apart a text to expose its many possible truths, to find the meaning that resonated with me, and to own and respect that resonance. I bring this experience and love of language to my own work as a writer, a vocation I've pursued since childhood. Most importantly, I've carried through from childhood the faith in the ability of language to capture experience, and a belief that in the expression of that experience through language, both writer and reader are transformed. This belief carries through to my clinical work, in which I have experienced first-hand the transformational power of the right words at the right time.

The question "Where is my place in the world?" is one that has pursued me since childhood. Despite the traditional rabbinic warning against studying Kabbalah unless one is over 40, married, and male, I began exploring it in my 20s. I was drawn to the idea of a meaning beyond me that might offer me a greater perspective on my own life, however, I found the Kabbalah to be elusive and incomprehensible. After reaching the age of 40, I took it up again, and aided by a flurry of new scholarship on Kabbalah (Drob, 2000a, 2000b; Green, 2004; Idel, 2002; Matt, 2004a, 2004b, 2006; among others) discovered that I was better able to begin to grasp some of its more compelling concepts without getting a headache.

The writings of the Kabbalah can be frustrating to read from a rational point of view. The texts are often ambiguous, fragmented, and extremely metaphorical. It's easy to lose your way. However, it's precisely this ambiguity that opens them to interpretation and makes possible a renewed relevance to modern life. As they move between clarity and obscurity, they mirror the human psychological experience of insight and perplexity. The characters of the Kabbalah make heavy use of elaborate metaphor.[1] The nature of metaphor, indeed its beauty, is that it hints at truths that are not easily accessible through rational language. Metaphor holds the key to unlocking meaning. The unlocking of meaning is also at the heart, and is the art, of the psychoanalytic endeavor.

---

[1]For example, the Kabbalah depicts the Torah as a living, divine, feminine presence, participating in a mutually enlivening and enhancing relationship with those who study her. The relationship between text and interpreter is portrayed as a relationship between two subjects who are each transformed by the encounter (Green, 2004). There are resonances here with the contemporary relational psychoanalytic view of the mutuality of the analytic relationship.

The problem of transformation is a compelling one. As clinicians, we often hear from our patients, "I *know* this intellectually, but I don't *feel* it. What do I have to *do* in order to change?" As patients, many of us have likely asked our own therapists this very same question. How do people change? Freud wrote of the arduous task of working through, of the need for the analyst to be patient, and to allow the process to take its course. Bion wrote of the need to remain in mystery and doubt, to be open to experience, to *being*, rather than *knowing*. Contemporary relational psychoanalytic models maintain that it's the *relationship* between patient and analyst, the collaborative striving for understanding in the context of a relationship of mutual recognition and connection that facilitates change. I believe that all these are true, and that they imply a stance of faith.

To be clear—in my use of the word "faith," I am not referring to religious faith or belief in God as an omnipotent being directing the course of natural events. Rather, the faith I'm referring to is an inner orientation toward unfolding potential, the attempt to live one's life with meaning and purpose. In the context of self-transformation, including in the psychoanalytic endeavor, faith is a stance characterized by a willingness, for the sake of discovering one's emotional truth, to face that truth in all of its aspects: to plunge fully into doubt and uncertainty, to be open to what emerges, and thereby engage in an ongoing creative process of being and becoming.

The Hasidim refer to the necessity, when confronted with doubt, of leaping into the abyss and standing in faith. From a psychoanalytic perspective, entering the abyss can be read as feeling what one has been avoiding, accepting responsibility for one's life in its totality, and perhaps the hardest thing of all, giving up the idea that one *has to know what will happen next*. In the kabbalistic formulation this means attaining, at least for a moment, the attribute of *chachma*, wisdom, in which one lives in the potential of what is and waits for what will come and what will be.

The abyss of which the Hasidim speak is a mode of experience alluded to by mystics and poets, as well as psychoanalysts. The Kabbalah conceptualizes it as *ayin*, *no-thing*, the emptiness from which being emerges; the Zen masters as the "don't know mind" (Epstein, 1995, p. 36); and T. S. Eliot (1968) as "the still point of the turning world" (p. 3). Psychoanalytic thinkers call for maintaining "the tension between the need for discovery and the need for closure" (Ghent, 1992, p. 155), and for remaining in the "nothingness which resides between the poles of paradoxical opposites" (Kumin, 1978, p. 482). Faith requires us to embody paradox. It impels us to tolerate uncertainty, to venture beyond what is known into the void of the unknown; and at the same time, to experience the stillness of the present moment and to accept its truth. This is not an easy task. There is an active, animating quality to my formulation of faith. It comprises both a receptive attentiveness to what Ghent (1990) calls the "passionate longing to surrender" (p. 115) and also an enflaming commitment and dedication to its realization. Analyst Michael Eigen (1981), quoting the *Sh'ma* ("Listen"), the ancient prayer that is the centerpiece of Jewish liturgy, called it "a way of experiencing which is undertaken with one's whole being, all out, 'with all one's heart, with all one's soul, and with all one's might'" (p. 413). Faith is our way of leaning into life.

I have taken Rilke's (1934) words to a young poet to heart, to

> be patient toward all that is unsolved in your heart and . . . try to love the questions themselves like locked rooms and like books that are written in a very foreign tongue. . . . And the point is, to live everything. Live the questions now. Perhaps you will then gradually, without noticing it, live along some distant day into the answer. (p. 35)

My interest in both psychoanalytic process and Jewish mystical thought springs from this love for the questions themselves. This scholarship is my way of living the answers into being.

Kabbalah

Kabbalah is an ancient term coined over 800 years ago to describe the Jewish mystical tradition. Passed down orally from teacher to student, the knowledge contained within Kabbalah was originally kept hidden from all but a very select few individuals deemed worthy of receiving it. The word Kabbalah itself means "received" and/or "tradition," reflecting the care that was taken to keep it secret and rooted in *halacha*, Jewish law and religious practice.

The original flowering of Kabbalah began during the Middle Ages, a period of fear and uncertainty for medieval Jewry. Faced with threats against their minority religion from Christian and Muslim authorities, the Jews were forced to constantly defend their traditions, which were also being challenged by new intellectual ideas such as Neoplatonism and Aristotelianism. They met these challenges by re-interpreting traditional Jewish teachings to incorporate these new ways of thinking. The form this re-interpretation took was the commentary, a legacy of the Talmudic age. The Talmud, or body of Jewish law, is itself a commentary on the Torah. (For a clear introduction to the Kabbalah and its central text, the Zohar, see Green, 2004.)

The Kabbalah is a highly creative commentary, rooted in traditional Judaism. Its creative exegesis is a mystical interpretation of biblical and rabbinic literature that tackles the big questions: How and why was the world created? How does the universe work? What is evil and why does it exist? (to name just a few). The kabbalists viewed language as the medium through which the world was created, considering the letters of the Hebrew alphabet to be the building blocks of the universe. To them, language was a reflection of the fundamental, spiritual nature of the world, a window into the soul of the human and the divine. The kabbalists raised the interpretive process to new heights of creativity, believing that they could derive unifying, cosmic structures from the words of the Torah. In fact, the Torah itself was believed to be the divine in word, a linguistic manifestation of God. The Torah was conceived as a living organism, containing within it an infinity of meanings (Scholem, 1969).

Most strikingly, the kabbalists vividly articulated the radical view of a mutual relationship between the human being and God as partners in creative process. By introducing the notion of tikkun olam, repair of the world, which emphasizes the unique contribution of the individual to the larger whole, they infused meaning and purpose into acts of traditional Jewish practice, which had become dry and overly intellectualized. The kabbalists developed a psychological system based on the concept that the microcosm mirrors the macrocosm. They interpreted the biblical passage in Genesis (1:27), stating that God made the human being in God's image, to mean that the creative and transformational processes of the cosmos are reflected in, and are affected by, those of the human psyche. In other words, the kabbalists sought to know God through knowing themselves—they believed that God is found not in Heaven, but by looking inward into the soul. Even more controversially—the kabbalists believed that through the individual's effort to know the self more deeply and to be transformed, God Himself is transformed (Green, 2004).

What follows next is an abbreviated version of the Kabbalah's metaphor of Creation, which is the basis for the concept of tikkun olam. In the 16th century, Rabbi Isaac Luria proposed that the infinite God began the process of creation by contracting, thereby forming a void expectant with potential. Into this potential space, God revealed Himself through the emanation of the ten divine attributes or *sefirot*, dynamic potentials that permeate all planes of existence, including the human psyche. In Luria's metaphor, the sefirot were envisioned as vessels, or containers for the divine light. The vessels were not strong enough to contain the light, and so they shattered. As the shards of the vessels fell, they entrapped sparks of light in their shells. Some of the light returned to its source, beginning the process of tikkun olam. The process of tikkun continues through the restoration of the remaining light, trapped in the shards, to its source. Most strikingly, only the actions of the human being, informed by intentionality, can continue the process of tikkun. It is through human acts that the light is restored, the shattered fragments reorganized into wholeness, and repair of the world made possible. In this framework, which is quite radical for a theosophical system, God and humanity are partners in an ongoing creative-reparative process (Scholem, 1995).

The Zohar,[2] the central text of the Kabbalah, describes "a spark of impenetrable darkness" flashing within the Infinite. Historian Gershom Scholem (1995) called this the "crisis" that spurs God to creation. What precipitated this crisis? Quite remarkably, the Zohar characterizes God's motivation for Creation as His longing for recognition by and connection with humanity— God's desire to enter into relationship with His own creation. In turn, the individual draws nearer to God in relationship through his efforts to perceive the divine spark clothed within his own soul. This interplay of seeking-out-connection and mutual recognition is said to sustain the world, whose very existence depends on the open channels of influence between the human being and the divine. Psychoanalyst Emmanuel Ghent (1990) proposed the existence in the human being of "a 'force' toward growth," linking it to the "longing to be known," to be recognized by an other (p. 110). The Zohar explicitly identifies this "'force' toward growth" as the creative energy that animates all being, locating its source in God's burning desire to be known— to be sought out and recognized by humanity.

The moment of creation, the turning point of God's transformation, is conceived as passage through ayin, no-thing. No-thingness is a moment on the brink, the liminal juncture between the unknowable and the perceivable; it is identified by the Kabbalah as the point of faith. Thus the startling conclusion is that God's bringing the world into *being* from the state of *no-thing* is, in essence, a divine leap of faith! Applying this formulation to the workings of the human psyche, the Kabbalah characterizes faith as a moment on the threshold, a instant of pure receptivity where potential becomes manifest. It is experienced as a flash of wordless intuition that seeks articulation. Faith emerges in consciousness as a sense of truth that is

---

[2]The Zohar, written in Hebrew and Aramaic, was "discovered" in Spain in 1286 by Moses de Leon, who attributed its authorship to Shimon Bar Yohai, a 2nd-century rabbi. However, modern scholars believe that the author was de Leon himself. Essentially a commentary on the five books of Moses, the Zohar contains discourses on the process of creation, the nature of good and evil, the composition of the human soul, and the attributes of God. It is an enigmatic text, written in a highly esoteric manner. Therefore, rather than offering direct citations of the Zohar text, for the most part, I have provided references to the works of contemporary Kabbalah scholars who have explicated the text. For readers interested in undertaking the challenge of reading the Zohar itself, Daniel Matt (2004a, 2004b, 2006) has written an excellent English translation, which I also refer to here.

beyond reason—at the threshold of perception, we cannot yet define it or explain why we feel it is true. (See Starr, 2008a for a more detailed examination of the role of faith in psychic change.)

Transformation

Although the Kabbalah and psychoanalysis originate from very different perspectives, each gives deep consideration to the human potential for transformation in the context of relationship. For Freud, who considered himself to be a scientist making objective scientific observations, psychic change was quantitative. The goal of analysis was to overcome the irrational forces of the unconscious, to strengthen the ego to better equip the individual to cope with reality.

Yet long before Freud, transformation has been associated, in a more qualitative sense, with religious experience. Individuals are said to be transformed by their encounter with the divine. They emerge with a profound awareness of being only one small part of a greater reality, a more expansive perspective of life's possibilities, and a clearer intuition of their own unique purpose. In the Torah, such a transformation is often marked by a change in name. At the moment of entering into relationship with God through His covenant, Abram becomes Abraham (Genesis 17:5) and his wife Sarai, Sarah (Genesis 17:15–16), signifying that the elderly, childless couple will be patriarchs of a great nation.

The night before he is to meet with his estranged and presumably hostile brother Esau, Jacob wrestles with a mysterious figure until dawn (Genesis 32:22–32). From the narrative, it is never clear whether the mysterious figure is a man, angel, God, or an aspect of Jacob himself; the text is ambiguous and open to interpretation. Jacob's conflict does not leave him unscathed, but it does leave him richer for the experience. Jacob emerges from his encounter with a wound in his thigh and a life-long limp, but also with an expanded perception of himself and his relationship with his brother. He is given the name Israel—"wrestles with God"—to mark the struggle as well as the suffering that is the turning point of his transformation.

Jacob's new name also signifies the manner in which he has changed. When we are first introduced to Jacob, he is characterized as a simple man, a tent-dweller, a man who, at the moment of his birth, grabbed on to the heel of his twin brother Esau, and then in later years stole his brother's birthright through deceiving his elderly, blind father. His name, Yaakov in Hebrew, has as its root the word "heel"; the Zohar interprets its meaning as "deceiver" (Matt, 2004b, p. 270). Because of his treachery, Jacob lived in fear of being killed by Esau, who was much stronger and more aggressive than he. But on this day, Jacob set out to meet his brother face to face, not knowing what the outcome would be—whether he would live or die. The name Israel signifies an added dimension to Jacob's identity, encompassing a newfound willingness to come to terms with his prior actions, to grapple with their consequences, and to tolerate the unknown of a new way of relating. He is different, somehow larger, than he was before. Interestingly, it is the agent of Jacob's transformation, the mysterious figure who struggles with him, who gives Jacob the name Israel. By naming him, he helps Jacob to grasp the emotional essence of what he has just gone through and to understand that he has been changed by it.

In turn, Jacob puts words to his ineffable experience by giving the scene of his transformation a name. He calls the place Peniel—"I have seen God face to face." By naming it, he acknowledges the revelatory nature of his experience and seeks its affirmation through linking his changed inner reality to the concrete outer reality of place. In psychoanalytic terms, naming is Jacob's way of processing an experience that was most certainly traumatic—painful, but also numinous—putting his experience into words helps him not only to understand it but also to assign it a transformative meaning, enabling him to go forth a changed person. Through his struggle, Jacob has come face to face with God and, in the process, face to face with a heretofore-unexpressed aspect of himself. Or perhaps it is the reverse, through Jacob's knowing himself more deeply, God is revealed.

THE TRANSFORMATIONAL ENCOUNTER–A KABBALISTIC EXAMPLE

In Genesis (12:1), God commands Abraham, *"Lech lecha."* These two words of biblical Hebrew are traditionally translated as "Go forth." The plain, or simple interpretation of this passage (in the biblical exegetical framework, this mode of interpretation would be called the *p'shat*; in psychoanalytic terms we might refer to this layer of meaning as manifest content) is that Abraham is being called by God to "go forth" and journey to a new place—to leave his home, the place of his birth, the house of his father, and to travel to a land that God will show him. If we rely only on the simple interpretation of the biblical narrative, Abraham's journey can be characterized as exemplifying transformation through change of place. However, the Zohar offers another, deeper layer of meaning (in the biblical exegetical framework, this type of interpretation would be referred to as *sod*, "secret" or "hidden";

in psychoanalytic terms we might think of it as latent meaning) of this same passage. It interprets the phrase *"Lech lecha"* hyperliterally, as "Go to yourself, to know yourself, to refine yourself" (Matt, 2004a, p. 9). Like a psychoanalyst attuned to her patient's narrative with her "third ear" (Reik, 1948), the Zohar is keenly attentive to the allusions of hidden meaning suggested by the words in the text. The Zohar casts God's directive as a call for Abraham to embark on a process of inward reflection that will ultimately lead to an experience of transformation and growth. God is urging Abraham to leave behind that which is familiar to him so that he may journey toward a new paradigm of being.

The Zohar's commentary on this passage explains, "Every person must search and discover the root of his soul so he can fulfill it and restore it to its source, its essence. The more one fulfills himself, the closer he approaches his authentic self" (Matt, 2004a, p. 9). This explanation suggests that transformation is a matter not only of leaving the familiar for the new, but of return or turning toward.[3] The Kabbalah equates the human desire for transformation with the soul's yearning to return to its source in God. But unlike mystical traditions such as Buddhism, transformation is not a matter of negating the self (Epstein, 1995); rather, it involves the soul's fulfillment, via the authentic experience of self.

The Kabbalah views transformation as a two-party process—a responsive interplay between the human being and God. The desire for transformation is not a one-way street but a mutual longing between two subjects. Says the Zohar, "Once one has aroused arousal, then arousal above is aroused" (Matt, 2004a, p. 7). The meaning of this obscurely phrased commentary is that God is not calling to Abraham from "out of the blue," as it would appear from the simple translation of the Torah text. Instead, God's longing ("arousal above") has been stirred by Abraham's internal awakening ("arousal"). In the kabbalistic formulation, God's directive to Abraham to "go to yourself; know yourself" is given in *response* to Abraham's internally felt imperative for personal transformation. In fact, it seems God has been waiting for this very moment.

The Kabbalah speaks of the divine spark clothed within a person's soul, longing to be perceived and enflamed, but veiled from conscious awareness. From a psychoanalytic perspective, the divine spark is evocative of Winnicott's (1964) "vital spark . . . this urge towards life and growth" (p. 27), which is cultivated in the emotional intimacy of the analytic relationship. While the psychoanalytic literature has engaged extensively with the subject

---

[3]Notably, the Hebrew word for transformation via repentance (or turning toward God) is *teshuvah*, which means "return," "turning toward," and "response."

of authenticity in terms of the individuality or multiplicity of the self, the Kabbalah offers us a unique perspective. It formulates authenticity not in terms of a static core self, nor in terms of the genuineness of a person in a given interaction, but as the *unique creative potential of that person and no other* as expressed across space and time. As potential, it can be made manifest only by being lived out in material reality through the individual's actions and interactions with others in her daily life. In the kabbalistic formulation, the divine spark is an aspect of God that can only be articulated by a human being in the material world. Hence living out one's authenticity in a life of meaning and purpose has both personal and cosmic implications; it is a singular manifestation of God that can find expression exclusively in the life of that person, and no other.

The journey toward self-understanding and self-realization is conceptualized as tikkun, repair, the process by which the particular spark unique to one's soul is restored to its source, bringing God Himself into balance! Conceived as the movement toward God in relationship, tikkun is the individual's specific and indispensable contribution to creation, and thus necessary to sustaining the world. The experience of at-one-ment with one's divine spark—coming into contact with the truth of one's soul—is not a static achievement, but an ephemeral moment that may recur throughout a lifetime, resulting in ever-deepening levels of awareness. It is conceived as meeting with God in the area of faith.

IMPLICATIONS FOR THE PSYCHOTHERAPEUTIC PROCESS

Bronheim (1994) noted that according to Jewish mystical tradition, the honest examination of the truth about one's self in the context of relationship is the leap of faith, the movement toward God.[4] It is what compels Adam, after he has eaten from the Tree of Knowledge and attempted to hide himself from God, to respond to God's question "Where are you?" by giving an honest account of his existential position—"I was afraid and I hid myself." In psychoanalysis we too, continually ask our patients, "Where are you?" encouraging them to reveal themselves, to expose their most intimate

---

[4]The material in this section is excerpted from the article "Faith as the Fulcrum of Psychic Change" (Starr, 2008a), originally published in *Psychoanalytic Dialogues*, and later in *Repair of the Soul: Metaphors of Transformation in Jewish Mysticism and Psychoanalysis* (Starr, 2008b, pp. 73–75). It is reprinted with the publisher's permission.

fears and feelings of shame when they admit "I was afraid and I was hiding" (Bronheim, 1994, p. 682). The analytic relationship of seeking out and finding, of being sought out and found, nurtures the emergence in the patient of a sense of identity and purpose. As she makes herself known and feels herself seen, she gradually formulates a meaningful answer to the question of where she is in the world.

Psychoanalysis has long grappled with the notion of the true self and how it may be nurtured within the psychoanalytic relationship. For Winnicott (1965), the true self is visible in the infant's spontaneous gesture and unfolds in relationship with its mother. Drawing upon Loewald (1960), Greenberg (1996) wrote that it is developed within the context of a deep and profound love. The mother who is empathically attuned to her child and at the same time aware of a future that the child cannot yet imagine is capable of "love that depends upon awareness and appreciation, in the moment, of actuality and potential, of the tension between the two, and of the possibilities for some resolution" (Greenberg, 1996, p. 892).

In the kabbalistic metaphor, the relationship within which one's truth is sought out and developed is between the individual and God, and so at first glance, doesn't translate easily into a consideration of psychotherapeutic technique. However, I believe that by bringing God into the equation, the kabbalists were free in a way that psychoanalysts haven't typically been, to articulate a dimension of psychic change that is most accurately described in terms of transcendent experience. The Kabbalah offers us something new. Instead of defining authenticity in terms of an essential true self or viewing it as a social construction, the Kabbalah depicts it as a flicker of unique creative potential within each of us that resonates with, and is essential to, the larger creative energy that animates the world. In so doing, it emphasizes the singular value of a human life, the unique contribution of the individual to the larger whole, as expressed through the creative process of self-exploration. Further, it instructs us as to the ineffability of the human being, to our inability to know all that is to be known about another person, even about ourselves. Although we may reflect multiple facets, the truth of who we are is not contained in any one of them, but transcends them in a unity that remains beyond sensual perception. The uniqueness of the individual is elusive, requiring something other than intellect to discern it.

Strikingly, the Kabbalah insists that the sacred is to be found not in heaven but on earth. The Zohar is populated with wandering characters who come upon delights of concealed meaning in the course of their travels. In the Kabbalah, as might be said about psychoanalysis, the secret lies not at the end of the journey but rather in how one negotiates what is met on the way. En route, the traveler unexpectedly discovers the sacred within the ordinary, the meaningful within the mundane, the divine within the human. This theme lies at the heart of the kabbalistic view of transformation, and indeed, of life itself. If the kabbalist can be said to have a goal, it is to cultivate a refined perception capable of recognizing the sacred within the commonplace, and reciprocally, of infusing everyday acts with meaning, thereby elevating them to the level of the sacred.

In formulating transformation in terms of the individual's relationship with God, the Kabbalah offers us a more expansive perspective from which to view the therapeutic undertaking. It suggests that the relationship of patient and therapist is deeply embedded in and facilitates the larger relational matrix between the individual and the universal. It implies a sacred significance to the therapeutic endeavor, suggesting that when we encounter ourselves in the heart of an empathic other, we at the same time approach God in relationship. In the meeting of minds of the therapeutic dyad we open to the larger possibility of a mutual encounter with God. In this potential space, which the Kabbalah characterizes as faith, we ask God the same question He asks of us—"Where are you?"—then listen closely for the answer that whispers within us. We discover that we are held in the embrace of the ineffable and unknowable God who has been longing from the Beginning for this meeting to take place. We emerge transformed, having attained paradoxically, a sense of union with a larger whole as well as a heightened subjectivity, an expanded awareness of our individual identity that we may then purposefully, and with renewed energy, carry with us into our everyday lives.

CASE EXAMPLE: JONAH

I offer the following clinical vignette as an illustration of how the kabbalistic metaphor of tikkun informed my thinking about my work with a patient who was engaged in a spiritual struggle to find meaning in his life, his work, and in himself. During our therapy sessions, I often found myself wondering how I could help my patient discern his "divine spark," or in psychoanalytic terms, to connect with a sense of his own creativity, vitality, and agency, and to feel that he could have an impact in the world. As it happens, my "spiritually informed intervention" had very little to do with God, and everything to do with human potential and responsibility. Some might call this tapping the divine within the human; others might call it faith in human possibility.

My patient was raised in a White, upper class, Catholic family. His parents' investment in religion appeared to have been linked solely to the elevation in status it would provide them, in the eyes of their wealthy, church-going community. The patient himself did not believe in God. His only memory of childhood religious practice was of being forced by his mother to serve as an altar boy at church. He recalled stifling the impulse to scream, as the wax dripping down from the candle he was made to hold burned his hands. I've given him the name Jonah because of the resonances for me, with the biblical prophet of the same name. The biblical Jonah tried to run away from his spiritual responsibility, was tossed by a storm at sea, and found himself swallowed up in the dark belly of a whale. This seems an apt metaphor with which to describe my patient's experience.

Jonah, an adjunct professor and doctoral candidate in history, suffered from a severe depressive episode, marked by his inability to write his dissertation. He spent hours at home, isolated and alone, attempting to craft the perfect paragraph, only to unravel it at the end of the day. Worse, his struggle with writing had leaked into the classroom. Although he greatly valued his role as a teacher, he had lost confidence in his ability to teach. Jonah found himself fixated on the sound of his own voice, becoming more and more anxious, trying to pack more and more material into his lecture, only to realize he had lost his students' interest.

Jonah hated himself. He told me of the harsh, internal, ever present voice in his mind that called him useless, a loser. Whenever he sat down to write, the voice became louder, leading him to delete the sentences he had so painstakingly written. Jonah's self-recrimination was relentless, fueling his pervasive feelings of hopelessness and despair. Our therapy sessions mirrored his struggles with writing. His sentences trailed off, unfinished, as if it were useless for him even to try to speak his thoughts aloud. I struggled to find a way in, to locate any aspect of Jonah's identity that could anchor him to a sense of his own goodness or his own agency. Nothing I said seemed to penetrate his self-defeating narrative. His world was in ruins, and all he could do was sift through the ashes.

Jonah revealed that his only pleasure came at the end of the day, when he left his apartment and drank with the regulars at the corner bar. Drinking was the closest he'd ever come to having a spiritual experience. His pain slipped away and life was beautiful. When he drank, rather than feeling alienated and alone, he felt like he belonged to the world. He was a member of the human race. That is, until morning, when hung over and ill, Jonah berated himself for drinking himself into oblivion, and the cycle of self-loathing began anew.

It soon became clear to me that Jonah was a lifelong alcoholic. When I confronted him, he admitted he had started at age 13 and never stopped. I pointed out that his drinking was unraveling any progress we made in therapy. He needed to detox, or he would never get better. If he continued to drink, neither of us could know who he was or who he had the potential of becoming.

Jonah was stunned by my directive. His parents knew about his drinking, as did his friends. Yet no one had cared enough to get him to stop. Soon after, Jonah admitted himself into a detox program and, after some weeks of painful struggle, got sober. He attended Alcoholics Anonymous (AA) meetings religiously, but hated AA, stymied by its directive to turn his will and his life over to a higher power. Even though he had been raised Catholic, or perhaps because of it, Jonah was a staunch atheist. AA's language, filled with references to God, felt alienating to him. Yet he was hungry for spiritual change. "I want to transform myself," he told me, fists clenched, his tone a toxic mix of desperation and self-hatred. "I need to work harder at letting go." Unfortunately, Jonah's fervent desire to change himself only fueled the fire of his harsh self-criticism. "I can't even do AA right," he lamented. I asked about ways he might interpret the phrase "higher power" that would be personally meaningful for him. Setting aside the notion of God, was there something beyond him that resonated with him, something he could believe in that was bigger than him?

Jonah's thoughts turned to his work, years ago, as a social activist. He had been passionate about political theory and about the transformative potential of political movements. He was interested in revolutionaries such as Gandhi and Martin Luther King, Jr., whose calls for political change were imbued with the imperative for spiritual transformation. He had embarked on his doctoral studies because he wanted to teach these ideas to the next generation. As he spoke, Jonah had the revelation that the topic he had been trying to write about for his dissertation had nothing to do with what had brought him into the field in the first place. It had been his advisor's idea, not his.

For the first time, I noticed a glimmer of life in Jonah I had not seen before. He was animated and excited. Eager to enflame the embers of the "spark" I was beginning to discern, I invited him to teach me about what interested him. At first haltingly, and then with increasing confidence, Jonah taught me about political theory and revolutionary movements. We discussed the theories of Louis Althusser, Karl Marx, and Walter Benjamin, and their relevance to his interest in Islam and Islamic history. Jonah was intelligent, patient, and thoughtful, even articulate. In my mind's eye, a different version of Jonah was gradually coming into view.

The backdrop to our therapy at this moment was the increasingly polarizing political discourse leading up to the 2016 presidential election. Muslims were being cast as religious extremists and potential terrorists. Jonah was becoming increasingly concerned about the escalation of anti-Muslim hostility. The Paris bombings thrust him out of his depressive spiral, bringing him abruptly into the present. Many of his students were Muslim and had already been targets of harassment. Concerned about his students, Jonah was unsure how to address these current events in his classroom. Should he adhere to his lesson plan? Or was it his responsibility to sound the alarm—to educate his students about the dangers of xenophobia and nationalism? If he did so, how could he ensure that his classroom felt safe for all his students, even those with divergent political views? He expressed feeling paralyzed, stuck, unable to take action. Even if he did act, what difference could he possibly make?

I suggested to Jonah that he seemed to be caught between two conflicting versions of himself—the loser or the activist. By his own account, he longed for spiritual transformation, but had no idea how to attain it. The way I saw it, the answer was right in front of him. I shared with him the kabbalistic notion of tikkun olam, repair of the world. I explained that this theosophical system placed great value on the unique contribution of the individual to the larger whole, no matter how seemingly insignificant this contribution might seem in the moment. What was important was being true to one's values and living out those values in everyday life. It was not the end result—which was unknowable in any case—but the effort itself, that mattered. Might it be possible that he, too, had a unique contribution to make in repairing the world?

Jonah decided to act. Suspending his lesson plans for three consecutive classes, Jonah conducted a "teach-in," educating his students about Islam and Islamic history. When it was over, Jonah believed he had made the right choice. He felt that, at least for now, he had succeeded in humanizing those who were being demonized. He felt a little less hopeless and a little bit better about himself. Instead of spinning around in his own head, he had acted in accordance with his values and newly connected with a sense of himself as having an impact.

Heartened by this sign of life in Jonah, I suggested that perhaps, for him, teaching was a form of spiritual practice. He may not believe in God, but there were certainly principles he believed in. Might he be able to harness his passion for political theory into making the lessons of history more relevant to his students' everyday lives? Could he help them think more critically about current events by applying what they learned in the classroom? Given all the injustice in the world, might it possible for one person to make a difference? Our therapy became an opportunity for us both to consider these questions. As we talked about Jonah's options for individual intervention in the face of larger political forces that increasingly felt beyond our control, I privately reflected on mine. As he wondered what he could do to make a difference, I wondered, what could I?

The shocking outcome of the 2016 presidential election and the ensuing flurry of executive orders emanating from the White House lent urgency to these questions. Several of Jonah's students who had traveled to visit family during the winter break were caught up in the Muslim travel ban. They were blocked from returning home for the start of the spring semester.

Jonah was stirred to action. Taking on my challenge, he overhauled his syllabus to include, in each class, a discussion of how what they were learning about historical political movements could be applied to current events. Jonah was candid about his own political views but was careful to make the classroom a safe place for respectful dialogue that could encompass multiple viewpoints. His students responded positively, grateful for the opportunity to have these discussions. At the end of the semester, several told him his class had changed the way they thought about the world.

In responding to my invitation to teach me about what mattered to him, Jonah was able to reconnect with an aspect of himself that was vital to him, but with which he had lost contact. In psychoanalytic terms, he was able to access a sense of aliveness and agency—in kabbalistic terms, his "divine spark"—that had heretofore so frustratingly eluded him. In turn, my work with Jonah had a positive effect on me. I came to realize that in helping Jonah put his values into practice, I was putting mine into practice as well. It made me feel a little less hopeless in response to political forces that felt beyond my control. Our therapy created a small ripple of change, sparking a creative-reparative process that—who knows?—may lead to a larger one. Social activist and psychoanalyst Andrew Samuels (2017) suggested that helping our patients be "citizen-therapists for the wider world" is a manifestation of tikkun olam (p. 687), and in addition to repairing the world, it may be good for the analyst's soul. In the case of my work with Jonah, I believe this to be true.

REFERENCES

Aron, L. (1996). *A meeting of minds: Mutuality in psychoanalysis*. The Analytic Press.

Aron, L., & Starr, K. (2013). *A psychotherapy for the people: Toward a progressive psychoanalysis*. Routledge. https://doi.org/10.4324/9780203098059

Bion, W. R. (1977a). Attention and interpretation. In *Seven servants: Four works by Wilfred Bion*. Jason Aronson.

Bion, W. R. (1977b). Transformations. In *Seven servants: Four works by Wilfred Bion*. Jason Aronson.

Bresler, J., & Starr, K. (Eds.). (2015). *Relational psychoanalysis and psychotherapy integration: An evolving synergy*. Routledge. https://doi.org/10.4324/9781315747422

Bronheim, H. E. (1994). Psychoanalysis and faith. *The Journal of the American Academy of Psychoanalysis, 22*(4), 681–697. https://doi.org/10.1521/jaap.1.1994.22.4.681

Drob, S. L. (2000a). *Kabbalistic metaphors: Jewish mystical themes in ancient and modern thought*. Jason Aronson.

Drob, S. L. (2000b). *Symbols of the kabbalah: Philosophical and psychological perspectives*. Jason Aronson.

Eigen, M. (1981). The area of faith in Winnicott, Lacan and Bion. *The International Journal of Psycho-Analysis, 62*(Pt 4), 413–433.

Eliot, T. S. (1968). *Four quartets*. Harcourt.

Epstein, M. (1995). *Thoughts without a thinker: Psychotherapy from a Buddhist perspective*. Basic Books.

Freud, S. (1968). The future of an illusion. In J. Strachey (Ed. & Trans.), *The standard edition of the complete psychological works of Sigmund Freud* (Vol. 21, pp. 1–56). The Hogarth Press. (Original work published 1927)

Ghent, E. (1990). Masochism, submission, surrender—Masochism as a perversion of surrender. *Contemporary Psychoanalysis, 26*(1), 108–136. https://doi.org/10.1080/00107530.1990.10746643

Ghent, E. (1992). Paradox and process. *Psychoanalytic Dialogues, 2*(1), 135–159. https://doi.org/10.1080/10481889209538925

Green, A. (2004). *A guide to the Zohar*. Stanford University Press.

Greenberg, J. (1996). Loewald's transitional model. *Journal of the American Psychoanalytic Association, 44*(3), 886–895.

Idel, M. (2002). *Absorbing perfections: Kabbalah and interpretation*. Yale University Press. https://doi.org/10.12987/yale/9780300083798.001.0001

Kumin, I. M. (1978). Developmental aspects of opposites and paradox. *The International Review of Psycho-Analysis, 5*(4), 477–484.

Loewald, H. W. (1960). On the therapeutic action of psycho-analysis. *The International Journal of Psycho-Analysis, 41*, 16–33.

Loewald, H. W. (1978). Instinct theory, object relations, and psychic-structure formation. *Journal of the American Psychoanalytic Association, 26*(3), 493–506. https://doi.org/10.1177/000306517802600302

Loewald, H. W. (1980). *Papers on psychoanalysis*. Yale University Press.

Loewald, H. W. (1988). Psychoanalysis in search of nature: Thoughts on metapsychology, "metaphysics," projection. *The Annual of Psychoanalysis, 16*, 49–54.

Matt, D. C. (2004a). *The zohar: Pritzker edition* (Vol. I). Stanford University Press.

Matt, D. C. (2004b). *The zohar: Pritzker edition* (Vol. II). Stanford University Press.

Matt, D. C. (2006). *The zohar: Pritzker edition* (Vol. III). Stanford University Press.

Mitchell, S. A. (2000). *Relationality: From attachment to intersubjectivity*. The Analytic Press.

Reik, T. (1948). *Listening with the third ear: The inner experience of a psychoanalyst*. Farrar, Straus and Giroux.

Rilke, R. M. (1934). *Letters to a young poet* (M. D. Herter, Trans.). Norton.

Samuels, A. (2017). The "activist client": Social responsibility, the political self, and clinical practice in psychotherapy and psychoanalysis. *Psychoanalytic Dialogues, 27*(6), 678–693. https://doi.org/10.1080/10481885.2017.1379324

Schachter, Z. M., & Hoffman, E. (1983). *Sparks of light: Counseling in the Hasidic tradition*. Shambhala Publications.

Scholem, G. (1969). *On the kabbalah and its symbolism* (R. Manheim, Trans.). Schocken Books.

Scholem, G. (1995). *Major trends in Jewish mysticism*. Schocken Books.

Starr, K. E. (2008a). Faith as the fulcrum of psychic change. *Psychoanalytic Dialogues, 18*(2), 203–229. https://doi.org/10.1080/10481880801909781

Starr, K. E. (2008b). *Repair of the soul: Metaphors of transformation in Jewish mysticism and psychoanalysis*. Routledge.

Winnicott, D. W. (1964). *The child, the family, and the outside world*. Penguin Books.

Winnicott, D. W. (1965). *The maturational processes and the facilitating environment: Studies in the theory of emotional developments*. Routledge.

Winnicott, D. W. (1967). The location of cultural experience. *The International Journal of Psycho-Analysis, 48*(3), 368–372.

8

"THE NAME OF GOD IS MERCY"

Reflections on Suffering, Healing, and Growth From a Roman Catholic, Contemplative, Mystic Psychoanalyst

THERESA CLEMENT TISDALE

The relationship between psychoanalysis and religion had an inauspicious start when Freud (1927/1961c) declared that "religion is the universal obsessional neurosis" (p. 42) and "a personal God is, psychologically, nothing more than an exalted father" (Freud, 1910/1957b, p. 122). Over the years, a number of works have explored possible reasons for this rather adamant dismissal, including connecting this disavowal with his family, culture, and historical context (Cooper-White, 2018; Rizzuto, 1998, 2004, 2009). Freud's influence on this topic cast a rather long shadow over psychoanalytic theory and practice. As Sorenson (2004b) discovered, there was a marked increase in psychoanalytic publications dealing with religion after Freud's death in 1939. What follows are some broad brushstrokes that highlight the sea change.

Fairbairn (1952), Winnicott (1965, 1971, 1975), and Guntrip (1971) were among the first to address religion or religious metaphor in their writings. Their works, along with Freud's (1962–1966), informed one of the first empirical studies on the topic, published in Rizzuto's (1979) book *The Birth*

The title of this chapter is drawn from Pope Francis (2016).

https://doi.org/10.1037/0000276-009
Spiritual Diversity in Psychotherapy: Engaging the Sacred in Clinical Practice,
S. J. Sandage and B. D. Strawn (Editors)

of the Living God. Rizzuto's qualitative study that explored how God representation is formed spurred several other empirical investigations into the connection between relationship with God, self, and others (Brokaw & Edwards, 1994; Tisdale et al., 1997). Other studies have explored similarities and differences between attachment patterns and styles when relating to God and others (Kirkpatrick & Shaver, 1990, is one example from more than 450 entries in PsycInfo on the topic).

Over time, interest in the religious or spiritual life of psychoanalysts led to the publication of articles and books about Winnicott (Hoffman, 2004; Parker, 2012), Fairbairn (Hoffman, 2004), and Dobbs (2009). Books relating psychoanalysis to particular religious traditions, including Buddhism (Safran, 2003), Judaism (Aron & Henik, 2010), Islam (Akhtar, 2008), Hinduism (Vaidyanathan & Kripal, 2002), Catholicism (Wolman, 1995), and Christianity (Bland & Strawn, 2014; Hoffman, 2010; Sorenson, 2004b), also began appearing in the literature. Evolutions have also included analysts of different religious traditions reflecting on the influence of their religious faith on their work as a psychoanalyst and the influence of their psychoanalytic theory and practice on their religious beliefs and practice (Aron, 2004; Fayek, 2004; Rizzuto, 2004; Sorenson, 2004a). All of these trends as well as continuing empirical investigations[1] strongly suggest a steadily growing and abiding interest and focus on religion and spirituality in psychoanalysis.

This chapter continues in the spirit and vein of the literature that describes the mutual, reciprocal influence between beliefs and practice. Wright et al. (2014) previously underscored the importance of particularity that illuminates the complex and unique ways in which traditions are embedded and embodied in context for every practicing clinician. I trust that this chapter is responsive to that exhortation.

SPIRITUAL, EXISTENTIAL, RELIGIOUS, AND THEOLOGICAL TRADITIONS INFORMING MY APPROACH

My approach to every aspect of my life (including my work) is informed by the Roman Catholic Church. For more than 2 millennia, the Church has been rooted and grounded in the person and work of Jesus Christ, His life, death, burial, resurrection, and ascension into heaven. There is a wealth of spiritual, religious, and theological wisdom and practices that have been

---

[1]APA PsycInfo includes more than 250 entries in a search of "psychoanalysis and god"; Psychoanalytic Electronic Publishing includes more than 500 entries.

handed down since the 1st century that equip Catholics to live a faithful and fruitful life and to meaningfully engage with the existential challenges and questions that life inevitably brings. My orientation to life has also been enriched through engagement with members of Jewish, Muslim, and Buddhist communities of faith.

Religious Identity and Context

I am what is referred to as a cradle Catholic: someone born and raised in the Roman Catholic faith. I attended Catholic schools through junior high and weekly religious education at our parish during public high school. As a family, we attended Mass on Sundays and Holy Days, prayed the Rosary together several nights a week, and received the Sacraments of Baptism, First Holy Communion (Eucharist), Reconciliation (then called Penance), and Confirmation. Religious education, receiving the Sacraments, parish life, and family spiritual practices inculcated in me a sense of awe and wonder about God. I loved Bible stories and learning about the saints. In Roman Catholic theology (Sollier, 1908), the communion of saints is all those past and present who are united in a shared faith in Christ. Those who have died are believed to exist in a state of consciousness that includes being accessible for intercessory prayer. Canonization is bestowed on those who demonstrated exemplary devotion to God, often including martyrdom and miracles related to their intercession.

For me, guilt and suffering were prominent themes of Catholic education at school and home. These teachings were more often sources of confusion than comfort. What is the purpose of suffering? What does "offering up suffering as a sacrifice" mean? Does God allow or cause suffering? Can guilt be relieved or removed? These were ponderous questions for a young mind.

It is often the case that one or more children in a Catholic family will be named after a saint. As an expression of gratitude for her intercession that resulted in my healthy birth, my mother decided to name me after Saint (St.) Thérèse of Lisieux, a French Carmelite nun. In her spiritual autobiography first published in 1898 (Thérèse of Lisieux, 1898/1975), she described her daily life as "the little way of spiritual childhood" (p. 17). Simplicity, unwavering trust in God, ardent devotion, and selfless service to God and others were hallmarks of her faith and life. In the decades following her death, as millions began imitating her little way, St. Thérèse was declared "the greatest saint of modern times" by Pope Pius X (Society of the Little Flower, n.d., para. 1). She was canonized in 1925 and, in 1997, was named Doctor of the Church, a distinction reserved for those saints whose life and writings have influenced Catholic theology and spirituality. She inspires me daily.

Although I remain Roman Catholic, as an adult I have been enriched by the diversity of theology and spirituality in a number of Christian church contexts. *Streams of Living Water: Celebrating the Great Traditions of Christian Faith* by Richard Foster (1998) has enlarged my understanding of the depth and breadth of ways Christians since the time of Christ express devotion to God. These ways include prayer, cultivating virtue, engaging in service, proclaiming the Gospel in action and word, working for social justice, and embodying spirituality in ordinary life.

Essentials of Catholic Theology

In 1994, *Catechism of the Catholic Church* (Libreria Editrice Vaticana, 1994) was published, having been commissioned then by Pope John Paul II. The *Catechism* summarizes the Church's teachings in four parts: The Profession of Faith, The Celebration of the Christian Mystery, Life in Christ, and Christian Prayer. The *Catechism* serves as a reference book and is used in religious education programs in parishes around the world. The sources for the *Catechism* are The Scriptures and Sacred Catholic Tradition. *Sacred Catholic Tradition* refers to the application of God's revealed Word in The Scriptures as well as to what Jesus taught the apostles, which has been faithfully and reliably written and handed down since the time of Christ. Rather than remaining static, Sacred Catholic Tradition in each age is animated by the Holy Spirit. The essentials of Catholic theology and belief are expressed through two ancient Creeds: The Apostles' Creed and The Nicene Creed. One of the two is always part of Catholic Mass liturgy.

Contemplative and Mystical Catholic Spirituality

Contemplation and mystical union with God are sources of vitality in my spiritual life. The focus of contemplative Catholic spirituality is cultivating sustained communion with God. I was drawn to contemplative spirituality through a desire for deeper connection with God in every aspect of my life. St. Thomas Aquinas (ca. 1265–1273/1981) believed that the contemplative life is one that is oriented to the practice of contemplation above any other preoccupation, intention, or pursuit. The chief aim of life becomes to know and love God. Aquinas defined *contemplation* as the soul's loving gaze focused *on* God, which is different from intellectual knowledge *of* God (p. 10). Early exemplars of the contemplative life are the Desert Fathers and Mothers of the 3rd and 4th centuries. A contemplative life is developed and sustained through meditation and prayer.

Contemplation involves intentional pursuit of communion with God. Mystical union, on the other hand, is a supernatural experience that is surrendered to rather than sought. Examples of Catholic mystics are St. Julian of Norwich (1373/1974), St. Teresa of Avila (1577/1961), St. John of the Cross (ca. 16th century/2003), and St. Faustina Kowalska (ca. 1920s–1930s/1981). I was drawn to mystical spirituality through suffering. A spiritual crisis in young adulthood was a turning point when I sought healing prayer offered weekly at my church. During these times of prayer, I encountered God in profound ways by surrendering to the experience of a Presence. For almost 40 years, mystical union has been unexpectedly graced to me during healing prayer, personal devotions, celebration of the Eucharist at Mass, events surrounding the death of my parents, contemplation of the communion of saints and global Catholic community, and meditation on the life of Jesus during Holy Week as well as viewing icons from St. Catherine's Monastery in Egypt.

Contemporary Exemplars

One contemporary exemplar whose life and work demonstrate devotion to God through contemplation, service, and perseverance through suffering is St. Mother Teresa of Calcutta, who founded the Missionaries of Charity headquartered in India. Her radical love of God and devotion to the poor, sick, and outcast people in society move me deeply. In 1982, although in poor health, she risked her life to broker a cease-fire in war-torn Lebanon so she and her Missionaries of Charity sisters could rescue 100 disabled Muslim orphans who had been abandoned by their caregivers when armed conflict drew too close to the orphanage. She received the Nobel Peace Prize in 1979 and was canonized a saint in 2016 (Bordoni, 2020; Noun, 2016; Sanness, 1979).

Pope Francis, who inspired the title of this chapter, is another exemplar who captures my mind and heart. Elected Pope in 2013, he is the first from the global south (Argentina) and the first to take the name Francis (for St. Francis of Assisi). In his initial address to the world, Pope Francis closed by asking people to pray for him (National Public Radio, 2013). He quickly became known as "the people's Pope" through his demonstrations of humility, solidarity with the poor, care for the environment, and pastoral responses to questions about complex social issues. He took decisive action to address the scourge of sexual abuse in the Church. He reorganized the governing body of the Catholic Church and closely reviewed and revised financial practices at the Vatican. While remaining grounded in Catholic theology and teaching, he consistently extends pastoral care and sensitivity to women; lesbian, gay, bisexual, transgender, queer + people; and others who feel disenfranchised by the Church (De Carolis, 2019; Pilkington, 2013; Winfield, 2020). His living witness is compelling and is a source of inspiration to me every day.

The Transforming Power of God's Mercy

Pope Francis consistently speaks and writes about God's mercy. In April 2015, he issued a proclamation that an Extraordinary Jubilee Year of Mercy would begin December 8, 2015, and end on November 20, 2016 (Francis, Bishop of Rome, 2015). He chose the theme of mercy with the intention of drawing people into deeper communion with God through contemplating the face of Jesus as the expression of God's mercy to humanity.

Contemplating the face of Jesus is likened to the loving gaze between a mother and child. Pope Francis proclaimed that the mercy received from God should be generously given to others, particularly through the spiritual and corporeal works of mercy. Spiritual works of mercy include instructing, advising, consoling, comforting, forgiving, and bearing wrongs patiently. Corporeal (embodied) works of mercy include feeding the hungry, sheltering the homeless, clothing the naked, visiting the sick and imprisoned, burying the dead, and giving alms to the poor.

When interviewed about the proclamation, Pope Francis (2016) said,

> Yes, I believe that this is a time for mercy. The Church is *showing her maternal side, her motherly face, to a humanity that is wounded.* She does not wait for the wounded to knock on her doors, she looks for them on the streets, she gathers them in, she embraces them, she takes care of them, she makes them feel loved . . . I am ever more convinced . . . our era is a *kairos* of mercy, an opportune time . . . etymologically, mercy derives from *misericordis*, which means *opening one's heart to wretchedness.* And immediately we go to the Lord: *Mercy is the divine attitude which embraces . . . God of mercy, merciful God . . . this really is the Lord's identity.* (pp. 6–9; italics added)

I embrace and desire to embody this extraordinary expression of God's presence with humanity.

PSYCHOTHERAPEUTIC THEORIES INFORMING MY APPROACH

Psychoanalysis is a theoretical and clinical approach to understanding human motivation, development, suffering, growth, and change. First introduced to the world by Sigmund Freud (1900/1952), psychoanalysis as a field has been alive and well and evolving for more than 120 years. Psychoanalytic thought has been the focus of interdisciplinary studies in a range of fields, including literature, politics, religion, government, social sciences, and cognitive neuroscience. Psychoanalysis has been the foundation and enduring source of influence in my professional life as a clinical psychologist and psychoanalyst. At the same time, I have also been introduced to, and benefited from, learning other theories and clinical approaches, such as behavioral, cognitive, cognitive behavior, and existential, and more recent evolutions of blended approaches, such as dialectical behavior therapy and eye movement desensitization and reprocessing. Because psychoanalysis is the foundation from which I work, it is the focus of this section.

Psychoanalysis in General

Although there have been many evolutions in psychoanalysis across a 120-plus year history, a number of theoretical and clinical constants have endured. These constants include unconscious mental life (what is outside conscious awareness but influences sensations, perceptions, affect, and behavior), transference (the ways patients relate to the analyst that are reminiscent of or replay unresolved unconscious internal and interpersonal conflicts), countertransference (all the ways the analyst experiences the patient), defenses (ways the mind protects from knowing what is not ready to be known), resistance (the human inclination to preserve homeostasis), and dream interpretation (the ways mental life during sleep reflects and reveals unconscious processes). These constructs remain fundamental to psychoanalytic theory and practice, although the ways in which they are conceptualized, articulated, and used in treatment vary across schools of thought. I find these fundamentals, and the permutations of them, relevant and useful in my work with patients.

In every branch of psychoanalysis, the relationship between patient and analyst is at the focus of the therapeutic process and facilitates working through intrapsychic conflicts; healing developmental deficits; strengthening self-cohesion; and resolving repetitive, unreflective interpersonal patterns that are rooted in unconscious processes and inhibit the capacity for mutual, reciprocal, healthy relating with others. How an analyst embodies their theoretical and clinical proclivities will influence their use of self in treatment. Psychoanalytic theories provide a psychologically comprehensive way of thinking about human nature, motivation, development, psychopathology, change, and treatment. Psychoanalytic practice focuses on addressing the root(s) of physical and psychological symptoms and suffering, which often have spiritual implications. I draw from the whole range of psychoanalytic theories when understanding the complexity of each patient's unique context, personality, and suffering.

Object Relations in Particular

I was drawn to psychoanalysis through the work of the British independent tradition of object relations. Shifting away from Freud's focus on biological drives as fundamental to motivation, development, and behavior, these analysts were oriented to the essential need for human relatedness. Two early architects of this evolution of psychoanalysis were Fairbairn (1952) and Winnicott (1965, 1971, 1975).

For Fairbairn and Winnicott, human nature is basically good, and what leads to psychopathology are failures in the environment, particularly during the early years. For Winnicott, early life is profoundly influenced by "the environmental mother" (Winnicott, 1971, p. 80), who is the person most closely related to providing the infant's biological and emotional needs. Healthy development is a result of "good enough mothering" in the context of a "facilitating environment" (Winnicott, 1965, p. 96). Winnicott, a pediatrician who later trained as a child and adult psychoanalyst, developed his ideas based on decades of experience with mothers and babies. He observed that stability, reliability, the anticipation of physical needs, capacity for attunement, and responsiveness to mutual cueing between mothers and babies contributed significantly to healthy development. When, for whatever reason, primary caregivers (usually mothers during Winnicott's era) lacked these capacities and instead needed responsiveness from their growing infant, this impinged on the child's capacity to evolve a true self comprising unique potentials, gifts, abilities, and creative expressions that would be affirmed and nurtured by good enough (although not perfect) mothering. Too much impingement resulted in development of a false self, which is an adaptation of the child to the caregiver that arises out of necessity, sacrificing the true self to obtain even minimal levels of responsiveness needed for survival. Winnicott's theoretical work often reads like poetry, which stirs my imagination about preverbal and early life experience. His clinical essays inspire me with rich examples of ways to respond to patients who suffer from early life deficits.

Fairbairn (1952), while resonant with Winnicott's (1975) notion of relational rather than biological drives as the basis of human nature and motivation, emphasized repressed (unremembered) bad objects and corresponding patterns of relating as sources of human suffering. Understandably, Winnicott's theory reflected his experiences as a pediatrician and with mothers and children separated during wartime. Fairbairn worked in relative isolation in

Scotland, and much of his clinical work was with traumatized war veterans. Fairbairn (1952) posited that traumatic/bad experiences, unremembered yet exerting influence on perception and relating, thwart the capacity to develop healthy connections. These unconscious there-and-then dynamic relations between fragmented aspects of self and others divert energy away from investing in relationships with others in the here and now. The unconscious internal dramas are lived out over and over. One notable evidence of this was the predictability that children would return to an abusive parent rather than be faced with the terror of having no parent; he opined that a bad object is better than no object. Interpersonal patterns tell the tale of the unconscious unresolved relational dynamics.

Because Fairbairn (1952) believed that treatment must address these unconscious conflictual relational constellations, the analyst and patient need to bear the return of these unremembered traumatic dynamics because they will inevitably and necessarily be expressed in the clinical relationship. Working through these previously unconscious relational dynamics frees the patient to develop healthy, mutual, reciprocal relationships in the here and now. Fairbairn's conceptualization and mapping of the intrapsychic drama has had the greatest impact on my clinical work because the dynamic he describes is ubiquitous; a version of it is evident in the life of every one of my patients over the past 25 years.

Synthesis of Multiple Theories Into Useful Methods

One analyst working today who has masterfully synthesized the breadth of psychoanalysis without sacrificing distinctives of each school of thought is Martha Stark. I first met Martha in the mid-1990s and discovered her book in 2009.

In *Modes of Therapeutic Action: Enhancement of Knowledge, Provision of Experience, and Engagement in Relationship*, Stark (1999) organized numerous theories according to the need–response dynamic between patient and analyst. Each of three modes is used in the context of moment-by-moment attunement by the analyst to the patient and is related to the conceptual model guiding the understanding of the process, the focus of encounters, the analyst's use of self, the understanding of etiology/sources of symptoms, the use of interventions, and intended outcome. The three modes are not linear nor are they mutually exclusive. All three modes of responsiveness are necessary within every session over the course of treatment.

In what Stark (1999) called Mode 1, the conceptual model is organized around resolution of intrapsychic, structural conflict between impulses (id) and external controls (superego/conscience). This mode reflects classical and neoclassical theory. The capacity for understanding and mediating internal conflicts is weak. From the perimeter of the patient's experience, the analyst engages as an observer of how conflicts are expressed through symptoms and transference. What is uncovered through the analytic relationship, often via interpretations, are conflicts about biological drives related to sex and aggression (Freud, 1923/1961b) and psychological drives related to love and hate (Klein, 1964). Insight and the release of affect that has been bound up in the unresolved conflict(s) lead to self-awareness and facilitate the resolution of structural conflict as well as lead to the development of ego strength, which is the capacity to live life in a reflective rather than reactive way.

In Mode 2, which is conceptually oriented to compensating for developmental deficits, the focus is on what was missing in a patient's early relational experiences. Stark (1999) referred to the primary source of psychopathology as "the absence of good" (p. 74). Winnicott's (1965, 1971) work is included in this mode because he underscored the impact on healthy development of an unreliable, insufficient, or unstable early life environment. In Mode 2, the analyst uses themselves to intervene in the realm of the patient's developmental needs and provides the responses and experiences that will facilitate growth. Stability, reliability, constancy, and attunement are among the essential provisions. Heinz Kohut's (1971, 1984) work is also included in Mode 2.

For Kohut (1971, 1984), empathic attunement in early life leads to robust self-cohesion and stable self-esteem. Conversely, if necessary experiences of mirroring and needs to idealize and join with or imitate caregivers are missing, development will be hindered. For both Winnicott and Kohut, the analyst's provisions are not seen as gratification because they are meeting a crucial developmental need without which a patient cannot grow and mature. The analyst's use of self is therapeutic when they facilitate movement from dependence to interdependence and evolving of the true self (Winnicott, 1965, 1971, 1975). The analyst attunes to the patient through mirroring the patient's experience and welcomes the patient's need to idealize the analyst as well at the patient's need to join the analyst's strengths with the patient's weaknesses (a self-object function) until the patient has internalized the therapeutic relationship in a way that facilitates developing self-cohesion and self-esteem (Kohut, 1971, 1984). In the course of treatment, the analyst will inevitably fall short of perfect attunement. For both Winnicott and Kohut, these failures, when they are gradual and not too prolonged, are important for the patient's maturation, self-cohesion, and stable self-esteem because the patient grows in the capacity to be resourceful in meeting their own needs. Provision is internalized and used for developmental growth.

Mode 3 (Stark, 1999) is conceptually organized around the work of Fairbairn (1952), intersubjectivity theory (originally conceived by Stolorow et al., 1994), and contemporary/relational theory (inaugurated by Greenberg & Mitchell, 1983). What is therapeutic about this mode is "authentic engagement" (Stark, 1999, p. 56). From this perspective, a patient's repetitive, unreflective instability in relating with others is the result of "the presence of bad" (Stark, 1999, p. 74) in early life. Physical, emotional, verbal, and sexual abuse are all examples of traumatic experiences that are internalized, repressed, and then lived out in relationships.

In treatment, the analyst is drawn into the patient's conflictual pattern, which often happens without conscious awareness or intention on the part of analyst or patient. These encounters are referred to as "enactments" because the dyad is experiencing the dynamic in the moment. The analyst's ability to remain sturdy and steady in the midst of aggression, anger, and rage is essential. Enactments often lead to ruptures in the analytic relationship, which are inevitable and necessary. Ruptures present the opportunity for repair, which is the heart of the authentic engagement needed by the patient to resolve repetitive conflicts. Repair includes the analyst's acknowledging their role in the rupture, affirming the patient's experience of the analyst, and restoring connection through empathy and understanding. As a result, the patient grows in their capacity to engage in healthy, mutual, reciprocal, and satisfying relationships. The unknown, intrapsychic drama has become known and worked through. The tale has been told in a context in which a new outcome is possible.

When I first encountered Stark's (1999) book, I experienced a eureka moment. Her theoretical breadth and clinical depth are breathtaking, exhibiting extraordinary bandwidth for holding complexity. Her comprehensive grasp of the expanse of psychoanalytic theories provides a wealth of references I use when conceptualizing my work with patients. The modes, which she illustrates through extensive clinical examples, inspire me with a range of ways to consider when engaging with my patients in the present moment.

SPIRITUALLY INTEGRATED PSYCHOTHERAPY: EMBODIED AND EMBEDDED IN CONTEXT

I believe that spiritually integrated psychotherapy (SIP) involves both models and methods. Theoretical models provide ways to think about human nature, motivation, development, the mind, psychopathology, change, the patient–analyst relationship, and diversity. Clinical methods/examples illustrate ways to listen, respond, and intervene throughout treatment. Each clinician implicitly or explicitly has a unique model and method that are informed and influenced by their particular embodied spiritual, existential, religious, theological, theoretical, and clinical traditions.

Both the Roman Catholic and psychoanalytic traditions are sources of influence on my SIP approach. Both inform my way of life, my orientation to vocation in all its forms, and my embodied presence in the world. This section of the chapter could easily fill a book. Pargament's (2007) *Spiritually Integrated Psychotherapy: Understanding and Addressing the Sacred* is a masterful example of a thoroughly explicated model and method. Given the parameters of this project, I highlight essentials of my model and method followed by the presentation of my work with a patient.

SIP: A Theoretical Model

Psychoanalysis is consistent, although not equivalent, with my theological and spiritual beliefs and values. In psychoanalysis, the focus is on discovering what is unconscious and bringing conflicts, affects, memories, relational dynamics, and fragments of experience into conscious awareness so that, in the context of relationship, what has been formerly unknown may become known, processed, reflected on, understood, and integrated into the person as a whole.

Catholic theology and spirituality emphasize the need for deepening understanding and awareness of self (Libreria Editrice Vaticana, 1994), and provide a metanarrative from which to contextualize and conceptualize all aspects life. The Catholic tradition grounds my understanding, and the psychoanalytic tradition contributes a wealth of ways to think about every aspect of life, human experience, and suffering as well as ways to understand and deeply engage in processes that lead to healing and growth.

Key Theoretical Concept: Mercy
Suffering humanity in need of God's mercy is a grounding belief and principle in my vocational life. Pope Francis declared his desire that the Jubilee Year of Mercy would be

> steeped in mercy, so that we can go out to every man and woman, bringing the goodness and tenderness of God! May the balm of mercy reach everyone, both believers and those far away, as a sign that the Kingdom of God is already present in our midst! (Francis, Bishop of Rome, 2015, p. 5)

The Church would show its maternal side by reaching out into every corner of society with expressions of God's merciful love. St. Mother Teresa embodied the mercy of God generously given. She sought out the least, the last, the lost. In *A Simple Path*, Mother Teresa (1995) wrote,

> The greatest disease in the West today . . . is being unwanted, unloved, and uncared for . . . the only cure for loneliness, despair, and hopelessness is love . . . many in the world are dying for a piece of bread but there are many more dying for a little love. The poverty in the West . . . is not only a poverty of loneliness but also of spirituality. There's a hunger for love, as there is a hunger for God. (p. 79)

Pope Francis and St. Mother Teresa of Calcutta are exemplars who embody mercy in action, and they inspire me to be mindful of God's mercy when I engage with patients.

Origins

My Catholic tradition precludes belief that humanity evolved from a lower species (Darwin, 1859), or that God and religion are illusions (Freud, 1927/1961c). According to Catholic theology (Libreria Editrice Vaticana, 1994), human beings were created by God in the image and likeness of God. In the beginning, humanity existed in harmony with God and creation. Because God desired authentic relationship, humanity was created with free will. By choosing to pursue life apart from God, humans broke from intended communion to a state of rupture in relation to God, self, and others—an event referred to as *the fall*. The fall resulted in all manner of suffering entering the world and human existence. The Catholic Church typically welcomes what scientific methods may reveal about the wonders of God's creation (Libreria Editrice Vaticana, 1994); however, the Church may not embrace the philosophical traditions that inform them when they pose contradictions to essential teaching.

Fundamentals of Human Nature

I embrace St. Augustine's simple yet profound statement about human nature. In *Confessions*, he wrote, "Thou hast made us for Thyself, O Lord, and our heart is restless until it finds its rest in Thee" (Saint Augustine of Hippo, ca. 400 C.E./1960, entry I.I.1 [Book I, Chapter I, para. 1]).

Being created in the image and likeness of God reflects the ontological reality of relationship. Trinitarian theology presents eternal God as One (essence) in three persons: Father, Son, and Holy Spirit (Libreria Editrice Vaticana, 1994). God is in God's self, relational. The rupture between God and humanity introduced into human nature *original sin*, which is the propensity to turn away from God. Although retaining the fundamental identity of being created in the image and likeness of God, the fall resulted in human nature consisting of conflicting desires for communion with, and independence from, God.

Source(s) of Motivation

In principle, Catholic theology grounds my beliefs. In theory and practice, both psychoanalysis and Catholicism inform my understanding of the complexities of human motivation. Catholic theology and tradition (Libreria Editrice Vaticana, 1994) depict human motivation arising from two competing desires: connection with God and independence from God. Grace received through the Sacraments strengthens motivation for communion with God. Freud (1905/1949, 1911/1958, 1915/1957a) posited that humanity is fundamentally motivated by biological drives, particularly for pleasure. Evolutions in psychoanalysis resulted in a paradigm shift to motivation for relationship. The continuum of psychoanalysis reflects human motivation arising from conscious and unconscious sources, which may be influenced by a complex constellation of biological and relational drives and needs.

How Development Unfolds

Both psychoanalysis and Catholicism contribute to my understanding of development and growth. According to Catholic teaching, physical life begins at the moment of conception and continues until natural death (Libreria Editrice Vaticana, 1994). By receiving grace daily from God, and through particular graces received during the Sacraments, Catholics are equipped in an ongoing way to grow in holiness and wholeness as well as participate in God's work in the world. During Mass, the elements of bread and wine are consecrated, and by God's action, they are transformed into the real presence of Christ. When a Catholic receives the Eucharist, they incorporate Christ into body, soul, and spirit. This incorporation is transformational. In addition to the Sacraments, growth and development also occur during religious education. Psychoanalysis provides a wealth of insight into complex processes related to every aspect of development, including physical, cognitive, moral, spiritual, sexual, and social. Constitutional, environmental, and relational experiences influence, enhance, or impede growth and maturation.

The Workings of the Mind

Catholicism and psychoanalysis are compatible with respect to understanding processes of mental life, so I draw from both sources. In the Catholic tradition, the capacity for thought and moral reasoning sets humanity apart from the rest of God's creation (Libreria Editrice Vaticana, 1994). God's indwelling

Presence, refreshed and renewed through the Sacraments and through Catholic spirituality and education, grows the human mind to increasingly yield to God and participate in God's movements in the world. Often, this growth entails bringing what is hidden into the light. In psychoanalysis, the human mind is the field where conscious and unconscious processes meet. I enjoy contemplating and using the many models and theories that provide useful perspectives for considering the complexity of the human mind as well as the mind–brain–body connection.

Etiology of Psychopathology

Catholic theology informs my fundamental understanding of psychopathology, and psychoanalysis contributes a rich expanse of ways to consider how it manifests in human suffering. At the time of the rupture between God and humanity, all manner of brokenness, sin, sickness, and death entered into human experience. Alienation from God resulted in alienation from self and others. Reconciliation with God through Jesus makes intrapsychic and interpersonal restoration possible. Psychoanalysis provides breadth and depth to my understanding of the limitless constellations of biological, psychological, and environmental factors that result in all manner of psychopathologies.

How Change Occurs: The Move From Futile to Fruitful Suffering

Both Catholicism and psychoanalysis contribute to my view of the change process as a movement from futile to fruitful suffering. According to Catholic tradition, yielding and responding to God's grace, especially in the Sacraments, lead to change and growth (Libreria Editrice Vaticana, 1994). A devotional life of meditation and prayer, education and study, and daily faithfulness to calling/vocation are also sources of grace, growth, and change. Formation and transformation are a process. In psychoanalysis, resolution of internal conflicts, remediation of developmental deficits, and authentic engagement in therapeutic encounters that facilitate interpersonal growth are also the result of a process.

Futile suffering is suffering without awareness or the capacity to love and live with purpose, creativity, and flexibility. Relationships are emotionally impoverished. Patterns of conflict repeat. Attempts to change the outcome are futile and end in failure and despair. Futile suffering is desperate, helpless, and hopeless. The accompanying shame and guilt are an agony. Pope Francis (2016) defined *mercy* as "opening one's heart to wretchedness" (p. 9). I believe this includes having a heart that is open to acknowledging my own wretchedness as well as that of others. I believe that when we encounter our own and others' brokenness, we are most in need of mercy.

Fruitful suffering has purpose. Entering into the depths of interior and interpersonal life, being open to knowing what has been unknown or unknowable, saying what has been unsayable, working through wounds of omission and commission, and grieving what was not and can never be involves suffering that leads to healing, change, and growth. The unfolding and ongoing process of awareness, understanding, working through, and integration is in the presence of another who will bear witness and show mercy and compassion in the midst of uncovering all that could not be known but only carried. This process also occurs in the Presence of an Other who desires healing, restoration, and redemption.

The Analyst–Patient Relationship

Both Catholic theology and psychoanalysis inform my focus on the therapeutic relationship as essential to healing, change, and growth. Because human beings are ontologically relational, meaningfully connecting with God, self, and others is central to Catholic theology and tradition (Libreria Editrice Vaticana, 1994). In psychoanalysis, the therapeutic relationship is the medium of change in the context of moment-to-moment attunement between analyst and patient (Stark, 1999). Relationship is the source of both hurt and healing.

Outcome of Treatment

The words of 2nd-century Church father St. Irenaeus of Lyons simply and profoundly express my prayer, hope, and goal for treatment, which is to become fully alive (Irenaeus of Lyons, ca. 175–189 C.E./2021). Irenaeus declared that to be fully alive glorifies God, and the vision of God holds the key to life. Thriving in life and becoming all God created one to be reflect God's glory to the world. To love God with one's whole heart, soul, mind, and strength and to love one's neighbor as one's self is the telos of Christianity.

My patients will not likely have Irenaeus' words and image in mind when they seek psychotherapy or psychoanalysis. However, experience has taught me that what often prompts someone to seek treatment are isolation, alienation, relational suffering, and inner turmoil that inhibit the capacity to be in life in fruitful and satisfying ways. Treatment outcomes in psychoanalysis include resolution of conflict, the healing of developmental deficits, and increased capacity to engage in healthy, mutual, and reciprocal relationships, which are all important ways to experience being fully alive.

Diversity Engagement

My passion to embrace diversity is inspired by the person and life of Jesus; by past and present exemplars, such as many of the saints as well as contemporary historical heroes, including Reverend Dr. Martin Luther King, Jr.;

and by biblical texts explicitly addressing diversity. The Gospels describe how Jesus sought out and embraced those who were marginalized. He welcomed those who had been rejected because of social class, sex, occupation, or personal history (*New American Standard Bible*, 1971/2020, John 4). In St. Paul's letters, he declared that former lines of division are brought together because, in Christ, whether Jew or Greek, bound or free, male or female, all are included in the family of God; there is no preferential status (*New American Standard Bible*, 1971/2020, Galatians 3:23). The book of Revelation, the last book of the New Testament, describes "a great multitude that no one could count, from every nation, from all tribes and people and languages" (*New American Standard Bible*, 1971/2020, Galatians 7:9) who are one in the body of Christ, the family of God. All of these biblical texts illuminate the expanse of diversity in humanity as well as the elevation of all human beings to a shared and fundamental identity of worth, value, and dignity by virtue of being created by God in God's image and likeness. Catholic tradition (Libreria Editrice Vaticana, 1994) across time has applied these fundamental principles and practices to every human person regardless of individual, cultural, or religious differences.

SIP: A Clinical Method

Theoretical models help me to think about and contextualize my work with patients. Clinical methods guide me in how to engage and intervene with patients. Both Catholicism and psychoanalysis inform the ways I engage in clinical encounters with my patients.

Key Concept: Contemplative Listening

From both Catholic and psychoanalytic traditions, I draw a relational/clinical posture of listening carefully, intently, and without judgment to words, phrases, metaphors, and images. Because communication is more nonverbal than verbal, tone, cadence, body language, and facial expressions are particularly important. As I take in all that patients are communicating, I am also aware of the Presence of God, who knows the complexity and depth of every person. This joint attentive and reflective awareness of temporal and spiritual realities becomes a sacred field within and between.

Key Concept: Embodiment

I embrace Roman Catholic theology that affirms the dignity and worth of all persons (Libreria Editrice Vaticana, 1994). I embrace what Pope John Paul II called "the culture of life" (Ioannes Paulus PP. II, 1995, p. 21) rather than "the culture of death" (p. 12). In *Man and Woman He Created Them: A Theology of the Body*, Pope John Paul II (1997) discussed a range of topics related to embodiment, including sexuality, marriage, celibacy, conception, and man and woman before and after the rupture with God. He emphasized the centrality of our physical bodies as the vessel through which we reflect the image and likeness of God. He made the compelling point that God is made visible to the world through embodiment. One of the implications of this teaching is that attending to the whole person is important in the context of treatment.

Consultation/Intake

Because I believe God is sovereign over life and creation (Libreria Editrice Vaticana, 1994), I am persuaded that God is involved in what draws patients to my practice. I regularly pray for past, current, and prospective patients. Roman Catholic theology regarding Divine sovereignty includes both certainty and mystery (Libreria Editrice Vaticana, 1994). In a treatment context, I embrace the certainty that our paths are crossing for a purpose as well as the mystery of the way(s) this has come about and will unfold. Although patients usually present with a particular symptom or problem, it is often related to a complex constellation of known and unknown physical, psychological, and spiritual factors. Each patient has a unique embodied and embedded life context.

As patients begin to tell their story, there is often a confessional tone to our encounters because they are sharing thoughts, feelings, experiences, memories, fantasies, and dreams that they have never shared with anyone before. I pray for the grace to embody the ministry of presence (Nouwen, 1986) through moment-by-moment attunement (Stark, 1999). As I listen, I am mindful that each patient's life has been and is unfolding in the wider context of the story of God's redemptive love through Jesus and the enlivening, animating presence of the Holy Spirit (Libreria Editrice Vaticana, 1994). This is part of the mystery.

Diagnosis

The *Diagnostic and Statistical Manual of Mental Disorders* (5th ed.; *DSM-5*; American Psychiatric Association, 2013) provides a classification system of disorders and symptoms that I use to guide my assessment of symptoms my patients report. However, the *DSM-5* contributes little to understanding etiology and treatment. The *International Statistical Classification of Diseases and Related Health Problems* (11th ed.; *ICD-11*; World Health Organization, 2019) is often required for managed care reimbursement purposes, so I include this information on statements after I have discussed the matter with my patient. The *Psychodynamic Diagnostic Manual: PDM 2* (Lingiardi & McWilliams, 2017) provides a thick, rich explication of psychological suffering based on both particularity and complexity. The *DSM-5* and *ICD-11* both identify diagnostic categories based on symptom cluster(s). This descriptive information does have a purpose; however, I find it quite problematic when classification of disorders by diagnostic category dictate decisions that prescribe the same treatment for every person with a particular symptom picture. Treatment that preserves and addresses the uniqueness of every person is more consistent with Catholic theology (Libreria Editrice Vaticana, 1994) and with a psychoanalytic sensibility.

Conceptualization

When conceptualizing a patient's suffering, I use a systemic epistemology that identifies individual, interpersonal, and sociocultural/environmental factors that contribute to their problems in living. Individual factors include biology, heredity, temperament, defenses, physical limitations, and personal spirituality. Interpersonal factors include attachment style as well as the nature and scope of relationships with family, friends, partner, spouse, and colleagues. Sociocultural/environmental factors include race; religion; ethnicity; socioeconomic status; education; daily life setting(s); geographic context; country of origin; historical context; religious or other communities; and significant events, such as traumas or natural disasters. These factors are not static in their influence but are in mutual, reciprocal, and dynamic relation, constantly shifting and changing. Internal and external systems are in motion in cycles of tension, collapse, and reorganization. Intervening in any aspect impacts the whole.

Treatment Planning and Goals

When considering treatment plans and goals, I begin by making space in my mind for the mystery of God's creative, restoring movements as they may unfold in the clinical relationship. I have no preconceived idea of how this will take place, nor do I expect that our conversation will explicitly include religion or spirituality. I develop treatment plans and goals collaboratively with my patients, and these inevitably evolve over time. I orient to what my patient desires from treatment and also offer recommendations that I believe are consistent with the patient's long-term goals. I note that there are many clinical approaches, and I am persuaded that understanding the roots of suffering will contribute to alleviation of symptoms. Symptom relief alone may not be lasting (Shedler, 2010).

Course of Treatment

I consider clinical work more of a journey of discovery than a means to a destination. Much of what takes place in the early months of psychoanalysis or psychoanalytic psychotherapy has to do with establishing rapport and a strong working alliance. This is the foundation from which we lean into deeper levels of engagement. Together, my patient and I uncover details about life experiences and discover the intricate workings of their mind, which are often revealed through dreams, free association, transference and countertransference dynamics, and fantasies. Remembering what has been forgotten, connecting threads that have been loose ends, beginning to articulate a life narrative, and pondering together complex meanings of experience are ongoing aspects of the process.

Often, with a treatment and working alliance more firmly established, defenses, impasses, and ruptures begin to emerge. I think it is a reality of the human condition that we long for change and also resist it. I recall a vivid depiction of this in an image of Sisyphus pushing the boulder up the hill, and on the other side of the boulder, he is depicted as pushing it back down the hill. Defenses are in place for a purpose and need to be respected and understood throughout treatment. Ruptures are inevitable because patients need the unknown to be known and because I will, in some way, hurt or offend them. These difficult encounters are the occasion for repair.

During latter weeks, months, or years, prominent themes related to grief and loss usually surface. I find that the ways my patients and I have responded to past endings will emerge in the relationship. Anger, cutoffs, and disappointments will be present to varying degrees. Termination may be a fruitful time of reflecting on change, healing, and growth that has taken place as well as sadness about unrealized hopes. It is an opportunity to experience endings in a different way—as a reality of life that may be talked about with honesty.

For the sake of clarity and discussion, I have presented the course of treatment in phases. In reality, engaging in discovery, contending with defenses, impasses, and ruptures, and processing grief and loss occur in various forms throughout the treatment relationship. In all methods of psychoanalysis, the evolving process presents occasions for new experiences and for modification of the ways the past is carried in our body, soul, and spirit. Working through intrapsychic conflicts (Mode 1; Stark, 1999), developmental deficits (Mode 2; Stark, 1999), and entrenched interpersonal patterns of conflict (Mode 3; Stark, 1999) is what facilitates the alleviation of futile suffering and contribute to healing and growth.

Freud (1930/1961a) believed that through psychoanalysis a person could move from neurotic suffering to ordinary, everyday unhappiness. My Catholic tradition offers a bit brighter picture. A life without suffering is not the promise. What is promised is Divine Presence in the midst of trials, tribulations, and traumas. I have found that communion with God and contemplating the sufferings of Jesus enlarges my capacity to discover meaning in suffering, which significantly contributes to experiencing deep healing and fruitful growth. Through communion and contemplation, I have discovered joy that transcends circumstances. Perspectives related to past, present, and future experiences may be transformed.

My Catholic tradition is a source of hope for me, which, perhaps paradoxically, enables me to enter into the suffering, helplessness, and hopelessness of my patients and remain there as long as is needed. Over the years, I have found that bearing witness to my patients' suffering often enables them to grieve and begin to imagine life beyond the misery and suffering they have endured.

Interventions: An Overview of My Approach
Interventions I use with my patients are informed by an internal reservoir of clinical and spiritual experiences. My work with all patients includes analytic methods of free association and dream interpretation. In addition, I have learned that daydreams, fantasies, and images patients hold in mind or seek out in print or via online sources often reveal deep longings and needs that are outside conscious awareness. Specific interventions I regularly use include clarification, observation, interpretation, integration, and confrontation as well as those that are unique to a patient's religious or spiritual tradition.

Interventions Particular to the Patient's SERT
Depending on my patients' spiritual, existential, religious, and theological (SERT) tradition, I use texts, stories, narratives, principles, and practices that are consistent with their beliefs. Having established during initial intake or consultation whether spirituality or religion is important and has any relevance for them in our work, I intervene accordingly to illuminate understanding of connections among physical, psychological, and spiritual dynamics. I am also attentive to the ways in which religion may be used as a means of protection from unwanted or disavowed affects, memories, or experiences.

Use of Self: Becoming Both the New Good and the Old Bad
When engaging with patients, the way I use myself is informed by the whole range of historic and contemporary psychoanalytic theories and clinical methods, which has been helpfully synthesized by Stark (1999). I am also inspired by the life of Jesus described in the New Testament Gospels.

When my patient needs insight and awareness about unconscious conflicts, I use myself as an observer and interpreter (Mode 1; Stark, 1999). When provision of experiences lacking in early life that have contributed to developmental deficits is needed, I endeavor to be responsive (Mode 2;

Stark, 1999). I am particularly mindful of providing a facilitating environment that includes stability, reliability, constancy, attunement, containment, and a regulating presence to hold overwhelming affects. Being a new good object is typically most resonant with a therapist's personal and professional identity. It is ego-syntonic to be helpful, kind, and compassionate. What is far more difficult is becoming an old bad object. Being misunderstood, accused, rejected, or the focus of rage and anger is ego-dystonic and consequently much more difficult to bear. However, I have discovered that patients need authentic engagement with a sturdy and steady other who can withstand the (re-)enactment of relational dynamics that originated in experiences of any form of abuse. Enactments are necessary to repair destructive cycles so that patients may be free to develop mutual, reciprocal, healthy, and satisfying relationships with others (Mode 3; Stark, 1999). The realization that we hurt our patients is painful as is the process of repair.

As my analyst often reminds me, psychoanalysis is not for the faint of heart (as a patient or as an analyst). To enter into deep and transformational engagement requires insight, patience, constancy, fortitude, humility, forgiveness, nondefensive listening, and the ability to curb the human inclination to retaliate. In the Gospels (Matthew, Mark, Luke, John), Jesus' example of skillfully revealing unconscious motives, His willingness to offer provision of love, acceptance, and care to marginalized persons, and His capacity to authentically engage and bear the frustration, anger, rage, disappointment, disillusionment, and hatred that led to His death inspires me every day.

CASE EXAMPLE: DANIEL–TO MARRY OR BECOME A MONK?

At the time we met, Daniel[2] was in his late 20s. He is Caucasian, male, cisgender, and heterosexual. He was referred to me by a friend of his who happened to know I am Roman Catholic and a psychoanalyst. Daniel is Catholic and wanted a therapist from the same tradition because his faith and spirituality are central to his life. At the time, Daniel was seeking help for three main concerns: his relationship with women, anxiety and panic attacks, and questions about whether to pursue ordained life as a brother

---

[2]Daniel, although not his actual name, is a former patient of mine. I provide enough detail to illustrate key aspects of my spiritually integrative approach, However, I have intentionally left out or disguised certain aspects of our work to protect his privacy and anonymity.

or priest. During our initial phone contact, I listened and prayed silently for discernment. I suggested we meet for a consultation session to mutually discern whether to work together. *Discernment* is a concept from our shared Catholic tradition that involves listening for Divine guidance.

In the course of the consultation, I explained the type of therapy I offer and how it is different from other approaches. Daniel affirmed that he wanted to work in a depth- and insight-oriented way so that he could understand himself better and be more confident in his vocational choices. I recommended we meet at least once a week and twice a week when possible. Our work continued for almost 2 years.

In the early months of treatment, our focus was on Daniel relaying to me the particulars of his early family life, his past and present relationship with his parents and siblings, his past and present relationships with women, his experience of school, his professional life, and his religious and spiritual life as a Catholic. Within the first 6 months, we began to discover links between the here and now and the there and then, and we were increasingly able to find images, words, and metaphors that brought what had been unknown or unsaid to light.

Over the next 12 months or so, we encountered some rocky terrain as dynamics characteristic of his relationships with women emerged in our work. During the final months, we both leaned into the joys of the healing and growth Daniel experienced as well as into the sorrow of saying goodbye. Rather than present a case narrative, I relate themes of our work and provide examples of interventions that represent application of my approach to SIP.

Themes Throughout the Treatment

One of Daniel's chief concerns was his relationships with women, particularly recurrent patterns in dating. He would meet a woman, become very enthusiastic about the relationship, and then begin to feel as though he were in a prison in which he could not think, speak, or act. This pattern had gone on through high school and college until he reached a point of crisis, at which time he experienced a renewal in his Catholic faith and committed to celibacy.

Another theme that continued throughout our work was sexuality. Daniel was introduced to sexual contact at a very young age, not all of it welcome. In elementary school, he engaged in watching pornography and mutual masturbation with a friend. From that time on, viewing pornography became an ongoing struggle.

A third theme that permeated our work was related to Daniel's life as a Catholic. Since his renewal, Daniel maintained a consistent devotional life of prayer and contemplation. He often attended retreats during which he received healing prayer. At the time we met, he had recently moved into a house with several other men who were interested in forming a lay community and developing commitments about life together. Daniel participated actively in the Sacraments of Reconciliation as well as Eucharist at daily or weekly Mass. He also followed the liturgical year, which moves through seasons that are oriented to the life of Jesus. Because of his love for ministry and the Catholic tradition, Daniel was considering ordained life in one of the monastic orders. He knew that painful dating experiences contributed to this inclination. His vision of marriage did not include thriving in life. Discerning between the vocation of marriage and ordained life in a monastic order was an ongoing aspect of our work.

Psychoanalytic Interventions

Daniel was very eager to work in a psychoanalytically oriented way. We usually sat face to face; however, on several occasions he used the couch when he was feeling weary or tired. He also used the couch when he wanted to access deeper sensations, thoughts, or feelings by letting his mind wander and tuning into his body. Although he felt a mix of shame and regret about his actions, he was very honest about his dreams, fantasies, and pornography addiction. During a session early in our work while he was relating some of these painful details, he paused and said, "When you looked at me, you had a piercing gaze. I thought of God looking at me, not looking away. Like God was saying, 'I am not going to reject you.'" I followed up on his use of the word *piercing*: "Is there anything about my gaze that is painful?" He answered, "No, it is that you see me." We would later learn that Daniel was actually ambivalent about being seen and known by a woman.

Throughout our work, when Daniel would describe feeling "helpless and paralyzed," I would invite his thoughts. He frequently associated to his early life, episodes with his father breaking household items, arguments with his parents. He tried to intervene but was yelled at himself. Early on, I sensed Daniel carried a lot in his body. He was often tired, weary, and fatigued. He had a pervasive sense that his fate was decided, and he was helpless to change it. So, we began to track his sensations and perceptions—what and where was he experiencing them in his body during our sessions and throughout the day.

Freud (1923/1961b) noted that the first ego is a body ego, the way we first comprehend our existence and separateness. Because Daniel often felt that emotional boundaries with women were nonexistent or that they did not respect his and because he noticed that it seemed his mind and body faded away when he was relating to particular women, it seemed he lacked a grounding in his existence and identity. This had obvious implications for our relationship, so whenever he described these dynamics in relationship with other women, I would inquire about his experience of our relationship.

As Daniel and I uncovered more and more about the suffering he experienced in trying to relate to women and his thoughts and feelings about marriage, I offered an interpretation that perhaps women, sexuality, and ordained ministry were related. At this point, our work took a turn as we began to explore connections between his struggle between married or monastic life as a vocation and how that related to his sexuality. Throughout his dating life, at no time could Daniel imagine a marriage in which he would feel fully alive and thriving. He continually reverted back to images of self-sacrifice; service became blurred with what began to sound like obliteration of the self. He felt confused trying to parse out self-extinction from giving of self and serving others. Because so much of his suffering was carried in his body, our work was intentionally slower paced so that the dynamic of his mind or body—or both—receding to the background did not overshadow our work. When he did sense this happening, we explored what was happening in the moment.

Daniel needed all that psychoanalysis has to offer in terms of therapeutic engagement. He needed insight, self-awareness, and release of affect with respect to intrapsychic conflicts related to sex and aggression (Mode 1; Stark, 1999). These conflicts emerged when we explored his relationship with his mother, images in fantasy and pornography, his dating life, and our relationship. When this content or process emerged, I would be an observer and interpreter. I would notice with him patterns, phrases, images, metaphors. The "unthought known" (Bollas, 1987, p. 4) could come to conscious awareness and be processed and integrated.

Daniel also needed provision of a stable, reliable, safe, secure relational experience (Mode 2; Stark, 1999) in which he could share his deepest pain, shame, anger, and confusion without fear of rejection or abandonment or the breaking of a fragile maternal other. I was very aware at these times of Daniel's need for a new, good object who would be providing for him rather than "sucking him dry," which was a phrase he used often in connection with dating relationships with women. Daniel's self-esteem and self-cohesion were also undernourished and underdeveloped, so I endeavored to provide experiences of mirroring, idealization, and twinship/being alike (Kohut, 1971, 1984). I realized our shared Catholic tradition was an important source of twinship for him.

Daniel also needed authentic engagement that could withstand the emergence of his rage and anger toward women (Mode 3; Stark). When he spoke of what angered him about women he dated, I would inquire whether he ever felt that in our relationship. On one occasion, we had a rupture over a comment I had made about him not needing to take care of me. He was able to tell me he felt extremely angry. "Yes, you do need me! I pay for you! I own you!" There and then exploded into the here and now. Daniel's fear of needing a woman and the security he gained from feeling more powerful in taking care of them, the allusion to money and his association with paying for sex, and his desire to overpower a woman because he felt chronically overpowered by them: It was all there in living color for us to sort through together—the good, the bad, and the ugly.

SERT-Informed Interventions

Daniel and I shared a common SERT (Catholicism); however, I did not at all assume that meant we experienced our tradition the same way. I was interested to learn all the particulars of Daniel's life as a Catholic. He was eager to share thoughts, feelings, and practices related to his daily devotional and interpersonal life.

Following the Church calendar provided us a way to reflect on seasons of his life that paralleled seasons of the liturgical year. Advent begins the year with a celebration of the coming of Jesus and the anticipation of Jesus' Second Coming. During this season, we would reflect on the ways in which Daniel was desiring, waiting for, or anticipating the Presence of Jesus in an area of his life. Christmas and Epiphany gave us a language to speak of the birth of new discoveries, awareness, and new experiences with God, self, and others. During Lent and Easter week, we often focused on his sorrow related to brokenness and the solace he received through unburdening his heart and spirit with a priest during the Sacrament of Reconciliation. Meditating and reflecting on the sufferings of Jesus offered him comfort as he considered the ways Jesus suffered in His humanity and could therefore be with him in his suffering.

Because I have had an empirical, clinical, and academic interest in the connection between experience of God, self, and others, I would weave into our conversations wonderings and inquiries about what Daniel felt and thought about God's responses to him in the midst of his struggles, especially with pornography. We explored together how Daniel felt as well as what he believed and noted that, at times, these were fairly far apart. Daniel often felt confused, discouraged, ashamed, tired, and frustrated about the patterns in his life; what was motivating him; and how difficult it was for him to imagine ever feeling differently about himself, women, and marriage. As this theme permeated our work, I began to sense some images and words emerging.

One day, I remarked to Daniel that a picture forming in my mind was a mass of tangles, and I asked if this reflected his experience. He readily resonated with the image. I then asked him whether he was aware of the painting that Pope Francis had called Catholic attention to; the painting is entitled, "Mary, Undoer or Untier of Knots." In the Baroque-style painting, the Blessed Mother is shown untying a long cord of knots. Daniel said he had seen it. I then wondered with him what it might be like for him if we held that image, both inviting the intercession of the Blessed Mother as we were about the work of untying the knots of his life. Daniel was very comforted by this image and idea, and our associations would return to it several times over the course of our work.

Other interventions related to the life of saints and mystics who wrote about suffering, such as John of the Cross and Teresa of Avila. Daniel, at times, did feel himself to be in a dark night of the soul and also desired God to illuminate all the areas or rooms of his life. Daniel was often in touch with shame and guilt, particularly related to sexual addictions.

Frequently, I sensed his feelings of wretchedness and introduced the topic of God's mercy. I asked Daniel if he was familiar with the diary of St. Faustina Kowalska (ca. 1920s–1930s/1981) who had detailed her encounters with God as a God of profound mercy. He said that he was familiar with her. I shared my association to *The Chaplet of the Divine Mercy* (a sequence of devotional prayers from p. 476 of Kowalska's diary) and the feelings that weighed down his body, soul, and spirit, and that I wondered if he might be comforted to envision God's deep love and mercy for him. Daniel was comforted by this connection and would often let out deep sighs in response to reflections on God's mercy for him. This was another reference we would return to numerous times.

Jesus as a servant was also in our conversations because of Daniel's confusion about what the Catholic teaching on serving others meant for him. He would remark that Jesus gave his life for others, and should not he do the same? Were boundaries of self-care in relation to others selfish? This came up a number of times, and I would invite him to share his thoughts and feelings. Part of him believed that self-care was good, and he also believed in serving others, but he would get confused trying to sort it out. I made a few observations about Jesus for him to consider. One is that Jesus made clear that he was laying down His life willingly; no one was taking it from Him (*New American Standard Bible*, 1971/2020, John 10:11–18). He was clear about His purpose, and although, in His humanity, He asked, "If it is possible, let this cup pass from me" (*New American Standard Bible*, 1971/2020, Matthew 26:39), it was His choice. I contrasted this with how Daniel often described his serving as dutiful and draining, and how he experienced losing himself in other people. He saw the connection right away.

I also noted that the Gospels describe Jesus as very sure of His identity and purpose. He had a strong sense of self, and from that foundation, He could live the life God called Him to live while on earth. I contrasted this with Daniel and the ways he often felt confused about who he is and how he felt pushed and pulled by other people's expectations of him as well as by an internal critical chorus of voices spouting negative commentary. Daniel readily saw this connection as well. The first time this came up, Daniel said, "Oh! So, this means I should share my thoughts and feelings with others rather than disappearing into the background." "Right!" I replied.

Diversity Considerations

Diversity is a single word that sums up a vast array of human differences, including race, culture, ethnicity, religion, age, natal sex, gender, sexual orientation, education, disabilities, and socioeconomic status; the list could go on. For me, what unites all diversity is commitment to ethics of respect, worth, dignity, and esteem that is a right of all persons by virtue of being created by God. The complexity of diversity is continually expanding as each nuance of human difference is discovered, articulated, and explored at social, religious, empirical, political, and personal levels of experience. In my work as a clinical psychologist and psychoanalyst, I am guided by central principles drawn from my Roman Catholic tradition as well as by the ethics of respect, dignity, worth, and esteem for all persons. I highlight and give examples of how I endeavor to embody and express these principles and ethics in my clinical work with respect to SERT differences.

Extending Mercy to All

My Roman Catholic theological and spiritual beliefs and commitments lead me to hold in mind the reality that "bidden or not bidden, God is present,"[3] and I prayerfully discern how to meaningfully enter into my patients' experience, embodying mercy by opening my heart to know them in all the dimensions of their unique and complex context. Because I am unwaveringly persuaded that Jesus is the face and form of God's mercy to all humanity and because I believe that my embodied presence in the world is the means

---

[3]This quote is often attributed to Carl Gustav Jung, who had the original Latin inscribed on a plaque over the door of his home. It has been discovered that Jung read this in the writings of Erasmus (Gillespie, 2017).

through which I express my vocation in the care of souls, my implicit spiritually integrated approach with all patients is a constant.

What changes is whether and how religion and spirituality are explicitly acknowledged, articulated, or addressed. I ask every new patient whether they were raised in any particular religious or spiritual tradition, whether it is part of their life now, and whether it is important to include their SERT as part of treatment. The responses to these questions inform the ways our clinical encounters unfold.

Engaging With Those of Uncertain or No Religious Belief
When working with patients who do not identify theology, religion, or spirituality as significant in their life, our conversations do not include this language. However, existential questions of meaning and purpose are salient in some way for every patient. I have discovered that many patients who report uncertain or no belief have a painful history with one or more spiritual or religious traditions. Although each person's story is unique, some collision between family, cultural, and religious values led to a crisis of faith that resulted in a drift into uncertainty, liminality, or complete rejection of any religious or spiritual connection. These painful and alienating experiences, memories, and possible traumas become part of all that is remembered, worked through, and integrated into their evolving life narrative.

At other times, I have encountered patients of uncertain or no religious tradition who describe themselves as spiritual, which may refer to a sense of connection to the whole of humanity, feeling at one with nature, or living according to life principles that have no obvious or conscious connection with religion or theology. In all clinical relationships, I orient myself to the ways my patients describe their experience.

I recall a young scientist I worked with some years ago. He presented with a desire to deepen his relationship with a woman he was dating. I engaged with him in the ways I have described, and our conversation did not include any explicit dialogue about religion or spirituality. However, I clearly remember one session: From what seemed like out of the blue, he looked at me and said, "You are a very spiritual person, aren't you?" I was a bit stunned and also intrigued to learn what had led him to that observation. Rather than inquire about the question, for some intuitive reason I responded, "Yes, I am" to which he replied, "I thought so. I can tell." We then went on to explore his comment. In the moment, I am not always entirely sure why I intervene in a particular way. In his case, I realized I intuitively responded to his tendency to question his perception of reality because he received little affirmation and validation in early life. In the moment, it was important to provide a new experience (Mode 2; Stark, 1999) and what Aron and Atlas (2019) would refer to as an affirming and creative generative enactment.

Engaging With Those From Christian Traditions Different From My Own
At the conclusion of the Second Vatican Council, the Church's commitment to ecumenical dialogue was reaffirmed and further defined (Abbott, 1966). The principles I embrace and desire to embody that relate most particularly to my clinical work are humility, charity, respect, genuine desire to understand different Christian traditions and to be enriched by them, acknowledgment of the value of diverse Christian customs, and affirmation of the historical contributions of all branches of Christianity. These ethics inform and infuse my desire to understand each patient as an individual. Our relationship may lead me to adopt the patient's language, or we may develop a lingua franca that bridges our shared, although distinct, Christian experience. Although we have Christian faith in common, I make no assumptions that I know about a patient's particular context or experience even if I happen to be familiar with their church or denominational affiliation.

Engaging With Those From Religions Different From My Own
In terms of interfaith or interreligious dialogue, I embrace and desire to embody the values articulated at the close of Vatican II, which were humility, genuine curiosity, and respect for each religion's honest search for God (Abbott, 1966). Productive dialogue is the fruit of those within each religion being rooted in their particular faith beliefs while simultaneously remaining open and receptive to others. Helping one another grow closer to God and be more compassionate toward humanity were identified as superordinate goals. Cooperatively engaging with those of other religions in preserving human dignity and addressing social ills are ways to build bridges of respect and understanding. These principles, values, and ethics inform my engagement with patients from religious traditions different from my own.

I was asked to consult on a case involving a young Muslim man who was seen in the clinic where I was interning. He had a history of persistent mental illness and was having troubling hallucinations and delusions. One of the staff psychiatrists contacted me, saying, "I think I remember learning you have a specialty or interest in religion, so I am wondering if you have any thoughts about this case." I was eager for the opportunity to help this troubled young man and perhaps advocate for taking religious beliefs seriously. After hearing the particulars of his current suffering, I offered observations and recommendations. I suggested that those caring for him discover whether he was attending a local mosque and what response or reaction members of the community had to his illness. If the community was supportive and kind, I recommended they ask the young man whether he would like them to consult with the Imam at his Mosque to explore ways they could partner in helping him. As to his hallucinations and delusions, I noted that these are highly contextual and suggested we approach understanding them in light of his Muslim faith. As a starting point, I related to the psychiatrist the five pillars of Islam: profession of faith, prayer five times daily, alms giving to the poor, fasting during Ramadan, and pilgrimage to Mecca. We explored whether the content of his hallucinations and delusions might, in some way, relate to desires, longings, hopes, anxieties, concerns, or fears he had about his ability to be a faithful Muslim. All of the recommendations I offered were warmly received by the attending psychiatrist, who planned to relay them to the treatment team. I was delighted to collaborate with other professionals about the importance of patients' faith.

CONCLUSION

I am grateful for the opportunity given to me by the editors of this book to participate in this meaningful conversation, which has begun through these chapters and hopefully will continue in other contexts. Leaning deeper into the richness of diversity is being recognized across every sector of American society and around the world. In the spirit of Vatican II and the commitment to ecumenical and interfaith dialogue, I pray that conversations between members of every faith may continue in an open and respectful way so that all may feel welcome at the table of our shared humanity.

REFERENCES

Abbott, W. M. (Ed.). (1966). *The documents of Vatican II* (Very Rev. Msgr. J. Gallagher, Trans.). American Press.

Akhtar, S. (2008). *The crescent and the couch: Cross-currents between Islam and psychoanalysis*. Jason Aronson.

American Psychiatric Association. (2013). *Diagnostic and statistical manual of mental disorders* (5th ed.). https://doi.org/10.1176/appi.books.9780890425596

Aquinas, St. Thomas. (1981). *Summa theologica* (Vols. 1–5; English Dominican Province, Trans.). Christian Classics. (Original work published ca. 1265–1273)

Aron, L. (2004). God's influence on my psychoanalytic vision and values. *Psychoanalytic Psychology, 21*(3), 442–451. https://doi.org/10.1037/0736-9735.21.3.442

Aron, L., & Atlas, G. (2019). Dramatic dialogue: Dreaming & drama in contemporary clinical practice. *Psychoanalytic Perspectives, 16*(3), 249–271. https://doi.org/10.1080/1551806X.2019.1653660

Aron, L., & Henik, L. (Eds.). (2010). *Answering a question with a question: Contemporary psychoanalysis and Jewish thought*. Academic Studies Press.

Augustine of Hippo, St. (1960). *The confessions of Saint Augustine* (J. K. Ryan, Trans.). Image Books. (Original work published ca. 400 C.E.)

Bland, E. D., & Strawn, B. D. (Eds.). (2014). *Christianity and psychoanalysis: A new conversation*. InterVarsity Press.

Bollas, C. (1987). *The shadow of the object: Psychoanalysis of the unthought known*. Columbia University Press.

Bordoni, L. (2020, September 4). Mother Teresa: A saint for all. *Vatican News*. https://www.vaticannews.va/en/church/news/2020-09/saint-mother-teresa-kolkata-annivesary-canonization.html

Brokaw, B. F., & Edwards, K. J. (1994). The relationship of God image to object relations development. *Journal of Psychology and Theology, 22*(4), 352–371. https://doi.org/10.1177/009164719402200420

Cooper-White, P. (2018). *Old and dirty gods: Religion, antisemitism, and the origins of psychoanalysis*. Routledge/Taylor & Francis.

Darwin, C. (1859). *On the origin of species by means of natural selection*. John Murray.

De Carolis, A. (2019, December 21). Pope to the Curia: Changes are necessary to better serve humanity. *Vatican News*. https://www.vaticannews.va/en/pope/news/2019-12/pope-to-the-curia-changes-are-necessary-to-better-serve-humanit.html

Dobbs, T. M. (2009). *Faith, theology, and psychoanalysis: The life and thought of Harry S. Guntrip*. James Clarke & Company.

Fairbairn, W. R. D. (1952). *Psychoanalytic studies of the personality*. Basic Books.

Fayek, A. (2004). Islam and its effect on my practice of psychoanalysis. *Psychoanalytic Psychology, 21*(3), 452–457. https://doi.org/10.1037/0736-9735.21.3.452

Foster, R. J. (1998). *Streams of living water: Celebrating the great traditions of Christian faith*. HarperSanFrancisco.

Francis, Bishop of Rome. (2015, April 11). *Misericordiae vultus: Bull of indiction of the extraordinary jubilee of mercy*. http://www.vatican.va/content/francesco/en/bulls/documents/papa-francesco_bolla_20150411_misericordiae-vultus.html

Freud, S. (1949). Three essays on sexuality. In J. Strachey (Ed. & Trans.), *The standard edition of the complete psychological works of Sigmund Freud* (Vol. 7, pp. 123–246). The Hogarth Press. (Original work published 1905)

Freud, S. (1952). The interpretation of dreams. In J. Strachey (Ed. & Trans.), *The standard edition of the complete psychological works of Sigmund Freud* (Vols. 4–5). The Hogarth Press. (Original work published 1900)

Freud, S. (1957a). Instincts and their vicissitudes. In J. Strachey (Ed. & Trans.), *The standard edition of the complete psychological works of Sigmund Freud* (Vol. 14, pp. 117–140). The Hogarth Press. (Original work published 1915)

Freud, S. (1957b). Leonardo Da Vinci and a memory of his childhood. In J. Strachey (Ed. & Trans.), *The standard edition of the complete psychological works of Sigmund Freud* (Vol. 11, pp. 57–138). The Hogarth Press. (Original work published 1910)

Freud, S. (1958). Formulation on the two principles of mental functioning. In J. Strachey (Ed. & Trans.), *The standard edition of the complete psychological works of Sigmund Freud* (Vol. 12, pp. 215–226). The Hogarth Press. (Original work published 1911)

Freud, S. (1961a). Civilization and its discontents. In J. Strachey (Ed. & Trans.), *The standard edition of the complete psychological works of Sigmund Freud* (Vol. 21, pp. 57–146). The Hogarth Press. (Original work published 1930)

Freud, S. (1961b). The ego and the id. In J. Strachey (Ed. & Trans.), *The standard edition of the complete psychological works of Sigmund Freud* (Vol. 19, pp. 1–66). The Hogarth Press. (Original work published 1923)

Freud, S. (1961c). The future of an illusion. In J. Strachey (Ed. & Trans.), *The standard edition of the complete psychological works of Sigmund Freud* (Vol. 21, pp. 1–56). The Hogarth Press. (Original work published 1927)

Freud, S. (1962–1966). *The standard edition of the complete psychological works of Sigmund Freud* (Vols. 1–24; J. Strachey, Ed. & Trans.). The Hogarth Press.

Gillespie, J. P. (2017, November 8). Vocatus atque non vocatus Deus aderit [Bidden or unbidden, God is present; Blog post]. The Church of St. Albert the Great. https://www.saintalbertthegreat.org/content.cfm?page_content=blogs_include.cfm&blog_id=383

Greenberg, J. R., & Mitchell, S. A. (1983). *Object relations in psychoanalytic theory.* Harvard University Press. https://doi.org/10.2307/j.ctvjk2xv6

Guntrip, H. (1971). *Psychology for ministers and social workers* (3rd ed. rev.). Allen & Unwin.

Hoffman, M. (2004). From enemy combatant to strange bedfellow: The role of religious narratives in the work of W.R.D. Fairbairn and D. W. Winnicott. *Psychoanalytic Dialogues, 14*(6), 769–804. https://doi.org/10.1080/10481881409348806

Hoffman, M. T. (2010). *Toward mutual recognition: Relational psychoanalysis and the Christian narrative.* Routledge.

Ioannes Paulus PP. II. (1995). *The gospel of life: Evangelium vitae* [Encyclical letter]. http://www.vatican.va/content/john-paul-ii/en/encyclicals/documents/hf_jp-ii_enc_25031995_evangelium-vitae.html

Irenaeus of Lyons. (2021). *Against heresies* (J. J. Wales, Ed.; A. Roberts & W. H. Rambaut, Eds. & Trans.). Christian Classics. (Original work published ca. 175–189 C.E.)

John of the Cross, St. (2003). *Dark night of the soul* (E. A. Peers, Ed. & Trans.; from the critical edition of P. Silverio de Santa Teresa). Dover Publications. (Original work published ca. 16th century)

Julian of Norwich. (1974). *The revelations of divine love of Julian of Norwich* (J. Walsh, Trans.). Abbey Press. (Original work published 1373)

Kirkpatrick, L. A., & Shaver, P. R. (1990). Attachment theory and religion: Childhood attachments, religious beliefs, and Conversion. *Journal for the Scientific Study of Religion, 29*(3), 315–334. https://doi.org/10.2307/1386461

Klein, M. (1964). *Contributions to psychoanalysis.* McGraw-Hill.

Kohut, H. (1971). *The analysis of the self.* International Universities Press.

Kohut, H. (1984). *How does analysis cure?* University of Chicago Press. https://doi.org/10.7208/chicago/9780226006147.001.0001

Kowalska, F. (1981). *Divine mercy in my soul: Diary of Saint Maria Faustina Kowalska* (G. H. Pearce, Trans.). Marian Press. (Original work published ca. 1920s–1930s)

Libreria Editrice Vaticana. (1994). *Catechism of the Catholic Church.* Liguori Publications.

Lingiardi, V., & McWilliams, N. (Eds.). (2017). *Psychodynamic diagnostic manual: PDM-2* (2nd ed.). Guilford Press.

Mother Teresa. (1995). *A simple path* (compiled by L. Vardey). Ballantine Books.

National Public Radio. (2013, March 13). *Transcript: Pope Francis' first speech as Pontiff.* https://www.npr.org/2013/03/13/174224173/transcript-pope-francis-first-speech-as-pontiff

New American Standard Bible. (2020). NASB Online. https://www.literalword.com (Original work published 1971)

Noun, F. (2016, September 2). Mother Teresa, the war in Lebanon, and the rescue of 100 orphans and children with disabilities. *AsiaNews.it.* http://www.asianews.it/news-en/Mother-Teresa,-the-war-in-Lebanon-and-the-rescue-of-100-orphans-and-children-with-disabilities-38470.html.

Nouwen, H. J. M. (1986). *Reaching out: The three movements of the spiritual life.* Image Books.

Pargament, K. I. (2007). *Spiritually integrated psychotherapy: Understanding and addressing the sacred.* Guilford Press.

Parker, S. E. (2012). *Winnicott and religion.* Jason Aronson.

Pilkington, E. (2013, September 19). Pope Francis sets out vision for more gay people and women in "new" church. *The Guardian.* https://www.theguardian.com/world/2013/sep/19/pope-francis-vision-new-catholic-church

Pope Francis. (2016). *The name of God is mercy: A conversation with Andrea Tornielli* (O. Stansky, Ed. & Trans.). Random House.

Pope John Paul II. (1997). *Man and woman: He created them: A theology of the body* (M. Waldstein, Trans.). Libreria Editrice Vaticana.

Rizzuto, A.-M. (1979). *The birth of the living God: A psychoanalytical study.* University of Chicago Press.

Rizzuto, A.-M. (1998). *Why did Freud reject God? A psychodynamic interpretation.* Yale University Press.

Rizzuto, A.-M. (2004). Roman Catholic background and psychoanalysis. *Psychoanalytic Psychology, 21*(3), 436–441. https://doi.org/10.1037/0736-9735.21.3.436

Rizzuto, A.-M. (2009). One hundred years after Freud declared that religion was a universal obsessional neurosis. In J. A. Belzen (Ed.), *Changing the scientific study of religion: Beyond Freud? Theoretical, empirical, and clinical studies from psychoanalytic perspectives* (pp. 35–55). Springer. https://doi.org/10.1007/978-90-481-2540-1_2

Safran, J. D. (2003). (Ed.). *Psychoanalysis and Buddhism: An unfolding dialogue.* Wisdom Publications.

Sanness, J. (1979). *The Nobel Peace Prize 1979, Mother Teresa: Award ceremony speech* [Transcript]. The Nobel Prize. https://www.nobelprize.org/prizes/peace/1979/ceremony-speech/

Shedler, J. (2010). The efficacy of psychodynamic psychotherapy. *American Psychologist, 65*(2), 98–109. https://doi.org/10.1037/a0018378

Society of the Little Flower. (n.d.). *The greatest saint of modern times!* http://www.thelittleflower.org/MODERN%20TIME.htm

Sollier, J. (1908). The communion of saints. In *The Catholic encyclopedia* (Vol. 4). Robert Appleton Company.

Sorenson, R. L. (2004a). Kenosis and alterity in Christian spirituality. *Psychoanalytic Psychology, 21*(3), 458–462. https://doi.org/10.1037/0736-9735.21.3.458

Sorenson, R. L. (2004b). *Minding spirituality.* The Analytic Press.

Stark, M. (1999). *Modes of therapeutic action: Enhancement of knowledge, provision of experience, and engagement in relationship.* Jason Aronson.

Stolorow, R. D., Atwood, G. E., & Brandchaft, B. (Eds.). (1994). *The intersubjective perspective*. Jason Aronson/Rowan & Littlefield.

Teresa of Avila, St. (1961). *Interior castle*. (E. A. Peers, Ed. & Trans.). Doubleday. (Original work published 1577)

Thérèse of Lisieux. (1975). *Story of a soul: The autobiography of St. Thérèse of Lisieux* (3rd ed.; J. Clark, Trans.). ICS Publications. (Original work published 1898)

Tisdale, T. C., Key, T. L., Edwards, K. J., Brokaw, B. F., Kemperman, S. R., Cloud, H., Townsend, J., & Okamoto, T. (1997). Impact of treatment on God image and personal adjustment, and correlations of God image to personal adjustment and object relations development. *Journal of Psychology and Theology, 25*(2), 227–239. https://doi.org/10.1177/009164719702500207

Vaidyanathan, T. G., & Kripal, J. J. (2002). (Eds.). *Vishnu on Freud's desk: A reader in psychoanalysis and Hinduism*. Oxford University Press.

Winfield, N. (2020, November 11). Pope Francis vows to end sexual abuse after McCarrick report. *AP News*. https://apnews.com/article/sexual-abuse-by-clergy-sexual-abuse-pope-francis-prayer-17191e15292dff26fae1fe01739d92d1

Winnicott, D. W. (1965). *The maturational process and the facilitating environment: Studies in the theory of emotional development*. The Hogarth Press and The Institute of Psycho-Analysis.

Winnicott, D. W. (1971). *Playing and reality*. Tavistock Publications.

Winnicott, D. W. (1975). *Through paediatrics to psycho-analysis*. The Hogarth Press and The Institute of Psycho-Analysis.

Wolman, B. B. (1995). *Psychoanalysis and Catholicism*. Jason Aronson.

World Health Organization. (2019). *International statistical classification of diseases and related health problems* (11th ed.). https://icd.who.int/

Wright, R., Jones, P., & Strawn, B. D. (2014). Tradition-based integration. In E. D. Bland & B. D. Strawn (Eds.), *Christianity and psychoanalysis: A new conversation* (pp. 37–54). InterVarsity Press.

PART **II** SPIRITUALLY
INTEGRATED
PSYCHOTHERAPY
WITH SPECIFIC
DIVERSITY
DYNAMICS

9

APPROACHING INTERSECTIONS OF SPIRITUALITY, RELIGION, AND NONTRADITIONAL GENDER IDENTITIES IN PSYCHOTHERAPY

RUBEN A. HOPWOOD

This chapter highlights clinical work with gender diverse people and the intersections of nontraditional gender identity, religion, and spirituality with the goal to support healing, restoration, and resilience. This work includes restoration of relationships with whatever or whomever the individual considers holy. Case examples are used for illustration.[1] I begin with definitions to help orient the reader and then provide a description of my approach to spiritually integrated psychotherapy (SIP) and how it is informed by my context, spiritual, and religious traditions.

DEFINITIONS

The following descriptions of nontraditional gender identities and the concepts of religion and spirituality are of necessity short and inexhaustive. Concepts and terminology represent current conceptualizations and understanding

---

[1]All cases are composites of multiple people. All identifying information, names, and situations are altered to protect privacy. Any resemblance to a singular person is coincidental and unintended.

https://doi.org/10.1037/0000276-010
Spiritual Diversity in Psychotherapy: Engaging the Sacred in Clinical Practice,
S. J. Sandage and B. D. Strawn (Editors)

while recognizing that gender identity, gender diversity, and developmental research and categories are not static across time (Zosuls et al., 2011).

Nontraditional Gender Identities: Gender Diversity

"Gender diverse," "transgender/trans," and "nonbinary" are a few terms within an evolving lexicon referring to a constellation of individuals for whom their sex assigned at birth does not correctly or completely describe their internally experienced gender. Traditionally, a person is expected to experience congruence between sex assigned at birth (e.g., male or female) and gender identity (e.g., man or woman). Within U.S. culture, this experience is also commonly expected to be constrained only to binary male or female options. For a small percentage of people, their sex assigned at birth—based solely on a visual inspection of the infant's genitals—may not align with their experienced and internal gender identity (Mueller et al., 2017). Sex designation of male or female is assigned at birth irrespective of the actual chromosomal/genetic sex of an individual. The sex assigned by genital appearance may be unrelated to, opposite, or unable to be defined by, typical sex designations[2] (Blackless et al., 2000).

It is clear when we learn more about variations in genetic sex how tenuous the connection is between visible genitals, chromosomal sex, and gender identity. So, although sex assigned at birth based on the appearance of external genitalia is strongly correlated to genetic sex and gender identity, genital configuration by itself is not causative of genetics or gender identity (Goldstein et al., 2017). There is no absolute relationship between them, and the belief that genitals alone determine gender and/or sex (e.g., essentialism) becomes impossible to sustain when faced with the reality of human biologic complexity.

Gender diverse individuals may or may not adopt specific descriptive adjectives (labels) that signal their nontraditional experiences of gender identity related to sex assigned at birth. When used, identity terms may include "trans," "trans* [trans-star]," "transgender," "transsexual," "nonbinary," "gender queer," "two-spirit," "neutrois," "gender neutral," "gender fluid," "gender expansive," "gender awesome," and many others. People who do not experience gender incongruence with their assigned sex may be called

---

[2]To learn more about intersex conditions or disorders of sex development, see the Intersex Society of North America website (https://isna.org); the website for InterAct: Advocates for Intersex Youth (https://interactadvocates.org); and Blackless et al. (2000), Richter-Appelt (2008), and Rodriguez and Follins (2012).

cisgender or nontransgender. There is no one way to experience gender and no singular way to manage the experience of gender incongruence or gender dysphoria (Hopwood, 2018).

Religion and Spirituality

Spirituality and religion have been defined a myriad of ways over time. It is beyond the scope of this chapter to examine the many understandings and expressions of the world's religions and spiritualities (Barnes, 2011). Spirituality is commonly associated with activities, such as meditation, prayer, silence, and ritual behaviors, that people may describe as helping them feel connected to something larger, to other people, or to life more globally and that may or may not be part of a formal religion or religious community activity. Religion is commonly associated with specific or organized and named groups (e.g., Christian, Jewish, Buddhism, Sikh, Islam) and their shared rituals; structured gatherings; formal or informal tenets of belief; and moral rules, behaviors, and restrictions. Sometimes spirituality takes on a colloquial meaning of experiences that are "pure" or "free" from the constraints or rules of religion. Some individuals may separate spirituality from religion to distance themselves from negative experiences with religious communities, for example, by saying, "I'm spiritual, not religious." I resist the cultural tendency in postmodern Western thought to pit religion as an all-bad, alienating, organized institution of rules and codified ideologies against spirituality as an all-good, liberating, internal, individualized, unboundaried, and illuminating experience of pure awe and wonder. In this chapter, I hold in tension religion and spirituality as inseparable, overlapping, and interrelated.

The constructs of religion and spirituality are complex and interrelated with the human tendency to seek understanding, meaning, and purpose in life. Religion and spirituality can offer support and enhance resilience for many people. Both are shown in psychological research jointly to also have positive effects on outcomes of health and well-being in lesbian, gay, bisexual, transgender, queer, nonstraight, and gender diverse groups (LGBTQ+; Rosenkrantz et al., 2016). My main concern in this chapter, however, is addressing the negative impact of religion and spirituality on health and well-being of gender diverse people compared with people who experience traditional gender identities (e.g., cisgender; Levy & Lo, 2013; Rodriguez & Follins, 2012). Clinically addressing the negative effects on gender diverse people through SIP includes challenges and opportunities for improved well-being.

COMMON PROBLEMS

Effective SIP, indeed, effective mental health care, is limited—if not prevented—by avoiding the existential concerns and influence on overall health of cultural and personal spirituality and religious beliefs. The clinician's unexamined religious and spiritual beliefs about human purpose, meaning, and belonging (e.g., existential) can contribute to suffering and insider–outsider dynamics that harm transgender and nonbinary people (Oswald, 2001). In this chapter, I present vignettes of common problems that arise in clinical work with gender diverse people around misalignments of stated beliefs and values with behaviors and attitudes. I describe self-reflective questions and treatment path decisions I used to identify personal and client biases, and I recenter on visible and invisible connections between gender diversity and religious and spiritual pain.

The approach to clinical problems I present in this chapter can be adapted to other spiritual and religious traditions and is not meant to be exclusive to only one religion or theological set of beliefs. I, however, situate my discussion primarily within the religious tradition with which I have the personal history and academic qualifications to speak in a reasonably informed manner. I speak from my own location as a White, male-identified, non-Trinitarian Christian and Unitarian Universalist while I invite myself and others to engage in critical self-reflection on the religious and theological traditions and systems that influence and inform my/our overt and implicit attitudes and actions.

MANAGEMENT OF VISIBLE AND INVISIBLE CONTEXTS IN SIP

My context influences my practice of SIP. My context—my *self*—is, in fact, my only means to engage with others. My realities and experience combine in ways that are not easily disentangled or entirely disengaged from my clinical practice and the lens through which I listen and interpret others' narratives. I experience visible and invisible privileges—earned and unearned—power and powerlessness, existing together, overlapping and intertwined, and moving together like a ball of felted wool fibers—inseparable.

Context

I am the youngest of five children, one who died before my birth. I was raised by a father who was a Presbyterian minister, county welfare department director, and former parole officer in the rural northern Midwest, and a mother, herself a preacher's child, who was a social worker in a state hospital for those with intellectual and developmental disabilities in the 1960s, 1970s, and early 1980s. In my family are many Protestant ministers and missionaries in myriad traditions. By age 25, I had personally been a member of Presbyterian, Methodist, Southern Baptist, a nondenominational Pentecostal, Metropolitan Community, and Roman Catholic churches, and I had attended many other worshipping communities. By age 34, I had been rejected for ordination from one denomination because of my sexual orientation and another because of my non-Trinitarian (i.e., "heretical") Christian theology, all while being simultaneously affirmed by these same religious authorities as having been "called to ministry." I am theistic in my beliefs and orientation to my life, purpose, and responsibilities. I have experienced the effects of having identities outside the dominant religious, spiritual, and societal groups and have worked to create healing, value, purpose, and meaning within compassionate relationships of accountability, humility, and vulnerability.

I am Northern European by heritage, white-skinned, descended directly from people who arrived on the *Mayflower* as part of the uninvited colonization of the North American continent, college educated, a licensed psychologist, and middle class by national definition—although I live in subsidized housing, existing significantly below the median income in my geographic area despite my race, education, and gender. Along with my doctoral degree in psychology and religious studies, I have a graduate degree in Christian theology (Master of Divinity, or MDiv) focused on Judaic studies and social ethics from a United Methodist seminary. My spouse is Jewish, we have twins, and my family and I are active members of a Unitarian Universalist congregation. I identify as being part of gender diverse, queer, *and* straight communities.

Visible Privilege

Visible privileges arise from my race, male gender presentation, and, at times, from my social class and education, although the latter are not automatically visible. The most profound privilege I have is the ability to be unaware of my privileges or to hide within them and remain ignorant of disparities between my location and that of other people. The ability to be unaware of or hide within privilege conflicts with my beliefs and values while it also is reinforced by the dominant culture and by some psychotherapeutic traditions and approaches. However, in my worldview, healing relationships call for open engagement with another. I use this tension between awareness of and hiding within privilege to explore problematic relationships to roles I and my clients, by turn, comply with and resist.

Inhibition of Care

My visible privilege affects SIP and relationships to other people based on attributes whether invited, true, within my control, conscious, positive, or negative. For example, I answered a call from someone seeking supports for gender-affirming treatment. My male name and lower tone of voice became the "visible" context that the caller added to privileges she assumed I had (e.g., Whiteness), which then got in the way of my ability to offer, or her ability to receive, care. The caller yelled back to my offer of support and resources: "Why does a f—ing *White man* think he can help me?!" In that moment, I represented the systemic oppressive power in our culture. She could not imagine I would be any different than those who had already harmed her—men, White people, a "male" Deity, and so on. Her pain, worn as anger, worked to shield her from any potential harm I might inflict. Sadly, it also worked to inhibit her hearing about support available to her. She was unable to engage in even a cursory relationship with me on a telephone. The wounds were too deep to accept the potential risk from another White male in a position of power over her pathway to healing. Recognizing and respecting how one's context may limit or inhibit engagement in SIP is crucial. This is part of the humility necessary to engage in SIP.

Response and Responsibility

Visible or contextual privilege invites response and responsibility. Client responses to visible and assumed clinician privileges and the wounding our privileges represent may be masked or may appear overtly, as illustrated by one client at our first meeting. As she entered the room for a group I was coleading, she stated, "I don't want to work with you! I saw that 'MDiv' after your name, and I don't want *anything* to do with you or your religion!"

I continually grapple with how to moderate the effect of my context on others. I intentionally do not hide my theological degree from people despite it not being a clinical degree. I have learned it needs to be visible to reduce some of the potential harm if clients learn about it after we are in a clinical relationship. If I do not lead with the degree visible and they learn about it later, it is experienced too often as an ambush by another religious person, and my hiding that aspect of my context becomes weaponized inside them regardless of my intent. If I render it visible, I can sometimes provide an experience that partially corrects past wounds—that enables a degree of religious and spiritual healing. This is what happened with the client in the group. She was able to identify her own preemptive rejection of all religious people as harmful and was willing to take a cautious instead of wholesale rejecting approach in the future.

I am unable to eliminate most of my context, such as my race, education, religious upbringing, social class, sexuality, and gender. What I *am* able to change is my *way* of being—my behaviors and my attitudes—in response to my context and its impact on others. In my clinical work, I focus on openly creating nonharmful relationships. This necessitates attention and responsiveness to the negative effects on others from both my personal behaviors and the global effects of sexism, racism, religious discrimination, elitism, classism, heterosexism, ableism, and cisgenderism (e.g., prejudice against gender diverse people).

Assumptions of Harm

Clients may create narratives based in old, yet raw, wounds. Sometimes, on the basis of my visible identities, people assume my intention is to cause religiously based harm to LGBTQ people, to women, or to people of color. For example, based on experiences from her past with theologically educated people, the client who was upset with my MDiv degree voiced suspicion that I was merely posing as an LGBTQ-affirming clinician so that I could inflict spiritual harm, judgment, and shame as well as attempt to force covert conversion therapy on her.

Spiritual and religious harm may create uniquely painful wounds because of the existential nature of religious condemnation and rejection. The existential harm arises from the implication or the claim that religious judgment *is* direct rejection/abandonment of the individual by God. The resulting woundedness is otherworldly, supernatural, and outside one's control, and may include intense guilt and sadistic images of eternal inflictions of harm and suffering. I understood the client's reaction to my theological degree, and reactions like this by others, as a sort of religious and spiritual posttraumatic stress response. It is risky for someone who has experienced religious and spiritual (e.g., "Divine") rejection to trust another person who may use their power to judge them "good" or "bad" in the name of God or some deity.

Transparency in my SIP practice includes a preemptive response to commonly assumed intentions of harm with assurances that I have no agenda to influence clients to adopt or reject any particular belief systems or religious practices. This responsive and responsible approach openly acknowledges the potential for harm and abuse of power that exists while it makes a commitment to humility and respect of the client's context. Humility includes acknowledging and expressing compassion and shared sorrow—not pity—for any harm done to a person in the name of religion or God.

Self-Protection. It is not uncommon to encounter initially aggressive or off-putting tactics or prickliness from clients meant to protect them from potential emotional or physical violence, or to intimidate and neutralize threats preemptively. The prickles are indicators of hidden wounds and of vulnerability too intense to manage; it is suffering turned outward for protection in response to visible threat (e.g., the noticed real or presumed privileges of the clinician). My response to this spiritual and religious suffering is offering compassionate respect and reaching behind the pain in word and deed to say, "I see you. You are safe and respected here, and I will listen to you without judgment."

Invisibility. In working with gender diverse people, compassion, safety, and respect start with knowing/seeing who is in front of you and reflecting their identity back to them without excuses. Seeing a person means asking from the first contact who they are—what name and what pronouns they use—and then using their correct name and pronouns when talking with or about them. Assumptions about client identities is the most common barrier to effective treatment that gender diverse people experience. I cannot imagine providing treatment without knowing who is there with me in the room, and I cannot know without asking. Gender diverse clients are less likely to volunteer information about their nontraditional gender identity as a result of historically high rates of discrimination and mistreatment of them by health care providers (James et al., 2016). Treatment offered to an anonymous or hidden other is meaningless at best and has the potential to actively harm the client because the clinician cannot offer relevant help without knowing who the client says they are.

Collusion. Gender identity is not inherently visible. Disclosure of a nontraditional gender identity or history is not inherently welcome or safe. The clinician must inquire into any possible marginalized identities, including gender identity, to provide effective SIP to a whole person. The quandary, however, is that it can be self-protective for a client to hide within the privilege of assumed cisgender identity to avoid possible rejection or harm from the clinician. This situation necessitates awareness by clinicians that to ask about a client's gender identity when the clinician has nothing to lose personally (i.e., is cisgender, or assumed to be) is a tremendous privilege and is a position of power over the more vulnerable client. However, *not* asking *all* clients about their identities (e.g., gender, sexuality, ethnicity, spirituality) reveals a provider's bias and confirms to gender diverse clients that it is safer to stay invisible in treatment with *this* therapist. Forgetting or rationalizing why one does not ask about gender identity may be a way of hiding within the privilege being cisgender, the clinical role, or discomfort around challenging one's assumptions or feelings of inadequacy.

Clinicians hold the power in the room and the responsibility to be proactive in asking about gender and other identities to relieve client assumptions and fears about clinical harm. Assurances of the intention not to harm must be explicit along with an invitation for people to disclose new or shifting information about themselves without shame in the future. Asking who the person is, while also leaving room for the person to change how they experience themselves, expresses graciousness and creates safety. Asking can be as basic as introducing oneself (e.g., "Hello, I am Dr. Hopwood") and one's pronouns (e.g., "I use he/him pronouns") at the initial visit or contact. This is followed by asking all clients what name they wish to be called (e.g., "What do you want me to call you?" and "What pronouns do you use?") and asking if clients have any concerns or questions about their gender on registration forms.

Invisible Privilege and Discrimination

Invisible privilege and experiences of discrimination also influence my approach to SIP. A felt sense from spiritual and religious experiences of being accompanied (i.e., having someone with you for support or comfort in tough times) informs how I accompany people in SIP as they struggle with creating or finding meaning, and belonging, and as they build a personal sense of sacred self-worth.

Powerlessness
Experiences of powerlessness—transphobia, sexism, heterosexism, cissexism, sexual harassment, assault, homelessness, poverty, disability, and religious condemnation—connect invisibly with my visible privileges. The simultaneous intersection of contradictory invisible realities can be complex and difficult to integrate into clinical roles and cultural contexts. Their invisibility makes them challenging to describe; suspect when disclosed; and, at times, rejected as made-up defensive or one-upmanship maneuvers. This complexity is illuminated when hearing similar experiences to my own from some clients. The impact of invisible experiences of health inequities, medical mistreatment, loss of meaningful relationships, fear of violence, discrimination, and being a target with the simultaneous appearance of having none of these

experiences shows up in my practice of SIP as part of my context. My responsibility in SIP is to translate into observations and actions my own resilience and reclamation of power so the client can become empowered. This is the action of enabling the powerless to become powerful.

Use of Self

This incongruous reality of things invisible yet formative to my SIP practices raises important questions about how to use one's experiences to enable growth and healing in others while one avoids inappropriate self-disclosure within therapeutic relationships. Although I use my own experiences to engage my empathy and convey hope of healing to the client, maintaining clinical boundaries in the practice of SIP, or any therapeutic approach, necessitates engaging in healing practices in one's own life. I engage in my own religious and spiritual practices, learning, and community to maintain balance and stay grounded. Self-awareness of my own religious and spiritual limitations, my wounds, my internal biases around gender and sexuality, and my intentional work to create healing, growth, and self-compassion enables me to hear client narratives that parallel my experiences while I stay focused on the client instead of becoming lost in myself. Staying client focused is staying attentive to the client's narrative, asking questions about their interpretations of experiences, and adjusting one's assumptions and conclusions to reflect and respect the client's reality.

Transformation

The therapeutic relationship in SIP can convey the possibility of something more compassionate and holy beyond the painful experiences of the client. I convey compassion through my nonjudging actions and words by offering grace, advocacy, education, empowerment, and communication with humility. I explore the client's wounds and significant experiences, looking for hope and healing, strengths, and resilience in their narratives. For instance, if someone speaks about religious condemnation or rejection by church leaders and separation from a community of belonging, I might ask about hymns or spiritual music they find soothing to explore this painful separation and help them find ways to reconnect to the Sacred that are not mediated by rejecting messages. I examine the lyrics and the felt or implied meaning of that music to the client to help them counter or correct hurtful external messages, using reflection on internal experiences of grace and acceptance from whatever they consider Sacred. Underlying my work is a spiritual desire to enable reconciliation, redemption, and transformed relationships with sacredness, others, and communities.

A TRANS-ORIENTED, CHRISTIAN, UNITARIAN UNIVERSALIST PSYCHOTHERAPY APPROACH

I use psychodynamic skills combined with my skills from formal training in spiritual direction and companioning to assist people to explore psychological, behavioral, spiritual, and existential concerns. I integrate theoretical models of human cognition and behavior, spiritual and religious traditions and teachings, social location, and gender diversity. I use interpersonal and systemic frameworks to understand and help improve relationships and personal agency in systems of power and inequity. I conceptualize my work in SIP through the concept of *tikkun olam* (in the Hebrew, עולם תיקון)—that is, action that heals, repairs, or improves the world. My aim is to assist people to identify misalignments, uncover core beliefs, and reframe and resolve connected issues of functioning in roles related to the self, work or school, and relationships.

Challenging Misalignments: A Case Example

While I primarily use a client-centered, nonauthoritative approach to SIP, I also incorporate a rational emotive tact as needed. Using this more active approach at times, I may openly challenge people on misalignments between their espoused theological and spiritual values, personal morals or ethics, and their behaviors.

The purpose of these challenges is to assist people in observing and eventually resolving disruptions or inconsistencies in their relationships to themselves, to the Sacred/sacredness, and to others. In this process, I reflect to clients the misalignments I witness in their narratives. I invite the clients to examine the apparent opposites that exist between their thoughts or beliefs, or both, and their actions. With gender diverse clients, as with any client, there is not a singular issue at the forefront: that of gender only. Misalignments may intersect across multiple areas in a person's life, agency, and identity. Addressing general misalignments and struggles may offer an opportunity later to address specific misalignments related to gender diversity, expression, acceptance, and integration of the authentic self, or other related concerns when needed.

The following clinical exchange is with a man with a history of gender diversity who has been discussing ways he feels betrayed by his wife and his simultaneous belief that God planned their marriage as a "gift" to him during the time he was undergoing gender-affirming medical treatments. The exchange illustrates my approach using SIP to challenge a general misalignment of his stated beliefs and values with his behaviors and attitudes to repair a split in the client's relationship with his wife and with God—with whom he is also angry for giving him this "gift":

THERAPIST: I notice that you've been talking a lot about how you hate your wife and secretly wish she would just leave you or die. Tell me how you understand your relationship with your wife given your earlier conversations where you said she was a "gift from God"? What type of a gift is she?

CLIENT: (*Pauses*) I feel guilty wishing she was dead. Thinking that scares me. I also pray for her. But I can't stand being around her! What kind of a gift is that?!

THERAPIST: That sounds hard. What kind of a gift do you think she is?

CLIENT: Well, she puts up with me and all my bull—t. (*Speaks quietly*) She hasn't left me, even though there is plenty reason to, but (*speaks loudly*) I don't want to be in the same room with her!

THERAPIST: It sounds like you are angry with her—and maybe with God, too? Why would God give you *this* gift?

CLIENT: (*Sits in silence for a few minutes*) I hadn't put it together like that. She has been a constant example of grace and forgiveness. She accepts me for who I am. And I treat her like s—t. She's really been a saint in my life. But how can I like her when I don't want to be around her?

With continued work to identify the client's definition of "a gift from God" and his disappointment that the "gift" was not what he imagined, he began to identify implicit beliefs that "one must never be ungrateful for a gift from God" compared to his experiences of emotional betrayal in his marriage. With this insight, he identified his anger toward God displaced onto and joined with anger at his wife's failures in his eyes. He was able to separate rigid and disrupted theological beliefs from experiences of relational wounds. This allowed him to further accept his and his wife's humanity and imperfection in how they related to each other and to themselves individually. He could then shift his goals for his relationship toward reconciliation and away from destruction. Continued work using this insight into his misalignments of belief and action allowed the client to reflect on his gender-affirmation treatment challenges and work through grief and additional anger about why "God made [him] this way" (meaning gender diverse). Learning the skills to identify and realign the misalignments of one's behaviors and beliefs/values is integral to improved relationships, self-acceptance, and overall health. In addition, it involves work to discover those beliefs and values that are at the center of the individual's understanding of themselves and the world.

Uncovering Core Beliefs

An integral component of SIP is discovering the client's core internal beliefs about themselves and the meaning of their existence. This involves assisting clients to explore their interpretations of life and how their conclusions help shape the meaning they assign to events, and experiences, which, in turn, drive actions/behaviors and affect emotional and physical health. This discovery process includes exploring why the client is and chooses to stay alive,[3] who they are being in their relationships with others, and whether they envision their future by looking backward to repeat the past or forward in their life to create something new.

Exploration involves examining how present actions disclose and affirm or deny core values and beliefs as well as how choices or behaviors are informed by these core beliefs and create or destroy relationships, the self, and the future. In this process of exploration and discovery, the client also may uncover whether they feel they have inherent worth and value despite, or because of, their gender diversity or other intersecting marginalized or stigmatized identities. Core beliefs deeply inform how the client interprets life and whether or how they feel they belong regardless of whether they are conscious beliefs. Examples include: "God doesn't hear me." "I am worthless." "No one will ever want to be with me." "I am sick."

Interpretation of Life and Creation of Meaning

In my experience, most people seek to understand themselves and their lives within the contexts of their cultures, beliefs, and physiology—or physical body. People may use social comparison to recognize and label their own experiences as typical, atypical, good, unwanted, fearful, exciting, or unusual (Suls et al., 2002). In addition, people tend to act in ways that conform to the norms and beliefs of groups in which they already do, wish to, or may be required to, belong (Festinger, 1954). As people notice differences between their personal experiences, knowledge, beliefs, and behaviors compared with these group norms and beliefs, they may experience emotions ranging from amusement and curiosity to self-hatred and alienation.

---

[3]Average rates of attempted suicide reported by gender diverse adults is 40% across their lifetimes. The U.S. national rate as of 2019 was 4.6% (James et al., 2016).

Interpreting one's experience of a gender identity that is atypical or non-traditional according to contextual and cultural expectations may be confusing or even anguishing and psychologically damaging. Recurring experiences of invisibility, discrimination, confusion, and kindness shape and inform a person's conceptualization and internalized sense of self and their place in relationships, communities, cultures, and groups. Gender diverse people participate as actively in interpreting, reinterpreting, and constructing meaning from their experiences as do traditionally gendered people.

Spiritual and religious communities and belief systems may not reflect or recognize the existence, meaning, or value of gender diverse experiences or personhood (Kanamori et al., 2019). These systems may respond with rejection or harmful actions intended to force conformity to the tradition, beliefs, or norms of the group (Wood & Conley, 2014). The relationship of a gender diverse person to any particular spiritual or religious system or community is outside the professional scope of mental health clinicians to demand or direct. However, supporting gender diverse people in thoughtful exploration of the intersection of their minority gender status with their beliefs, meaning making processes, and membership in any community is central to effective SIP therapeutic work.

Belonging and Rejection: A Case Example

Working compassionately with gender diverse clients in SIP involves awareness of their experiences of risk and safety and belonging and rejection related to nontraditional gender identities, religion, spirituality, and cultural expectations. For instance, in the following exchange with a man with a history of medical gender-affirmation treatment, awareness of his visible and invisible experiences helped me explore his current religious and spiritual concerns. Looking behind what sounded like a typical postmodern American narrative of rejecting religious institutions to assess the client's recent isolating behaviors for a common feeling of otherness resulting from nontraditional gender identity uncovered a profound existential crisis. The crisis was more than routine religious disillusionment or U.S. cultural masculinity roles demanding isolation from others to connect to or defend from experiencing emotions and vulnerability:

THERAPIST: You said you had "given up on all that church stuff," "it wasn't for [you]," and you are just exploring spirituality on your own on hiking trips now. You seem sad.

CLIENT: Yeah, I guess a little lonely. I love being in nature and looking out over the lake, but I feel all alone.

At this point in the dialogue, I could take one of a few directions. Perhaps taking a friend along would help him feel less alone, or I could explore other routes to solitary or unstructured spiritual experiences. I could explore the observable sadness and assess for depressive symptoms and suicidality that are overrepresented in gender diverse populations. I could explore other times when he felt alone or what past experiences of hiking were like. I could explore the meaning of the lake he mentions or the meaning of water. Some directions are within SIP and some are more in line with routine psychotherapy, motivational interviewing, or cognitive behavior therapy. My awareness of the client's intersecting identities and experiences guided the focus to exploring a possible connection between gender diversity, feeling alone, and spiritual devaluation. This example highlights the necessity of asking about gender identity and development as part of the initial evaluation to effectively treat the person and avoid assumptions:

THERAPIST: You feel alone? It's interesting that you feel alone doing what you wanted to do for your spirituality. Why did you give up the "church stuff"?

CLIENT: I just didn't fit in. I don't belong there.

THERAPIST: What do you mean by "fit in" and "belong"? It sounds like you aren't feeling like you belong alone in the woods either.

CLIENT: Well, it's just—it's the men's group. I don't fit in. I'm different. They think differently than I do.

THERAPIST: Does your gender history have anything to do with your not feeling you belong or fit in with the men?

CLIENT: I thought I was fitting in, but some of the men were talking, and I got into an argument with them. Some guy said I sounded "just like his wife," and someone else wanted to know how I got all this "special insight" into how women feel and what they're like. I felt trapped, mad, and exposed, like I wasn't one of them. But I'm not one of the women either. I got mad and said I *did* know because I used to be female! (*Pauses*) That sure stopped the conversation. They yelled at me, "Freak" and to "get out!" The pastor called me later to tell me I couldn't come back unless I was "ready to repent." He said I was "disgusting," that I'm not "hot or cold"—not male or female—and God will "spit me out" [*New Revised Standard Version Bible (NRSV)*, 1989/2007, Revelation 3:16] because I'm neither! So, I have nothing! I am nothing.

> I am alone. Does God really think I'm disgusting? If God doesn't want me, who do I talk to? What do I do? I feel like I have to choose between myself and God. I feel alone.

The client disclosed this experience of spiritual harm and rejection in response to focused probing of inconsistencies in what the client said guided by knowledge of his gender diverse history. Feeling rejected at the core of one's being disrupts the ability to find meaning and purpose. It can also exacerbate or initiate suicidal ideation and actions as well as lead to existential despair that is difficult to resolve without work directly on the existential and spiritual crises. The hurtful names, accusations of deceit for not disclosing his medical history, and the declaration by religious leaders that he is "disgusting" and literally "spit out" by God have the impact of Divine rejection and devaluation of this man's inherent worth. It utterly devastated his sense of spiritual relationship with a Divine presence in his life. Thus, separated from a valuing, compassionate relationship with God, he quickly isolated himself from everyone and fell into despair, shame, and self-loathing. He struggled with active suicidal ideation. Our work shifted to repair of his relationship to himself and to what and who was holy in his life.

Attempting to treat the symptoms of depression, poor self-image, and self-destructive desires and actions without addressing and healing the core lost sense of self-worth and value connected directly to the intersection of religious and spiritual harm and gender diversity would have been ineffective and misdirected care. The cause of the damage must first be addressed, and, for gender diverse individuals, the cause of the damage is often the hostility from others toward the individual's nontraditional gender identity that seeks to deny the person their inherent worth and equal right to be loved and accepted. While issues of inherent worth and human value are correctly considered psychological issues, in my view, they extend deeper into dimensions that are intrinsically spiritual and existential.

Inherent Worth

I view psychotherapy as a way of helping another on a pathway toward personal and spiritual wholeness built on restoring or discovering a sense of inherent worth and value. I understand wholeness to be founded on spiritual, existential, religious, or theological well-being. Grounded in my own beliefs and combined Christian and Unitarian Universalist traditions, I include everyone as possessing inherent worth with the capability of experiencing well-being. Informed by my own values, I work to show the same love, understanding, and compassion to others that I show to myself.

This means I have an obligation to be loving and truly compassionate toward myself. I must continually restore and renew my own relationships to myself, the Divine, and others to help anyone else reach toward wholeness in their lives.

With gender diverse clients, I most often work to counter the damaging religious and spiritual messages from the culture that they are unlovable and meant to be lost—to be purposefully rejected as having no value. I gently work to restore or discover the message that the Divine never stops searching for anyone (*NRSV*, 1989/2007, Luke 15). The hardest work is not exploration or affirmation of gender; rather, it is in (re)instilling an internal felt sense of self-worth *as who they are*—not who others want them to be.

Restoring broken and blocked relationships with the Divine/sacredness can be supported by working through the incongruence between harmful, rejecting messages and experiences of feeling connected to, or in the presence of, something greater than oneself. For some clients, incorporating their tradition's sacred stories and metaphors may assist in connecting with internal self-worth. They become the metaphorical lost person who is *not* forgotten and, when found, is *not* met with Divine chastisement and punishment but with rejoicing and celebration (*NRSV*, 1989/2007, Luke 15). Indeed, it is my theological understanding that inherent worth and value mean there is no place a person can ever be so lost as to be outside the reach of love, compassion, grace, hope, and Divine desire for a restored relationship. Theologically, spiritually, I understand this as the impossibility to be lost— the impossibility to be without possibility of being found.

I ground my hope for clients in the indestructible object of the Divine who does not "lose" anyone even when other humans may wish this were the case or, worse, tell others that it *is* the case, such as one client who reported his sister's response to learning he was transgender. She told him, "God doesn't hear your prayers anymore. You're an abomination." While I follow the language and location of individual clients without imposing any particular worldview, spirituality, religion, or language on them, my view is that SIP offers a unique and effective clinical approach for many clients to achieve well-being in their lives. Through my actions of intentional acceptance and desire to find the whole person in front of me, I communicate my hope with clients that one cannot *cause* the Divine to stop seeking and loving them—or cause themselves to lose their inherent worth. SIP may help to correct an image of abusive and contingent, coercive, and controlling love to move toward inherent self-worth. My aim is to help the individual reframe, reconcile, and restore relationships with the self, the Sacred/sacredness, and others.

I conceptualize people to have within them the Spirit (i.e., *ruach*, or, in the Hebrew, רוּחַ), or breath, of God (*NRSV*, 1989/2007, Job 33:4). This not only imbues each person with inherent worth but with inescapable responsibilities and accountability for themselves and others. Inherent worth and responsibility in relationships cannot be separated from a radical acceptance of free will to choose one's actions or inactions. I have a decidedly Western worldview that people have a right to make their own effective and ineffective "good" and "poor" choices as well as a responsibility to accept the consequences of those choices and actions—barring mental incapacity to understand one's actions and the impact of same. A right to make and exercise choices is not to be contorted into support of selfish, narcissistic, and insensitive decision-making practices. Responsibility to accept the consequences is inseparable from the right to make choices.

Freedom and responsibility to make one's own choices are critical to growth and healing. This is true even though many of the choices all humans make are ill informed and are based on assumptions, incorrect and self-serving attributions, rationalizations, distortions of understanding, and painful memories (fears). Radical responsibility also means accepting that, when enacted, our choices sometimes cause irreparable harm to others: hence, human suffering and broken relationships. Accepting responsibility for one's actions makes it possible to work toward reconciling relationships, to respond to harm inflicted, and to take action to relieve suffering.

Healing Relationships

To examine one's context and impact on others is to wrestle with what it means to be human—a particular human—framed as the question, "Who am I?" This has been asked as long as people have existed. It is reflected in sacred texts (e.g., *NRSV*, 1989/2007, Psalms 8:4–8) and the work of SIP. The questions "Who am I?" and "Why was I made this way?" are often central to gender diverse clients. Exploring formative influences on a person's development over time is also inherently psychodynamic. Clients' answers to these questions form core beliefs and behavioral patterns, and impact their mental health and well-being. Others' answers to these questions regarding the client also affect health and well-being.

Separation and Wounding

Some clients describe shattered beliefs in Divine compassionate love as the result of destroyed trust from familial reactions that render them feeling worthless and unlovable. Nontraditional gender identity can engender a range of reactions, from positive to negative and from benign to murderous[4] (James et al., 2016). One trans-female client expressed her painful experience of rejection from her mother because of her identity as female:

> I told my mom I was a girl inside and needed to be a girl outside, too. She said she wished I had never been born and said I should go and kill myself so no one in the family would have to be around me anymore. She kicked me out of the house. I was only 15, but I was on my own.

The task in SIP is to shine lights into the darkness that remains when others isolate and alienate the gender diverse person from religious, spiritual, or any community and from Divine presence. Separated from religious community and told by religious authorities you are unwanted, are an abomination, and are better off dead, and that God does not hear your prayers (i.e., no longer seeks to find you) leave a person with little hope for reconciliation and add profoundly to suicidal thoughts and actions (James et al., 2016). This is a response that several gender diverse people have also reported hearing when calling suicide hotlines for help and after disclosing their gender diverse identity (e.g., trans, nonbinary). It is a reminder that religious or spiritual harm and dehumanization are not experienced exclusively coming from formal religious institutions or religious leaders.

Grief and Fear: A Case Example
The exploration of these deeply inflicted wounds, dehumanization, and human-induced separation from the grace of a Divine and loving presence is where I often focus my attention. The exploration of religious and spiritual trauma is trauma. This trauma requires a gentle probing with explicit permission of the client to change the subject or to take breaks along the way. SIP is not a form of brief treatment. It needs time and effort to establish trust and for the client to see the respect the therapist holds for them—a core value because the therapist plays the role of comfort and guide as they enter their own darkness to expose the existential fears hidden there.

One example of exposing and resolving an existential fear of ceasing to exist is seen in this exchange with a trans-male client who was distraught about old photos of himself that his parents displayed prominently in their home despite his sending them new photos. He feared this might mean he was "dead" in their eyes now:

THERAPIST: The photos make you both angry and sad. What stops you from talking to your parents about them? Is there anything else you're afraid of?

---

[4]The reader is invited to go online (https://www.glaad.org/tdor) to learn about the Transgender Day of Remembrance.

CLIENT: (*Long silence follows*) Well, I've been trying not to think about it. It's silly. In our family, people tend to hold grudges a long time. Sometimes it's like someone died—they just sort of disappear from conversation and family gatherings—they never change their pictures from the moment they stopped talking to them.

THERAPIST: So, they haven't changed your pictures, and you fear, if you ask them to and they don't, that it is confirmation that—to them— you are dead and you are only real in the old photographs. The real you who is living right now will be forgotten—has already been forgotten, perhaps—removed from the family.

CLIENT: (*Starts to cry*) I work really hard not to think about that. But I think about it all the time anyway! Why can't they take them down? I've given them new pictures! When I visit, I walk in, and I just want to scream, "That's not who I am!" I just want them to see me—really *see* me. It's like I'm a shadow—like I don't exist—like I'm some random visitor.

While part of his life was fully alive, another important part felt metaphorically and emotionally dead. The client experienced being invisible— a shadow who no longer existed—through the presence of old images and the absence of current photos of him in his parents' home. Being unseen— invisible—is to be stripped of existence and of humanity, and it can cause trauma and stress responses over time for any individual. Through SIP, the client explored this existential fear of ceasing to exist even when alive. He had to find courage to form new answers for "Who am I?" and embrace being a whole and valued person.

Courage

Facing the fear that one's life might simply disappear with no memory or record that one existed has been an enduring human anxiety since ancient times, spurring monuments; real and mythical crusades for fountains of youth and holy grails; and various modern attempts to suspend or replicate, reanimate, or create animatronic people who never truly die. This enduring fear of humans also shows up in ancient and modern philosophy and theology, and is central to religions and entire worldviews that work to answer the questions of purpose and meaning as well as "Do I exist?" and "What does it mean to exist?" There are no universally correct answers to these existential questions. Nevertheless, wrestling with existential questions in the context of an accepting relationship may be enhanced through SIP and may lead to improved self-understanding or increased well-being. I ask most clients to consider whether their lives and relationships *must* remain as they are now. Do they see themselves as helpless pawns in the hands of a capricious or sadistic Creator or other? Do *they* have the power to shape their future? Where do they draw power and hope from? Where can they act on their own lives?

Over several months in SIP, the client who was distraught about the old photos of himself gained courage to face the fear he would be excised from the family if he asked them to remove the old pictures and put up the new ones. He challenged his assumptions that he was already dead to them (existential fears) by acknowledging that he was regularly welcomed into their home, which was not how others who were rejected from the family at large were treated. He learned to challenge his fears and conclusions with the reality he experienced. When he had enough courage to ask, his parents were understanding and changed the pictures, having not known he felt unseen by them. They were able to form a deeper relationship, and he was able to ask about their fears of losing him and learn that the photos were their manifested fears that he was pulling away from them. These conversations, absent the existential fears of being forgotten, changed their relationships profoundly.

The client's courage and deeper integration and valuation of himself enabled him to develop internal confidence and strength. He resolved the intense fear that he would cease to exist if he boldly embodied who he is by affirming his gender. He began to see his worth as inherently within who he is and less externally based on whether and how others saw him. He created a stronger relationship with his parents by his willingness to risk existential annihilation by their potential disowning him. SIP helped him increase resilience and reduce the invisibility he felt, which had caused the heightened trauma and stress response he was stuck in. His work through SIP enabled his healing internally and in his relationships so he was open to an experience of comforting grace—the state of being fully known and accepted.

Balms of Healing

For some, the experience of healing and intimacy is reflected through music in hymns or spiritual songs, such as "In the Garden" and "Precious Lord."[5] Spiritual music depicting being comforted by a divine presence in one's greatest hours of need is prevalent. It can be helpful to incorporate lyrics

---

[5]"In the Garden" was written in 1912 by Charles Austin Miles. "Precious Lord" was written in 1932 by Thomas A. Dorsey after the death of his wife during childbirth (Sample, 1992).

from hymns and religious music in SIP treatment. Music has a way of bypass-ing some defenses and touching on both pain and routes to healing with minimal resistance. Religious and spiritual music from one's traditions of origin may provide existential hope and access to memories of belonging, pain, anger, and hurts that may need exploration to heal.

I occasionally ask clients about favorite hymns or religious and spiritual songs, and I read the lyrics. This includes songs the individual labels as "spiritual" that connect them to something larger, outside the self—something mysterious or comforting. For example, one client described how the children's song, "Jesus Loves Me, This I know," sustained him in times of greatest need, although he had left religious communities 30 years previously. Song lyrics can offer insights into clients' gut theology and offer glimpses of wounds and comfort. *Gut theology* refers to instinctual beliefs, whether conscious or based on formal theological teaching. Often, gut theology is experience or tradition based, as in "My mother always says . . .," and may conflict with stated theology/beliefs (Barrett, 1999). I have brought copies of song lyrics into sessions and asked the client to explore the meanings they draw from the words and where they see themselves inside the song. Are they singing? To whom? Are they being sung to? By whom? Does it switch around? It is possible in this way to approach thoughts, memories, and feelings in a less threatening way than the typically cerebral conversations of therapy. These conversations form a remarkably intimate way to see a person more deeply than the surface and reflect to them what you have witnessed.

Witnessing and Mirroring: A Case Example

I view wholeness, self-definition, and self-knowledge to be fundamentally relational and impossible to locate outside human relationships. The thera-peutic relationship is one that holds a possibility for healing when it con-tains the client's woundedness and reflects it in manageable ways that allow recovery and build resilience. The relational nature of healing shows up especially through mirroring and witnessing the reality of the other person. This has a direct, sometimes immediate, impact on gender diverse indi-viduals who may struggle to form adequate self-identities of worth in a world hostile to them and one that rejects, reviles, and harms them daily (James et al., 2016; Lev, 2004). The immediate and profound impact from being witnessed and reflected in work with gender diverse individuals is illustrated in the following exchange with a client in our first session. The client is female identified, although an assigned male, and is living currently as male socially:

THERAPIST: I see what name your insurance is listed under. Is there a particular name that you go by or would like me to call you in sessions?

CLIENT: No one's ever asked me that! (*Gives a wide-eyed look of surprise and shows other visible emotions*) I call myself Susan, but I've never shared that with anyone! (*Speaks softly and looks away*) Is that okay?

THERAPIST: Susan, that's a nice name. Tell me more about how you chose your name?

CLIENT: (*Starts to sob openly*) I—I'm sorry. I've never heard anyone call me Susan before. I've never heard my name out loud. It's so hard. No one ever sees me. Sometimes *I* have trouble seeing me through all this (*points to whisker stubble on face*). I cry and cry in front of the mirror when I have to shave several times daily. I never thought I would hear someone call me by my name. Thank you! Thank you! Thank you!

For many gender diverse clients, working with a therapist practicing SIP may be the first time they have ever experienced compassion and respect or been viewed as a whole person of inherent worth. While witnessing and reflecting another person are routine clinical (human) skills, they may also bring out the therapist's unexamined gender role expectations or religious or spiritual proscriptions. These may appear as shaming, discrediting, prohibiting, paternalizing, and invalidating gender diverse clients' experiences and identities. Examining one's own resistance to—and incomplete or distorted understanding of gender and biologic/genetic sex—is key to non-harmful treatment of this population. The task of the therapist engaged in SIP with gender diverse individuals is to truly *see* the person inside the external trappings of clothing, grooming, and physical body parts or visual cues and work to set them free.

PARTING REFLECTIONS

SIP offers an approach to explore wounds, questions, fears, and seemingly impossible pathways to healing, health, and improved relationships. I have offered one perspective on the intersections of spiritual, religious, existential, and theological complexities in the experiences of gender diverse people. I have illuminated ways assumptions and biased use of religious and theological authority harm these individuals and their relationships to themselves, to other people, to spirituality, to community, and to that which is holy. The psychotherapist working within an SIP framework has a unique opportunity to accompany and encourage a person on a journey of emotional and spiritual healing and restoration. The therapist must work from a gender-affirming approach, resisting pressures to believe that a majority experience of gender equates to the only reality—and certainly not a divinely sanctioned one for all.

Becoming a gender-affirming psychotherapist involves asking oneself the questions and working through the problems shown in this chapter and noted in the list in the following section. Wrestling with these issues helps clinicians become aware of and attuned to harmful religious and spiritual messages that tell gender diverse people they are outside the image of God and beyond the experiences any Divinity can comprehend; they are unseen, unheard, and without hope of being sought after they are lost or celebrated if or when found. Practicing SIP with gender diverse populations demands that the clinician address patterns of hiding within cisgender privilege and behind the overconfident belief in the certainty of human genetic diversity; question attitudes of scarcity of Divine love; and challenge assumptions of the power to decide—on behalf of God—who has inherent worth and value.

THE QUESTIONS

The following are some of the critical and self-reflective questions I ask myself and others—particularly Christian others—who are in positions of power and have influence over the well-being of anyone. The questions arise from common Christian comments and messages rooted in and from sacred texts. Used as self-reflective questions, they help me focus on listening for distortions and harmful theologies that may be integrated into a client's core beliefs. I sometimes use these as active questions in sessions to ask clients to reflect on religious and spiritual experiences in their lives and to challenge contradictory and rejecting messages. I find this process of clinical exploration effective in enabling insight, resilience, and empowerment:

• What does it mean to say humans are created in the image of the Divine given all the variations and medical issues (e.g., "deformities," variations in chromosomes and physiology) that occur? What exactly is *the* "image" of God? Do humans exist who are *not* created in the image of the Divine? Who decides this?

- Does the Creator who "knits us together in the womb" (*NRSV*, 1989/2007, Psalms 139:13)[6] and "counts the hairs on our heads" (*NRSV*, 1989/2007, Luke 12:7) make mistakes when knitting or lose count for some people (e.g., birth defects, genetic disorders, alopecia)?

- For Christians, what does it mean to say that Christ has suffered, or even experienced, everything and every temptation that *all humans* have or will ever face? What if you are told that this does not mean *your* experience?

- How do we decide which of the "lost" are worth looking for (*NRSV*, 1989/2007, Luke 15:3–10) and which ones we intentionally want to lose? Do we wish some did not return home after all (*NRSV*, 1989/2007, Luke 15:11–32)?

- What if we truly *are* loving our neighbors *in exactly the same way* we "*love*" ourselves? Who defines what love or caring for another looks like (*NRSV*, 1989/2007, Luke 10:25–37)?

- What do Christians make of the unambiguous statement in Galatians 3:28b that "*there is no longer . . . male and female*" (*NRSV*, 1989/2007; italics added) when they consider gender and sexual diversity?

REFERENCES

Barnes, L. L. (2011). New geographies of religion and healing: States of the field. *Practical Matters, 4,* 1–82.

Barrett, J. L. (1999). Theological correctness: Cognitive constraint and the study of religion. *Method & Theory in the Study of Religion, 11*(4), 325–339. https://doi.org/10.1163/157006899X00078

Blackless, M., Charuvastra, A., Derryck, A., Fausto-Sterling, A., Lauzanne, K., & Lee, E. (2000). How sexually dimorphic are we? Review and synthesis. *American Journal of Human Biology, 12*(2), 151–166. https://doi.org/10.1002/(SICI)1520-6300(200003/04)12:2<151::AID-AJHB1>3.0.CO;2-F

Festinger, L. (1954). A theory of social comparison processes. *Human Relations, 7*(2), 117–140. https://doi.org/10.1177/001872675400700202

Goldstein, Z., Corneil, T. A., & Greene, D. N. (2017). When gender identity doesn't equal sex recorded at birth: The role of the laboratory in providing effective health-care to the transgender community. *Clinical Chemistry, 63*(8), 1342–1352. https://doi.org/10.1373/clinchem.2016.258780

---

[6]All scriptural references are to Hebrew and Christian texts as found within a typical Christian biblical cannon. Translations and paraphrased versions of biblical texts may have differences in wording, grammar, and syntax. Catholic and Protestant Bible versions may contain different total collections of sanctioned books.

Hopwood, R. A. (2018). Supporting the transgender individual in deciding their pathway. In M. R. Kauth & J. C. Shipherd (Eds.), *Adult transgender care: An interdisciplinary approach for training mental health professionals* (1st ed., pp. 61–77). Routledge.

James, S. E., Herman, J. L., Rankin, S., Keisling, M., Mottet, L., & Anafi, M. (2016). *The report of the 2015 U.S. Transgender Survey*. National Center for Transgender Equality. https://www.ustranssurvey.org/reports#USTS

Kanamori, Y., Pegors, T. K., Hall, J., & Guerra, R. (2019). Christian religiosity and attitudes toward the human value of transgender individuals. *Psychology of Sexual Orientation and Gender Diversity, 6*(1), 42–53. https://doi.org/10.1037/sgd0000305

Lev, A. (2004). *Transgender emergence: Therapeutic guidelines for working with gender-variant people and their families*. The Haworth Clinical Practice Press.

Levy, D. L., & Lo, J. R. (2013). Transgender, transsexual, and gender queer individuals with a Christian upbringing: The process of resolving conflict between gender identity and faith. *Social Thought, 32*(1), 60–83. 10.1080/15426432.2013.749079

Mueller, S. C., De Cuypere, G., & T'Sjoen, G. (2017). Transgender research in the 21st century: A selective critical review from a neurocognitive perspective. *The American Journal of Psychiatry, 174*(12), 1155–1162. https://doi.org/10.1176/appi.ajp.2017.17060626

New Revised Standard Version Bible (First). (2007). National Council of the Churches of Christ in the United States of America. HarperCollins. (Original translation published 1989)

Oswald, R. F. (2001). Religion, family, and ritual: The production of gay, lesbian, bisexual, and transgender outsiders-within. *Review of Religious Research, 43*(1), 39–50. https://doi.org/10.2307/3512242

Richter-Appelt, H. (2008). Gender identity conflicts and psychological problems in adult subjects with different forms of intersexuality (disorders of sex development, dsd): The Hamburg Intersex Project. *Sexologies, 17*(Suppl. 1), S79. https://doi.org/10.1016/S1158-1360(08)72729-4

Rodriguez, E. M., & Follins, L. D. (2012). Did God make me this way? Expanding psychological research on queer religiosity and spirituality to include intersex and transgender individuals. *Psychology and Sexuality, 3*(3), 214–225. https://doi.org/10.1080/19419899.2012.700023

Rosenkrantz, D. E., Rostosky, S. S., Riggle, E. D. B., & Cook, J. R. (2016). The positive aspects of intersecting religious/spiritual and LGBTQ identities. *Spirituality in Clinical Practice, 3*(2), 127–138. https://doi.org/10.1037/scp0000095

Sample, T. (1992). [Lecture notes on practical theology]. Saint Paul School of Theology, Kansas City, MO.

Suls, J., Martin, R., & Wheeler, L. (2002). Social comparison: Why, with whom, and with what effect? *Current Directions in Psychological Science, 11*(5), 159–163. https://doi.org/10.1111/1467-8721.00191

Wood, A. W., & Conley, A. H. (2014). Loss of religious or spiritual identities among the LGBT population. *Counseling and Values, 59*(1), 95–111. https://doi.org/10.1002/j.2161-007X.2014.00044.x

Zosuls, K. M., Miller, C. F., Ruble, D. N., Martin, C. L., & Fabes, R. A. (2011). Gender development research in sex roles: Historical trends and future directions. *Sex Roles, 64*(11–12), 826–842. https://doi.org/10.1007/s11199-010-9902-3

10

SPIRITUALLY INTEGRATED PSYCHOTHERAPY WITH LGBQ INDIVIDUALS

SARAH H. MOON

The field of psychology and mental health treatment has shifted with regard to the increase in knowledge and acceptance of integrating spiritual and religious (S/R) dynamics in psychotherapy (Captari et al., 2018; Pargament et al., 2013; Shafranske & Sperry, 2005; Vieten et al., 2013; Worthington & Sandage, 2002). The field's struggle to incorporate important aspects of S/R in psychotherapy began with Freud, who provided analysis of religion as a defense and God as an illusion (Rizutto, 1998). There are more data to show that S/R issues are very important for people: About 73% of the U.S. population reported that religion was either "very important" or "fairly important" in their lives (Gallup, 2020), and psychological research has shown that clients value the inclusion of S/R issues in their treatment (Post & Wade, 2009; Rose et al., 2001/2008).

Committed religious and spiritual clients in psychotherapy have reported (a) having negative psychotherapy experiences, if they experienced the therapist as being resistant to discussing S/R issues or perceived the therapist to be in opposition to the client's religion (Cragun & Friedlander, 2012); and (b) tending to demonstrate much higher psychotherapy outcomes when the

https://doi.org/10.1037/0000276-011
Spiritual Diversity in Psychotherapy: Engaging the Sacred in Clinical Practice,
S. J. Sandage and B. D. Strawn (Editors)

work openly included the integration of S/R issues (Worthington et al., 2011). Not only does this demonstrate the need for therapists to develop the ability to understand the complexity and depth of S/R issues in clients' lives, it further strengthens the argument that S/R dimensions in clinical practice are integral parts of practicing culturally competent psychotherapy (American Psychological Association [APA], 2003, 2017; Shafranske & Malony, 1996). S/R dynamics are included in the APA (2003, 2017) and the National Association of Social Workers guidelines for ethical clinical practice. Although there appears to be movement in the field toward a more accepting and open posture for the inclusion of S/R issues, a framework for how to conceptualize S/R in psychotherapy and competent practice has been limited. Many therapists do not receive training or education during their graduate program, beyond those who attend programs that specialize in this area (e.g., Fuller Theological Seminary, Rosemead School of Psychology, Wheaton College), which leaves it up to the individual to seek their own supervision or consultation (Brawer et al., 2002; Schafer et al., 2011).

Similar to the growing efforts to consider S/R issues in psychotherapy, the inclusion of sexual and gender minorities in the mental health field has faced its own battles, given the field's long history of discrimination against LGBTQ[1] individuals (Bartoli & Gillem, 2008; Goldfried, 2001; Pachankis & Goldfried, 2013). Through the work of various civil rights movements and research completed on this topic, we are at a point where the field supports and affirms LGBTQ-affirmative therapies and calls for competency in this area (APA, 2003, 2012, 2017). An affirmative therapist "celebrates and advocates the authenticity and integrity of lesbian, gay, and bisexual persons *and their relationships* [emphasis added]" (Tozer & McClanahan, 1999, p. 736). Some still argue that the depth of affirmation by a clinician may be "shallow, over-simplified, and non-inclusive," where they are not sure or aware of how to practice in a meaningful way, thus, more training and knowledge in this area is needed (Bieschke et al., 2007).

Although both the LGBQ and S/R communities have been advocating for inclusion in the field of psychology and psychotherapy, and the separate groups have made progress, the intersection of these identities have brought

---

[1]In this chapter, I use the acronym LGBQ to encompass the various ways sexuality can be experienced and expressed by individuals and partners within this community and am intentionally omitting transgender and nonbinary identified individuals. I believe that attending to the unique topics and experiences of the transgender and nonbinary community deserves its own chapter and voice (see Chapter 9, this volume).

to the surface new sets of challenges. The intersection of these identities poses dilemmas around how to allow for both in the therapy room when they might appear to conflict (Bartoli & Gillem, 2008). With the long history of differing beliefs and values between religious institutions and the LGBQ community, the conflict historically has led to the oppression of and discrimination against LGBQ individuals (e.g., the practice of conversion therapy, laws prohibiting same-sex marriage, prohibiting individuals from taking on leadership roles within religious institutions). There can be varying levels of acceptance or affirmation that one might see within Christian institutions. Yakushko (2005), as well as Nugent and Gramick (1989) before Yakushko, provided a helpful framework for the various ways religious institutions have approached the "homosexuality debate":

1. the rejecting punitive stance, where "homosexuality" is considered morally and ethically wrong, and this stance is essential to the faith institution. Institutions who take on this approach are hostile and rejecting of the LGBQ community;

2. rejecting nonpunitive stance, where "homosexuality" is viewed as sinful but the church still welcomes and make attempts to care for LGBQ individuals;

3. qualified acceptance stance, where institutions perceive "homosexuality" as acceptable but inferior to heterosexuality. Institutions that take on this approach see a hierarchy of what is acceptable and unacceptable regarding sexuality, which often is seen in banning LGBQ congregants to hold leadership positions within the church; and

4. full acceptance stance, where institutions fully accept the LGBQ community and view same sex relationships and attractions as normative. (Yakushko, 2005, p. 133)

There are many cases in which a church might have a specific stance on this issue outwardly or in their doctrine, but not all congregants that are part of the church align with the church's stance. In other words, although the church's doctrine might not be fully affirming, some congregants that attend that church do hold affirming theologies.

The larger societal conflicts present themselves in the therapy room in various ways, and a therapist's awareness and competence in working with the intersection of LGBQ and S/R will likely help clients navigate these identities.

KEY DEFINITIONS

Before we move forward, it would be helpful to discuss how spirituality/religion and sexual orientation have been defined in this chapter. Sexual orientation is conceptualized as being on a continuum rather than distinct categories; the term, as defined by Fassinger and Arseneau (2007) in the *Handbook of Counseling and Psychology With Lesbian, Gay, Bisexual, and Transgender Clients*, refers to the affective, cognitive, and behavioral dimensions that "constitute an individual's sense of self as a sexual and intimately relational being" (p. 42). The authors also pointed to the problem of understanding sexual orientation by focusing primarily on the gender of the intimate partner; they argued that it is vital to conceptualize this in complex relational terms, such as considering one's orientation toward other social categories (i.e., race, age, ethnicity). As previously mentioned, I use the acronym LGBQ to encompass the various ways sexuality can be experienced and expressed by individuals and partners within this community and am intentionally omitting transgender and nonbinary identified individuals in this chapter. I believe that attending to the unique topics and experiences of the transgender and nonbinary community deserves its own chapter and voice (see Chapter 9, this volume).

The definition of R/S, according to Shafranske and Sperry (2005), points to two distinct ways one can relate to something or someone mystical or transcendent: (a) religion as dogma or belief system, and (b) spirituality as a personal connection. Religion and spirituality can be interconnected and overlapping (Bartoli & Gillem, 2008). Most psychology training programs better provide teaching and supervision on working with LGBQ clients but less around religious diversity.

In this chapter, I discuss some clinical considerations that therapists might consider as they provide spiritually integrated psychotherapy for LGBQ individuals, specifically clients that are trying to make sense of the intersection of their faith and sexuality. This also includes our role as therapists in this process. I offer the following three themes that I have found important in my work, and I encourage readers to consider when working with religious LGBQ individuals and LGBQ individuals who have a religious history. The central point to these themes is that therapists must be willing to engage clients in depth around both (a) S/R dynamics and (b) sexuality without trying to control the outcomes. The themes of authenticity, desire, and therapist choice and power are considered throughout the chapter and summarized as follows:

- *Authenticity* must be conceptualized through a cultural lens, one in which being "out and proud" is not privileged over purposeful privacy about one's sexual orientation, especially when it is not culturally or contextually appropriate. I address different ways authenticity can be considered when working with religious LGBQ individuals, as it is a complicated social and spiritual value.

• *Desire* is a complicated issue for religious individuals from Evangelical traditions, as it is often connected to teachings around restriction, tempering, or disowning desires (both sexual or otherwise) in order to place god at the central focus of one's life. I address how these teachings impact the conversation around sexuality as a whole, and consequently, issues around sexual orientation.

• *Therapist choice and power* to disclose their affirmative or nonaffirmative stance, when clinically appropriate, represents an important set of considerations, including the impact that this can have on their clients. The issue of power imbalance is crucial in this conversation.

LOCATING MY OWN SPIRITUAL/RELIGIOUS AND LGBQ VALUES

My social location (the intersections of my various identities) must be acknowledged as I discuss S/R and LGBQ dynamics, as it gives context to the voice and ideas that I share about in this chapter. I have inevitably been influenced by my various identities, but for the sake of brevity, I will focus on my S/R and sexual identity. First, there is a strong history of Christianity in South Korea, from which I emigrated as a young child. Although my parents had strong Catholic and Buddhist roots, my family found a sense of community and safety within the Evangelical Korean-immigrant church in the United States, and much of my identity growing up was centered around my faith. Furthermore, my graduate education at Fuller Theological Seminary afforded me the opportunity to study both Christian theology and clinical psychology.

At the time, I did not realize that going through this program would lead me to my own challenges of making sense of life questions, critically evaluating my theological views, and shifting my understanding of what is considered sacred. As I studied the history of the Christian church and teachings, and the historical context in which the Bible was written, I have come to believe in a progressive theology; that is, one that asserts that god affirms the fullness of LGBTQIA+ identities and romantic relationships. In other words, I believe that same-sex relationships and marriages should be regarded as sacred.

With regard to sexuality/sexual orientation, I identify as queer, and I have personally gone through the experience of seeking integration of my queer identity and my religious background. I recognize the complexity of navigating these identities on a very personal level.

This chapter focuses primarily on the experience of current or former Evangelical Christian LGBQ clients because I am using examples from my own clinical experience. These are the clients who tend to have the most difficulty finding coherence in their sexual identity and religion. This will be important to keep in mind as I discuss Christian ideas and teachings, because I recognize that Christianity includes diverse traditions and teachings, many of which are theologically affirming; however, I will be focusing on client experiences of religion that have been more harmful.

AUTHENTICITY IN CONTEXT

Authenticity is considered to be an essential part of well-being (Winnicott, 1965; Yalom, 1980), with various definitions of authenticity provided by scholars. From a philosophical perspective, there are essentialist and existentialist approaches to authenticity. The essentialist perspective would describe authenticity as a process-oriented path toward understanding the self, and subsequently, living in congruence with the self. The existentialist approach focuses on the choices made about one's life and commitments to live accordingly to these choices, with responsibility of being consistent in action as an essential aspect of this approach (Kernis & Goldman, 2006).

There are two primary approaches to authenticity in psychological research, both of which find their roots in Greek philosophy (Kernis & Goldman, 2006; Sheldon et al., 1997). The *trait* approach values consistency, in that self-concept aligns with one's personality, behaviors, and actions. Sheldon (2013) argued that this approach is problematic because the self can be fluid across various contexts and roles, which has been found to be true in various research studies especially in those examining cultural contexts and cultural dimensions (Boucher, 2011; Cross et al., 2003; Reinecke & Trepte, 2014; Sutton, 2018). The *coherence or organismic* approach views authenticity as a process-oriented path toward understanding the self, allowing for more space for individuals to experience or show different "selves" depending on the context. This tends to be true for individuals who hold one or more marginalized identities, where shifting one's self depending on the context is used as a healthy coping strategy. As Sutton (2018) noted, authenticity should be described as finding coherence rather than consistency—where the value is placed on understanding why different personality traits or actions are shown in various contexts rather than focusing on consistency across situations.

In my clinical work, I find that clients most often have internalized the trait approach rather than the coherence approach to authenticity. I believe there are two reasons for this: First, the mainstream culture of the LGBQ community is one that celebrates the idea of being "out and proud," which places pressure on sexual minorities to live out their sexual orientation in one particular manner—the Western individualistic approach. A great example of this is explained by Noman (2019), who critiqued the popular Netflix show *Queer Eye* for taking the American show to Japan. Ultimately, the show's Western approach to prioritizing outness was imposed upon a collectivistic community. She argued that the coming out process can be harmful to the individual and to their families in these communities:

> The paradigm of sexual identity tends to come in the form of a binary: One is either out of the closet or in it, proud or ashamed, open or repressed. Embedded in this paradigm is a righteousness, a belief that somehow there is a "right" way to be out. (Noman, 2019)

She went on to state that "acceptance especially in some intergenerational families and close-knit communities, can be powerful even when it doesn't come wrapped in a rainbow flag" (Noman, 2019).

Research shows that it might not always be helpful to disclose sexual orientation as well: LGBQ individuals were found to be more likely to be disclosing of their sexual orientation if they were with people who supported their autonomy, regardless of the person's gender, age, or sexual orientation (Legate et al., 2012). Disclosing was also correlated with lower levels of depression and anger and higher levels of self-esteem. In contrast, disclosing to people who were "controlling" or did not support the person's autonomy did not lead to higher well-being. The study showed that there might only be benefits of disclosing or coming out in supportive environments. It is a common and healthy practice for LGBQ individuals and couples to transition from privacy to outness multiple times throughout the day depending on the context, and one must not be shamed for doing so; being able to context switch might actually bring a person more freedom, peace, and coherence. I do not intend to mean that there isn't something beautiful and freeing about being open about one's sexual orientation, but rather, for many LGBQ clients who come from a more complicated cultural and/or familial background, it may be psychologically healthier to maintain privacy. Being able to move through spaces in a fluid way is extremely difficult, courageous, painful, and necessary for many.

The second reason I see the trait approach being internalized by many of my clients is due to the misuse of "truth-telling" in Christian contexts, where disclosing one's sexual orientation is pushed upon them as a form of healthy repentance. We, as therapists, can aid clients by helping them notice when they are conflating truth-telling with coming out, the former negates the importance of considering boundaries and privacy in the coming-out process. Let's take a look at some biblical passages that explicitly teach about the importance of truth-telling:

- 1 Peter 3:10: "For, Whoever would love life and see good days must keep their tongue from evil and their lips from deceitful speech" (Bible Gateway, 2021).

- Proverbs 12:22: "The Lord detests lying lips but he delights in people who are trustworthy" (Bible Gateway, 2021).

- Colossians 3:9: "Do not lie to one another, seeing that you have put off the old self with its practices" (Bible Gateway, 2021).

Many of my LGBQ clients have taken these passages, along with how their church preached on this topic, and generalized this message to their coming-out process without consideration of the consequences or personal/familial risks. Authenticity is a relational matter, which includes important situational and relational contexts to consider when disclosing aspects of the self. This is true for all people regardless of sexual orientation, but there is a layer of complexity for LGBQ individuals, such as considering where a family member is regarding their religious views on same-sex relationships, relational closeness to the particular family member, and the family member's emotional capacity for differentiation. These are just a few contexts that clients and therapist would benefit from processing when the client is considering disclosing their sexuality.

As an example, I met with C, a Taiwanese, gay, cis-male client, who grew up in the Presbyterian church and initially sought treatment to address his anxiety around informing his parents that he was in an ongoing romantic relationship with a man for 3 months. His case brought up the specific issue around how Christian churches encourage truth-telling or confession of sin in harmful ways in which there is a lack of boundary and safety, and how he generalized this message to navigate his coming-out process. C and I explored his anxiety by first processing his intention and motivation for coming out to his parents. My curiosity was piqued upon noticing his strong conviction and unwavering decision that he needed to tell his parents by the end of the month, because keeping the relationship a secret for 3 months was unacceptable to him. As we continued exploring, we came to an insight that this pressure was linked to experiences he had in his church youth group while growing up. He recounted a time during a prayer group where the youth leader asked everyone to go around and share the most challenging sin that they were dealing with at the current moment, so that each person could be prayed for. My client remembered experiencing an immense amount of shame and anxiety in the moment, not knowing if he should share that he had watched pornography the prior day. He felt deeply conflicted because he believed that sharing one's sin with another is what god and his church had wanted for him, but he felt uncomfortable and shameful about what he had done. The situation felt dangerous for my client because there were no appropriate boundaries set or containment provided by his youth leader to ensure safety, nor would his authenticity be supported in noncondemning ways. Of course, these were thoughts he did not have insight into at the time.

As we continued working together, this memory was tied back into his current anxiety about telling his parents about his dating relationship. My client had taken the biblical teachings about truth-telling and generalized them to all truths regardless of the situation or relational context. When he described his coming-out process to his friends, he stated that he found himself telling as many people as possible, which led him into a deep depression several years prior to our working together. He thought that failing to disclose these "secrets" was bad, and honesty was "good," so, therefore, he *needed* to come out to everyone, even if he knew they would not be affirming. Subsequently, his need to tell his parents about his new boyfriend was underlaid with the idea that keeping this "secret" meant that he was lying to his parents, which he was not able to tolerate.

This was when I began to discuss with him the coherence approach to authenticity. C seemed to find it helpful when I began to ask him about ways authenticity can be lived out in his life that felt congruent to what he was feeling, while keeping context in mind. As I mentioned previously, we explored important situational and relational contexts that would help him decide when and how he would come out to his parents. He was able to slow down his thought process and decrease his anxiety, as he deeply processed what he felt ready for and what he wanted in his relationship with his parents.

C also shared that it was helpful when I stated that privacy was not antithetical to authenticity. In one of our sessions, I made a distinction between privacy and secrecy by sharing that authenticity through privacy can be held as a way to honor and respect his own process and boundaries. There were many aspects of his current context that needed to be processed and explored before making the big decision of coming out to his parents. C's experience provides us with an example of a clinical situation where clients need the space to work through the internal conflict around disclosing their sexual orientation, and process the positive or negative consequences of doing so. This would be both for their own mental health and well-being as well as the impact that disclosing will have on others. For C, his religious and East Asian cultural values were two contexts in which he needed and wanted to process before coming out to his parents, as well as with others who did not know about his sexual orientation or relationship status. In our work together, we examined the benefits and risks of disclosing the nature of his relationship with his boyfriend from the perspective of his Asian immigrant family (some who were religiously conservative and some who weren't), Asian American friends from church who would or would not be affirming, Asian American friends who did not attend church, to name just a few. Within each of these social contexts, we discussed the risk of disclosing, as each context had particularities that made the issue more or less challenging. I also worked with C regarding the fear of not knowing—as much as we processed the risks and benefits, there was no way of predicting how others might respond.

The theme of grief and/or anticipated grief was processed heavily in these sessions. The process of coming out often includes a sense of loss, whether it be of specific people or internal and external parts of one's life. C and I spent many sessions grieving the loss of a religion he grew up believing so deeply in, a sense of security and certainty, the comfort and sense of belonging he felt when he entered into his church building, how "easy" it felt to be seen as straight, and the loss of friends that felt like family to him. The uniqueness of the tangible and not-so tangible losses that C experienced was explored, identified, and honored. Lastly, we worked toward solidifying the friendships he had that were supportive of his sexual identity by asking for help or support and by strengthening his confidence that he would be able to cope with and manage the negative responses or experiences.

The practice of repentance can lead some to disclose their sexual orientation or come out to family or friends prematurely, for the sake of being an honest and "good" person, without fully processing the benefits and risks of doing so. This demonstrates a singular/one-dimensional understanding of what might have been taught in church or read in the Bible, in that social and relational context matters are not considered enough when vulnerability is expressed. Failure to consider context can possibly lead to reckless disclosure that can cause pain and hurt. Shame might be a helpful theme to explore, in order to prevent shame from triggering an impulsive or premature disclosure, as well as understanding of how Christians might conflate the practice of "repentance" versus "disclosure." This is not to say that one should only disclose if they will receive a positive response, but rather, to disclose if they understand as much as they can as to the risk it might mean to disclose (e.g., losing family members or friends, being bullied or teased). Therefore, as therapists, it can be helpful to remind clients that remaining in the closet in some relationships, or maintaining privacy around romantic relationships, can be a true practice of authenticity.

EXPLORATION OF DESIRE

Within the Evangelical Christian tradition, there are messages that imply that merely having a thought or desire can lead to "idolizing" something or someone other than god, which would be deemed as "sin" or "sinful." In Exodus, Colossians, Galatians, and 1 Corinthians, the writers urge Christians to have no other "idols" other than god, and, furthermore, that Christians should be suspicious of "bodily passions" that might impede god's will or plan (Farley, 2006, p. 38). Religious clients that I have worked with, regardless of sexual orientation, often speak of these repressive theologies that has had damaging effects on their sense of self and relationship. They have shared that churches did not encourage them to explore their thoughts, wants, and desires because they did not want the focus to be on themselves in fear that it would be considered sinful. This reinforced the message that desires should be minimized or suppressed; not merely physical or emotional desires but also desires for success, money, or marriage, as an excess of desire would be making an idol out of those things apart from god. Matthew 5:28 is often quoted in these conversations: "But I tell you that anyone who looks at a woman lustfully has already committed adultery with her in his heart." Many of my religious clients have historically avoided thinking about or processing what they want and need, consciously or unconsciously, and this has been especially true when faced with topics around sex, sexual desire, or sexual intimacy. It is no surprise to me that many, if not most, of my LGBQ clients who identify as former or current Evangelical Christians indicate reluctance to discuss topics that identify their own wants, because they think it is selfish or they regard their own physical or sexual desire as sin in our sessions.

Furthermore, purity culture has also had negative impacts on religious LGBQ clients, for women especially (Valenti, 2009; Watkins, 2008). Purity culture was popularized in the early 1990s as a way to promote abstinence and sexual purity in conservative Christian institutions: Purity rings, purity balls, purity pledges, and books such as *I Kissed Dating Goodbye*, by Joshua Harris, *Why True Love Waits*, by Joshua McDowell, and *Passion and Purity*, by Elisabeth Elliot, were part of this movement. A culture of shame and controlling of bodies driven by these repressive theologies has had an immense impact on many of my religious clients who identify either as heterosexual or LGBQ.

I believe it is always important to consider the historical, sociocultural context from which Christian ideas and teachings are derived, in order to seriously critique and engage with concepts and teachings. According to Foucault (1976), sex and sexuality were openly discussed in early Western civilization, primarily around technique and how to derive pleasure. This shifted after the Enlightenment, as the Catholic Church began to incorporate values and practices from the monastic tradition pertaining to celibacy and practices of self-denial into their practices and teachings (Foucault, 1976; Wilchins, 2004). Consequently, sex became one of the focal points of the morality and ethics debate in religious communities. Not only were sinful actions and behaviors a focal point of teachings in the religious communities, but now the sinful ideas and thoughts themselves without action were of concern. Foucault asserted that sex and sexuality focused on confessing and repression, with an obsession of "self-examination and self-reporting about sexual experiences" in various contexts (Farley, 2006, p. 20). To this day, unfortunately, many religious institutions have kept to a similar process of speaking on what *not* to do or think about, rather than developing a healthy and authentic sexuality. Simply stated, many "Christians have learned and inwardly digested the repressive lesson that God is good and sex is bad" (Heyward, 1989, p. 89). For example, churches will often focus on negative aspects (i.e., sin, sinfulness) of premarital sex, masturbation, extramarital affairs, and pornography, rather than focusing on sexual growth, sexual intimacy, and the importance of knowing one's own body.

Another way to frame this is a sex-negative versus sex-positive approach. Schnarch (1991) similarly asserted that spirituality and sexuality are both developmental processes that should be approached from a self-affirmation stance rather than self-negation. Schnarch referenced Francouer's work stating that there are two frameworks within various religions to demonstrate the diversity within each tradition, as well as the similarities across religions, when it comes to discussing sexuality. Francouer called it the Type A and Type B sects: The theology of sexuality in Type A sects focuses on control of sexuality because sexuality is viewed as dangerous, whereas Type B sects focus on how religion enhances sexuality by allowing an individual's fullest potential to emerge. All religions have Type A and B sects, suggesting that there are within group differences. Schnarch argued for process theology, which emphasizes "becoming and emerging, rather than obeying" (p. 555).

I would encourage therapists to first address the broad topic of desire with your religious LGBQ client, to understand the ways in which they may or may not have been impacted by repressive theologies, and to what degree they have been impacted. This helps to set the frame and context before exploring the complex issues around sexuality, sexual orientation, or physical intimacy. The following questions demonstrate a few examples of how this might be done clinically:

- What explicit or implicit messages did you hear or learn about wants and desires?

- Do you trust your intuition and thoughts and perceive them as valid?

- What questions did you have about sexual desire or intimacy that you were too afraid to ask when you were younger?

- How has that impacted your romantic relationships and your relationship to your own body?

- Was purity culture present in your church context, and if so, how have these repressive theologies unconsciously or consciously impacted your thoughts, feelings, and actions?

Questions like these may allow for a deeper understanding and awareness of what consequences clients feared, if they were to explore desire with friend groups, parents, or church leaders. Some clients may need some guidance around how to talk about desire and sex, and some guidance in working toward affirming their desires. Unlearning and questioning the repressive theology might be a challenging, but important, process for the client in the therapeutic context. Engaging in this discussion could provide a relationally restorative and healing experience that could lead to a greater capacity for exploration, intimacy, and differentiation, with the purpose of facilitating growth for the client in their relationships. As Heyward wrote (1989): "Therapists are encouraged to help their clients explore a variety of religious sexual ethics in order to see if there are versions that may be congruent with their value system" and facilitate a reframing to an ethic that "affirms, rather than denies or attempts to qualify, the value of experiencing and sharing body pleasures" (p. 123).

THERAPIST CHOICE AND POWER TO AFFIRM IDENTITIES

The APA has been vocal about the organization's strong stance against conversion therapy. In 2009, APA's Task Force on Appropriate Therapeutic Responses to Sexual Orientation reported that evidence on efforts to change sexual orientation is lacking and that, therefore, it should not be a part of psychological treatment (APA, 2009). To this day, only 20 U.S. states have laws banning conversion therapy for minors (Movement Advancement Project, 2021). Although many therapists are against conversion therapy itself, there are many who maintain the theological view that having same-sex attractions and/or being in a same-sex relationship is sinful and is counter to what god intended for human relationships. We, as therapists, have the freedom in our clinical work to choose whether or not to disclose our theological stance. I have spent a significant amount of time in my own reflection and in consultation with colleagues about the best way to approach the theme of self-disclosure when working with LGBQ religious clients. I once had a conversation with a White, straight, cis-male therapist who was in the beginning process of deconstructing his faith and religious values, as he was seeing more queer clients in his practice but was still heavily involved in his conservative Christian church. He was trying to make sense of his previously nonaffirming perspective and his movement toward questioning that stance. As I provided consultation around his therapeutic work with a gay male client, I asked him whether the client had ever asked him if he was affirming. The therapist answered no and shared that he would be afraid if the client asked, and admitted that he has intentionally tried to avoid this topic. I think this is a dilemma that all therapists working with LGBQ individuals should process and understand for themselves—specifically, why they would or would not disclose their views on sexuality.

My practice as a social-justice-oriented therapist includes explicitly disclosing my affirmative stance regarding sexuality. I think it is a very personal choice around exactly how this disclosure is made by therapists, whether in explicit or indirect ways. The justification for this stance is partly from my reading of Root's (1990) model for biracial identity development, which I found to be helpful to the religious and sexual identity development process; that is, individuals who are exploring various identities will have a difficult time exploring identities that are not explicitly affirmed. If a client experiences a microaggression or subtle criticism for exploring an identity, or is unsure how the therapist will respond, clients might foreclose that process before fully allowing themselves to seek and explore. This can also be said for religious identities; our role as therapists is to provide a space where clients can navigate *both* their religious and sexual identities, while not feeling pushed to privilege one identity over another or to collapse the exploration of either identities prematurely. Too often, I see therapists, in an effort to be supportive of a client's sexuality, criticize and diminish the important role that the church has played in the client's life. Ultimately, it leaves the client feeling uncomfortable around sharing about the importance of religion/spirituality in their lives. If a therapist takes an affirmative stance, and chooses to disclose this, it is important not to privilege LGBQ identity over and beyond religious identity or belief, if that is not what the client is needing to feel supported. For example, my clients have reported that they fear talking about their faith with other LGBQ friends or former therapists who do not understand the immense difficulty of leaving the church and church community. They fear that the friend or therapist will suggest that they cut these relationships out to "set healthy boundaries."

I would like to expand upon this topic by sharing another case. I was meeting with L, a lesbian, Black, cis-female for weekly psychotherapy for 2 years, working through her process of grieving the loss of her church family. "Church members helped raise me—I have such fond memories of spending weeknights and weekends playing at the church with other kids while the adults prayed, cooked, and shared stories with one another." As she was processing her coming-out experience with a few people from her church, L described her experience with those folks as an out-of-body experience, where she felt pulled out of her own reality, especially when the argument that God does not affirm same-sex relationships was brought up. She recalled a moment when one of them went through each passage in the bible that condemned "homosexuality." L knew in her mind and heart that her attraction toward women was not a sin (she had worked through this theological shift before coming to see me), but every time she visited home and saw these same people, she would feel at times subtle and at other times violent ways they made her question whether she was a bad or flawed person. "These conversations make me question my own reality and make me feel crazy, Dr. Moon!" L felt even more confused because sometimes these friends would not explicitly say anything negative to her or the conversation might not even be about sexual orientation, but their presence felt oppressive because L knew how they viewed her. Over time, she came to the insight that having to hide such an integral part of herself from important people in her life felt as though they were asking her to deny her own reality.

I explored with L the real or anticipated losses that she may have. The theme of absence and presence was central to our work: absence and presence of god, absence and presence of family and friends, absence and presence of her own identities. The concept of absence and presence was not one that was understood in the physical context, but in an emotional and spiritual one. She once told me that the loss of her faith community was the most difficult thing she had ever experienced; she lost her sense of belonging and family, and also lost parts of herself when in the presence of her community. With issues of identity conflict, the theme of loss is often related to the anxiety and depression associated with this type of dilemma (Bartoli & Gillem, 2008).

From my clinical and personal experience, some of the more challenging dynamics are around how to navigate relationships with friends or family who are "supportive but not affirming," more-so than navigating outright homophobic family members or friends. Referring back to Yakushko's (2005) model, this would fall under the rejecting, nonpunitive stance. Someone who has a rejecting, nonpunitive stance might, for example, show love and care through action, but they have not done the hard work of confronting or questioning their own theological views around same-sex relationships. In conversation, they may respond with statements such as the following:

- "I would say that I'm affirming in practice, but I don't know how to back that up as well theologically."

- "I would attend a gay wedding, but I would not be their groomsmen or officiate the wedding."

- "If you introduced us to your partner, I would love them and love you because you are like family to me. But if you were to ask me where I stand theologically, I just haven't figured out how to reconcile what it says in the Bible."

- "I don't believe it's a sin to be queer, because no one's identity is a sin as god made all of us, but the relationships are the part that I'm working through."

- "I believe that being gay isn't god's intention for us, so because it doesn't fall in line with his original intent, it is as much a sin as any other in our lives. But I don't believe that it makes you any less or doesn't make me love you any less, or that god sees you any different."

I have found it useful to help LGBQ clients explore the issue of power, when they are discussing their sexual orientation with someone that is not fully affirming. Within this dyad, the person that holds the power is the religious person, both in terms of the historical oppression of LGBQ people and communities, as well as the stance that some conservatively religious people might have around the "truth" and "inerrancy" of the bible. Furthermore, the degree of ambiguity in these statements can add extra burden and stress on the LGBQ client to try to understand where the other might stand, or it may demonstrate the others' lack of commitment in figuring out their own beliefs. This adds to my justification around therapist self-disclosure, as it can be a mode of balancing the power dynamics in the therapy room. So many clients are in positions of lesser power when having difficult conversations with friends or family that are not affirming, making it even more important to share my affirmative stance.

This brings me to my final point, around how my affirmative stance might impact a religious LGBQ client who chooses celibacy. As a therapist, I honor and respect the clients who choose to remain celibate or pursue opposite-gender partners for the sake of holding onto their commitment to their nonaffirming theology. I have had close friends, colleagues, and clients choose to not pursue same-sex relationships, and I believe it is decision that it is complex and painful. This has and continues to pose internal dilemmas for me, as my desire for my client is to affirm their own sexuality as good and beautiful. However, I cannot impose my idea of what is good or beautiful onto the client. My role as a therapist is to help clients process what can be challenging and/or what kinds of negative impacts the decision to remain celibate or their heterosexual relationship/marriage might have on them. In my work with clients, my hope is to help them understand and process the loss and challenges they will face in making this decision. My role is not to choose this for them but to facilitate a decision-making process that feels coherent to the client. I continue to work on honoring the parts of the client that I might not fully align with. One might argue that I am not best fit to work with these clients because of my affirmative stance; however, I believe that it is because of my affirmative stance and my self-disclosure of this with the client at the onset *and* my honoring of their religious beliefs, that good work is facilitated. My intent is to practice with integrity by honoring my own values and beliefs, being open and honest with my client about these values, and allowing the process to unfold as we work together.

The therapeutic relationship can provide a safe and healing environment for clients to explore both S/R and LGBQ identities, but this requires a therapist's capacity to sit with tension while providing empathy and taking a posture of warm curiosity. I am not suggesting that therapists need to help clients find a resolution, as full integration of the identities may not be realistic or helpful. We should not be expecting a clean integration or resolution of all the tensions and dilemmas. Cohesion and coherence seem to be more accurate terms that acknowledge that exploring different parts of one's identity can illuminate its resonance and its conflicts. Using the term coherence honors the fact that navigating the intersection of these identities will always likely involve loss, tension, conflict, and ambiguity.

I have come to understand and believe that there is something sacred and transcendent about the experience of finding a more cohesive sense of self for religious LGBQ individuals—one where it leads people to a greater sense of living and being, along with a greater sense of fear and sorrow that grief and loss will be part of one's life. Reconciling these two realities is what makes this process both liberating and challenging; you learn to hold joy and pain together to differing degrees at different seasons of life.

FINAL THOUGHTS

As we help our clients navigate their sense of coherence in their sexual and religious identities, I offer this passage from Thomas Merton's (1961) book, *New Seeds of Contemplation*. In it, Merton points to the importance that reminds us and our clients that we are more in the likeness of god when we are most ourselves.

> A tree gives glory to God by being a tree. For in being what God means it to be it is obeying [God]. It "consents," so to speak, to [God's] creative love. It is expressing an idea which is in God and which is not distinct from the essence of God, and therefore a tree imitates God by being a tree. (p. 29)

What the client may "choose" at the end of the therapy process may not be final, and it may be what is best for their given narrative and circumstance in that moment. This, hopefully, relieves the pressure and anxiety for therapists to have to find the right answer in their work with LGBQ individuals (Bartoli & Gillem, 2008). Clinicians are encouraged to remember that a "resolution" for one client will differ from a resolution for the next client. Some may experience a decrease in depression and shame by leaving their religion, whereas others might feel that their religious community is too important for their well-being, and thus they seek out biblical texts and scholars that affirm their whole self and find an affirming community. For many of our clients, this process might be one that is ongoing. A dear friend shared with me,

> I am still in process of figuring out the complexity of religion and queerness, both as how they go together and how they don't go together. Identifying with both does not mean I understand both to the fullest, never mind how they are together.

My hope for my clients is that they will be able to experience moments of feeling most alive, as much of their lives has been deadened, twisted, and damaged by nonaffirming relationships and theologies. Alive, in this case, does not necessarily mean feelings of joy in isolation, but alive in the sense that they are able to experience a coherence within themselves that leads to peace and contentment amidst seasons of rest and struggle. The coming-out process and the acceptance of one's own sexual identity is one that is accompanied by both deep freedom and deep pain; it is immensely sacred and fraught at the same time. Therapists must hold these tensions with their clients, as the clients navigate feelings that seem impossible to coexist within themselves but exist together at the same time.

REFERENCES

American Psychological Association. (2003). Guidelines on multicultural education, training, research, practice, and organizational change for psychologists. *American Psychologist, 58*(5), 377–402. https://doi.org/10.1037/0003-066X.58.5.377

American Psychological Association. (2012). Guidelines for psychological practice with lesbian, gay, and bisexual clients. *American Psychologist, 67*(1), 10–42. https://doi.org/10.1037/a0024659

American Psychological Association. (2017). *Ethical principles of psychologists and code of conduct* (2002, Amended June 1, 2010, and January 1, 2017). http://www.apa.org/ethics/code/index.aspx

American Psychological Association, Task Force on Appropriate Therapeutic Responses to Sexual Orientation. (2009). *Report of the American Psychological Association Task Force on Appropriate Therapeutic Responses to Sexual Orientation.* https://www.apa.org/pi/lgbt/resources/sexual-orientation

Bartoli, E., & Gillem, A. R. (2008). Continuing to depolarize the debate on sexual orientation and religion: Identity and the therapeutic process. *Professional Psychology: Research and Practice, 39*(2), 202–209. https://doi.org/10.1037/0735-7028.39.2.202

Bible Gateway. (2021). *A searchable online Bible* (NIV Version). https://www.biblegateway.com/versions/New-International-Version-NIV-Bible/

Bieschke, K. J., Perez, R. M., & DeBord, K. A. (Eds.). (2007). *Handbook of counseling and psychotherapy with lesbian, gay, bisexual, and transgender clients* (2nd ed.). American Psychological Association. https://doi.org/10.1037/11482-000

Boucher, H. C. (2011). The dialectical self-concept II: Cross-role and within-role consistency, well-being, self-certainty, and authenticity. *Journal of Cross-Cultural Psychology, 42*(7), 1251–1271. https://doi.org/10.1177/0022022110383316

Brawer, P. A., Handal, P. J., Fabricatore, A. N., Roberts, R., & Wajda-Johnston, V. A. (2002). Training and education in religion/spirituality within APA-accredited clinical psychology programs. *Professional Psychology: Research and Practice, 33*(2), 203–206. https://doi.org/10.1037/0735-7028.33.2.203

Captari, L. E., Hook, J. N., Hoyt, W., Davis, D. E., McElroy-Heltzel, S. E., & Worthington, E. L., Jr. (2018). Integrating clients' religion and spirituality within psychotherapy: A comprehensive meta-analysis. *Journal of Clinical Psychology, 74*(11), 1938–1951. https://doi.org/10.1002/jclp.22681

Cragun, C. L., & Friedlander, M. L. (2012). Experiences of Christian clients in secular psychotherapy: A mixed-methods investigation. *Journal of Counseling Psychology*, *59*(3), 379–391. https://doi.org/10.1037/a0028283

Cross, S. E., Gore, J. S., & Morris, M. L. (2003). The relational-interdependent self-construal, self-concept consistency, and well-being. *Journal of Personality and Social Psychology*, *85*(5), 933–944. https://doi.org/10.1037/0022-3514.85.5.933

Farley, M. A. (2006). *Just love: A framework for Christian sexual ethics*. Continuum International Publishing Group.

Fassinger, R. E., & Arseneau, J. R. (2007). "I'd rather get wet than be under that umbrella": Differentiating the experiences and identities of lesbian, gay, bisexual, and transgender people. In K. J. Bieschke, R. M. Perez, & K. A. DeBord (Eds.), *Handbook of counseling and psychotherapy with lesbian, gay, bisexual, and transgender clients* (pp. 19–49). American Psychological Association. https://doi.org/10.1037/11482-001

Foucault, M. (1976). *The history of sexuality* (Vol. 1). Random House.

Gallup. (2020). *Religion*. https://news.gallup.com/poll/1690/religion.aspx

Goldfried, M. R. (2001). Integrating gay, lesbian, and bisexual issues into mainstream psychology. *American Psychologist*, *56*(11), 977–988. https://doi.org/10.1037/0003-066X.56.11.977

Heyward, C. (1989). *Touching our strength: The erotic as power and the love of God*. HarperCollins Publishers.

Kernis, M. H., & Goldman, B. M. (2006). A multicomponent conceptualization of authenticity: Theory and research. In P. Z. Mark (Ed.), *Advances in experimental social psychology* (Vol. 38, pp. 283–357). Academic Press. https://doi.org/10.1016/S0065-2601(06)38006-9

Legate, N., Ryan, R. M., & Weinstein, N. (2012). Is coming out always a "good thing"? Exploring the relations of autonomy support, outness, and wellness for lesbian, gay, and bisexual individuals. *Social Psychological and Personality Science*, *3*(2), 145–152. https://doi.org/10.1177/1948550611411929

Merton, T. (1961). *New seeds of contemplation*. New Directions Publishing.

Movement Advancement Project. (2021). *Conversion "therapy" laws*. https://www.lgbtmap.org/equality-maps/conversion_therapy

Noman, N. (2019, November 8). *Netflix's "Queer Eye: We're in Japan!" highlights a big problem with mainstream LGBTQ advocacy*. NBC News. https://www.nbcnews.com/think/opinion/netflix-s-queer-eye-we-re-japan-highlights-big-problem-ncna1078756

Nugent, R., & Gramick, J. (1989). In R. Hasbany (Ed.), *Homosexuality and religion* (pp. 7–46). Harrington Park Press.

Pachankis, J. E., & Goldfried, M. R. (2013). Clinical issues in working with lesbian, gay, and bisexual clients. *Psychology of Sexual Orientation and Gender Diversity*, *1*(S), 45–58. https://doi.org/10.1037/2329-0382.1.S.45

Pargament, K. I., Mahoney, A., & Shafranske, E. P. (Eds.). (2013). *APA handbook of psychology, religion, and spirituality: Vol. 2. An applied psychology of religion and spirituality*. American Psychological Association. https://doi.org/10.1037/14046-000

Post, B. C., & Wade, N. G. (2009). Religion and spirituality in psychotherapy: A practice-friendly review of research. *Journal of Clinical Psychology*, *65*(2), 131–146. https://doi.org/10.1002/jclp.20563

Reinecke, L., & Trepte, S. (2014). Authenticity and well-being on social network sites: A two-wave longitudinal study on the effects of online authenticity and the positivity bias in SNS communication. *Computers in Human Behavior, 30*, 95–102. https://doi.org/10.1016/j.chb.2013.07.030

Rizutto, A.-M. (1998). *Why did Freud reject God: A psychodynamic interpretation.* Yale University Press.

Root, M. P. P. (1990). Resolving "other" status: Identity development of biracial individuals. *Women & Therapy, 9*(1–2), 185–205. https://doi.org/10.1300/J015v09n01_11

Rose, E. M., Westefeld, J. S., & Ansley, T. N. (2008). Spiritual issues in counseling: Clients' beliefs and preferences. *Psychology of Religion and Spirituality, S*(1), 18–33. https://doi.org/10.1037/1941-1022.S.1.18 (Reprinted from "Spiritual issues in counseling: Clients' beliefs and preferences," 2001, *Journal of Counseling Psychology, 48*[1], 61–71. https://doi.org/10.1037/0022-0167.48.1.61)

Schafer, R. M., Handal, P. J., Brawer, P. A., & Ubinger, M. (2011). Training and education in religion/spirituality within APA-accredited clinical psychology programs: 8 years later. *Journal of Religion and Health, 50*(2), 232–239. https://doi.org/10.1007/s10943-009-9272-8

Schnarch, D. M. (1991). *Constructing the sexual crucible: An integration of sexual and marital therapy.* W. W. Norton.

Shafranske, E. P., & Malony, H. N. (1996). Religion and the clinical practice of psychology: A case for inclusion. In E. P. Shafranske (Ed.), *Religion and the clinical practice of psychology* (pp. 561–586). American Psychological Association. https://doi.org/10.1037/10199-041

Shafranske, E. P., & Sperry, L. (2005). Addressing the spiritual dimension in psychotherapy: Introduction and overview. In L. Sperry & E. P. Shafranske (Eds.), *Spiritually oriented psychotherapy* (pp. 11–29). American Psychological Association. https://doi.org/10.1037/10886-001

Sheldon, K. M. (2013). Authenticity. In S. J. Lopez (Ed.), *The encyclopedia of positive psychology* (pp. 75–78). Wiley-Blackwell.

Sheldon, K. M., Ryan, R. M., Rawsthorne, L. J., & Ilardi, B. (1997). Trait self and true self: Cross-role variation in the Big-Five personality traits and its relations with psychological authenticity and subjective well-being. *Journal of Personality and Social Psychology, 73*(6), 1380–1393. https://doi.org/10.1037/0022-3514.73.6.1380

Sutton, A. (2018). Distinguishing between authenticity and personality consistency in predicting well-being: A mixed method approach. *European Review of Applied Psychology, 68*(3), 117–130. https://doi.org/10.1016/j.erap.2018.06.001

Tozer, E. E., & McClanahan, M. K. (1999). Treating the purple menace: Ethical considerations of conversion therapy and affirmative alternatives. *The Counseling Psychologist, 27*(5), 722–742. https://doi.org/10.1177/0011000099275006

Valenti, J. (2009). *The purity myth: How America's obsession with virginity is hurting young women.* Seal Press.

Vieten, C., Scammell, S., Pilato, R., Ammondson, I., Pargament, K. I., & Lukoff, D. (2013). Spiritual and religious competencies for psychologists. *Psychology of Religion and Spirituality, 5*(3), 129–144. https://doi.org/10.1037/a0032699

Watkins, B. A. (2008). *Purity balls: Protecting a daughter's innocence while controlling her sexuality.* The University of Alabama.

Wilchins, R. (2004). *Queer theory, gender theory.* Magnus Books.

Winnicott, D. W. (1965). *The maturational processes and the facilitating environment.* International Universities Press.

Worthington, E. L., Jr., Hook, J. N., Davis, D. E., & McDaniel, M. A. (2011). Religion and spirituality. *Journal of Clinical Psychology, 67*(2), 204–214. https://doi.org/10.1002/jclp.20760

Worthington, E. L., Jr., & Sandage, S. J. (2002). Religion and spirituality. In J. C. Norcross (Ed.), *Psychotherapy relationships that work: Therapist contributions and responsiveness to patients* (pp. 383–399). Oxford University Press.

Yakushko, O. (2005). Influence of social support, existential well-being, and stress over sexual orientation on self-esteem of gay, lesbian, and bisexual individuals. *International Journal for the Advancement of Counselling, 27*(1), 131–143. https://doi.org/10.1007/s10447-005-2259-6

Yalom, I. D. (1980). *Existential psychotherapy*. Basic Books.

11

RELIGIOUS DIFFERENCES IN SPIRITUALLY INTEGRATED COUPLE THERAPY

STEVEN J. SANDAGE

Couple therapy involves helping couples develop capacities to connect and collaborate amid the vast array of differences that typically emerge in couples' relationships over time. The literature on attending to dynamics of difference and diversity in couple therapy, such as differences across gender orientation, culture, race, and sexual orientation, has been growing. However, there has been very limited attention to religious differences and religious diversity in couple therapy. Dynamics of religion and spirituality can be so highly nuanced within personalized meanings and contexts that we could say there are religious and spiritual differences at some level within every couple, even if both persons identify with the same religious or spiritual (RS) traditions or disidentify with religion and spirituality altogether. For some couples, RS differences are enlivening sources of healthy connection and resilience in difficult times, while other couples can experience these differences as conflictual, painful, and estranging.

This project was influenced and supported by a grant from the John Templeton Foundation on "Mental Healthcare, Virtue, and Human Flourishing" (#61603).
https://doi.org/10.1037/0000276-012
Spiritual Diversity in Psychotherapy: Engaging the Sacred in Clinical Practice,
S. J. Sandage and B. D. Strawn (Editors)

Couples have also become increasingly religiously and spiritually diverse across many parts of the world, and the rate of interreligious marriage has doubled in the United States over the past century (Putnam & Campbell, 2012). By "interreligious couples," I mean couples who differ in their religious identification either markedly (e.g., Hindu, atheist) or within a broader shared religious tradition (e.g., Conservative Jew, Reform Jew), though this second example is sometimes called an "interfaith couple" in the literature. Nearly half of marriages in the United States are between individuals who are interreligious in background, and around one third of marriages remain interreligious over time. (Note: The difference in these figures is based on religious conversion by one spouse.) This trend generally cuts across religious demographics, although some religious communities continue to show a higher preference for marriage within their religious tradition (e.g., Latter-day Saints, Jews, Evangelicals, Black Protestants, Latinx Catholics) relative to some other religious communities (e.g., Anglo Catholics, mainline Protestants; Putnam & Campbell, 2012; see also Pew Research Center, 2015). Therefore, it is fair to assume therapists in many contexts will continue to see rising levels of religious difference among the couples they work with.

In this chapter, I offer a brief overview of the clinical implications of research on religious differences in couples. I then describe ways my own spiritual and religious journey has influenced my approach to spiritually integrated couple therapy based on the relational spirituality model (RSM; Sandage et al., 2020), and I apply the RSM to two couple cases. However, I will first clarify my definitions of spirituality and religion.

DEFINITIONS OF SPIRITUALITY AND RELIGION

My colleagues and I have developed the RSM by defining *relational spirituality* broadly as "ways of relating to the sacred" (Sandage et al., 2020, p. 24; see also Worthington & Sandage, 2016). This definition builds on the work of Hill and Pargament (2003), who defined spirituality as related to "a search for the sacred." They used the term "sacred" to signify "a person, object, principle, or concept that transcends the self" (p. 65). The sacred can include "a divine being, divine object, Ultimate Reality, or Ultimate Truth" that is "set apart" as holy and beyond the ordinary (p. 65). The term "search" implies actively searching for sacred meaning. Connections with the sacred may come through specific rituals or practices but can also be part of everyday life for some people (Ammerman, 2020). My relational theoretical orientation to clinical practice has led me to foreground the relational dynamics of spirituality by attending to the varieties of ways people relate to whatever they consider sacred, and these relational styles can include trust, fearful avoidance, sacrificial service, hunger for mirroring, questioning, worship, mindful dwelling, disappointment, and many other relational dynamics. Clinically, this means I want to understand what is ultimately important and valuable (or sacred) to clients and how they relate to whatever they consider ultimate and valuable, also recognizing that some clients do not consider themselves "spiritual" or "religious" and would locate their deepest values within a secular framework.

There are many ways to differentiate definitions of *spirituality* and *religion*. Again, following Hill and Pargament (2003), I define both religion and spirituality as related to the "search for the sacred" (p. 65), with spirituality the broader construct that can potentially be expressed through religious (social and institutional systems) or other social contexts. Religious traditions influence the contexts and practices of relational spirituality for many people, at least implicitly, although a growing number in the United States self-identify as spiritual but not religious (Ammerman, 2020). Clinically, I also find that a client's RS self-identification does not always predict the extent to which they may want to process issues related to religion or spirituality. Some clients have painful or even traumatic experiences related to religious and spiritual communities they want to process, and others find pockets of ambivalence about religion and/or spirituality that emerge when working on other issues that activate existential questions. These dynamics become particularly complicated when doing couple therapy and needing to negotiate differing religious and spiritual dynamics within the couple while also attending to my own presence within the couple system. As a clinician, I typically enjoy the learning that occurs for me in trying to relate effectively across this range of client diversity, and I try to regain a sense of curiosity, humility, and empathy when my countertransference is provoked by differences with my clients in these areas.

In the RSM, we also acknowledge the importance of existential and theological dimensions that can be important to some clients, so this shapes our use of the spiritual, existential, religious, and theological (SERT; Rupert et al., 2019) heuristic for an inclusive orientation to client diversity. In this chapter, the focus is on religious differences in couples, but I will interpret these dynamics using RSM and SERT frameworks.

RELIGIOUS DIFFERENCES AND COUPLES

The social scientific and clinical literature on religious differences and couples is extremely limited and largely addresses heterosexual married couples from Christian, Jewish, and Muslim traditions. Some earlier research on inter-religious marriage in the 1980s (Chinitz & Brown, 2001; Glenn, 1982) had suggested religious similarity was a predictor of marital stability. However, as suggested earlier, a lot has changed in attitudes toward interreligious marriage (and couple relationships, more generally) in the last 4 decades. I will highlight some of the dynamics from the literature and my clinical experience that can affect religious differences in couples.

First, levels of religious commitment and social identification with particular religious traditions can influence attitudes toward religious diversity in couples (Cila & Lalonde, 2014; Sahl & Batson, 2011; Van Niekerk & Verkuyten, 2018). Religious differences may not be particularly problematic for couples where both partners have a low commitment or connection to a particular religious tradition, but the opposite may be true if religious commitment is high for one or both. It is also possible that the relevance of religious commitments and the associated challenges of difference may intensify at particular points in the life cycle (e.g., birth of a child, loss of family members; Greenstein et al., 1993; Singh, 2017). From a relational and systemic perspective, it is valuable to assess the life-cycle context and social networks of a couple struggling with religious differences, as can be seen in the case studies later in this chapter.

Second, a global perspective clearly shows that diverse social contexts around the world shape differing views of interreligious coupling (Gordon & Arenstein, 2017). For example, some countries are characterized by limited immigration and social or religious diversity, making interreligious coupling unlikely or even illegal. In strongly traditional and homogeneous contexts, family and social connections may serve to discourage coupling across religious and other forms of diversity, although there will be individual differences in openness to interreligious relationships in every context (Cila & Lalonde, 2014). Other countries are pluralistic and mostly secular, making it hard to accurately determine rates of interreligious marriage. Clinically, it is important to consider the sociocultural and political contexts and intergenerational backgrounds of interreligious couples who are struggling with religious differences (Singh, 2017).

Third, there is some evidence that gender can affect views of interreligious couples, at least in some Muslim contexts. For example, in a large study across 22 Muslim majority countries, attitudes among Muslims toward interreligious marriage were more negative if imagining a daughter marrying a Christian compared with a son doing the same (Van Niekerk & Verkuyten, 2018). This might reflect concerns about the intergenerational transmission of religion and the social reality that men in those contexts would generally retain authority over religious influences on their children, whereas Muslim women might be expected to defer to their Christian husbands. A study of Muslim Canadian young adults also found men were more open to interreligious dating and marriage than were women (Cila & Lalonde, 2014), perhaps reflecting different gender socialization about the importance of religious homogamy. As mentioned above, religion can often shape beliefs about gender that can influence various areas of couple functioning, including gender roles and power, sexuality, birth control, and childrearing, among others. This sometimes promotes a stronger sanction against religiously diverse coupling for women, which obviously contrasts with feminist and other socially progressive views of gender and sexuality among couples (Singh, 2017).

Fourth, views of race and racism can intersect with views of interreligious coupling. For example, Sahl and Batson (2011) found White parents reported greater opposition to interfaith dating and marriage of their children than did Black parents in a sample from the southern United States. These findings invite questions about the ways social views of religious homogamy among certain dominant groups might intersect with racism and other forms of social prejudice, and also the ways nondominant groups in certain contexts might develop more tolerant attitudes toward diversity due to flexible religious frameworks and pressures to assimilate.

Fifth, there is some research evidence that relationships tend to become more homogenous as the level of commitment increases from dating to marriage (Sahl & Batson, 2011). That is, certain contexts may tolerate higher diversity in couples who are dating but expect similarity across religion and other social categories as couples move toward marriage. Some couples presenting for therapy with religious differences may have experienced stronger support from family and friends prior to their engagement or marriage.

Finally, the modest literature on interreligious couples suggests that certain aspects of psychosocial or relational development might potentially moderate the outcomes of religious differences in couples. Parsons and colleagues (2007) studied predictors of marital satisfaction in a sample of interfaith married individuals in the United States and found (a) achieved identity development and (b) differentiation of self (DoS; i.e., capacities for self-regulation of emotions and interpersonal flexibility) to be positively associated with interfaith marital satisfaction, whereas foreclosed identity status was negatively related with the same. These findings suggest that couples may better negotiate religious differences with a healthy and flexible sense of selfhood and the abilities to manage the anxiety of differences, whereas individuals with low identity development and DoS may struggle with conflicts over even the most granular of religious differences with their partner. Thus, couple processes related to religious differences rest upon various relational development capacities to navigate differences and conflicts more generally (Caffaro, 2011; Chinitz & Brown, 2001). More research is needed in this area, but this fits my clinical experience with couples in that the content of particular differences is often less influential than the partners' developmental capacities for reflective self-awareness, perspective-taking, humility, and anxiety management, which are all correlates of DoS (Sandage et al., 2020).

MY SERT JOURNEY TO COUPLE THERAPIST

Before describing my approach to spiritually integrated couple therapy, I should locate myself and relay a little of how my own SERT journey has shaped that approach. I was born and raised in Iowa and grew up in the United Methodist Church (mainline Protestant). During my adolescence (1980s), the agriculture crisis in the Midwest produced tremendous stress for many families, including my own. The economic losses turned existential with a growing number of suicides in our wider social network. I was among part of my family that intensified religious commitments during this time by turning to the more conservative Evangelical and Pentecostal branches of Christian traditions. In retrospect, I am sure we were looking for more stable existential grounding and forms of religion and spirituality that were as experientially intense as the stress we were facing.

In my transition to college, I became interested in ministry as a possible vocation. I have a distinct memory of trying to attend a more progressive and intellectual Methodist church during my freshman year of college and, given my ministry interests, being invited to sit in on a meeting of the church leadership team. They seemed to spend the entire time discussing how to put up the storm windows around the church and other things I found quite banal to my 19-year-old religious fervency, so I made my way to a more Evangelical United Methodist church pastored by a passionate and reflective man from Sri Lanka. This unfolded at a time when I was becoming more aware of powerful religious differences within (a) my wider family system, (b) the different church groups I was attending, and (c) my surrounding community. Prior to college, I was mostly oblivious to religious differences beyond common versions of Christianity (e.g., Evangelical, Catholic, mainline Protestant), but college began to introduce me to a slightly wider spectrum, and I observed some incidents of religious bigotry and marginalization. I was majoring in psychology (since one of my Christian mentors told me the religious studies department at my university would be too liberal), and I am sure this mix of factors shaped my lifelong interests in the intersections of psychology, religion, and diversity. Although it would take many years to articulate, questions were developing about the various forms of relational spirituality that could serve to either bridge or estrange people across differences depending on how God and the sacred were imagined and engaged.

After college, I enrolled in an Evangelical seminary in Chicago to study theology and psychology of religion; however, I also took courses at a more progressive United Methodist seminary. I enjoyed and was troubled by both theological contexts. I found that some Evangelicals could be very parochial and disinterested in social justice concerns, whereas progressives could become highly intellectual and relativistic in ways that seemed removed from the existential uncertainty I had experienced. Looking back, I was working out a dialectical intuition that authentic spirituality should provide both grounding in deep commitments and also openness to a wider sense of community with those who are suffering. Refuge *and* diverse solidarity. This was reinforced through living and working on the grounds of a synagogue as part of an interfaith student-learning program during the latter half of seminary, in which I was exposed to the dynamics of community and openness in another religious tradition (Reform Judaism).

Seminary clarified for me that I wanted to be a psychologist, so I entered a PhD program in counseling psychology while also starting work as a correctional chaplain and then as a psychologist in juvenile detention facilities and prisons. These correctional settings showed me levels of religious and other forms of diversity I would have never encountered while working in churches, and I was struck by the variety of ways different expressions of spirituality and religion could contribute to well-being, pathology, or combinations of both. My pull toward working with couples and families moved me from correctional to outpatient mental health settings, and I was increasingly stretched by the systemic reality that every couple or family case included multiple perspectives on RS dynamics. Most of my training in psychology and theology had led me to think about individuals, but I was drawn to the challenge of thinking about RS dynamics from relational frameworks that attended to (a) the interactions between people and (b) the influences of differing systemic contexts.

Given the religious tensions in the early phase of my SERT journey, it seems appropriate I have split my career with the first half on the faculty of an Evangelical seminary and working clinically at Evangelical-owned clinics and now on the faculty of a progressive United Methodist seminary and clinical training staff at a pluralistic clinic. I identify as Christian, and my theological orientation is most strongly influenced by relational process, existential, and liberation theology traditions. I continue to resonate with many aspects of the Wesleyan theological roots that have influenced United Methodism, such as the strong emphases on relationships as sources of transformation, the necessity of working to integrate personal and social holiness, and the potential for grace and forgiveness to heal perpetual temptations toward perfectionism. These beliefs are also held with a contemplative and existential sensibility that growth often requires tolerating periodic movements into ambiguity and liminal darkness before regaining clarity.

RELATIONAL SPIRITUALITY MODEL OF PSYCHOTHERAPY

My colleagues and I have applied the RSM to psychotherapy (Sandage et al., 2020; Shults & Sandage, 2006), which builds on the relational definition of spirituality provided earlier. The RSM also integrates relational development and systemic theories with a relational and dialectical view of change. I will summarize some of the key tenets of the RSM that are most relevant for religious differences in couple therapy (for broader coverage of an RSM approach to couple therapy, see Sandage et al., 2019, 2020; Worthington & Sandage, 2016).

First, the RSM suggests that human development involves ongoing dialectical balancing of dwelling and seeking. "Dwelling" references the human need for grounding, orientating commitments and values, and sources of relational and community support that provide safe-haven functions for emotional and existential regulation of stress and anxiety. Spiritual and religious communities, traditions, and practices can represent resources for dwelling, although the need for dwelling is broader than spiritual and religion and represents the need for stabilization, security, and place. "Seeking" refers to the human need to explore, to grow, to encounter diversity and novel situation, and to make new meaning out of complex human predicaments. Seeking maps on to the secure base function of the attachment system, and exploration can be anxiety provoking, so it is important to have safe havens for regulation and recalibration.

Dwelling and seeking form a dialectic in both individual development and larger relational systems (e.g., couples, families, organizations), and these dynamics can be organized in ways that are opposing or they can be integrative functions. For example, in a couple system one partner could be oriented strongly toward spiritual dwelling with consistent involvement in a particular religious community, and it could generate conflict when the other partner moves beyond that religious community and starts seeking new spiritual experiences outside the prior system. In my view, systems need both stability and novelty; however, the process of balancing and integrating those two needs will be highly turbulent in some cases and may result in the dissolution of the prior relational system.

The RSM also focuses on three key developmental systems—attachment, differentiation, and intersubjectivity—that can have profound influences on relational spirituality (Sandage et al., 2020). These developmental systems are somewhat overlapping, yet each is also unique in developmental emphases, evolutionary functions, and ethical and spiritual goals. The attachment system focuses on establishing security, cultivating trust, and engaging in secure base exploration through relational regulation. The differentiation system focuses on ways self–other identity development ("Who am I?" and "Who are you?") interacts with (a) interpersonal flexibility of connection and autonomy to facilitate cooperation with others and (b) the self-regulation of emotions, particularly anxiety related to interpersonal differences. The intersubjectivity system focuses relational and triangular dynamics among self, other, and third spaces (i.e., space between persons) that can shape possibilities for intimacy and mutual recognition. The intersubjectivity system is also involved in the repair of relational ruptures in contrast to oppressive power imbalances of "doer" and "done to" (Benjamin, 2018). The RSM promotes clinical assessment of these three developmental systems with treatment planning shaped and sequenced based on the primary developmental challenges for a particular couple.

Spiritual, religious, and existential struggles are common human experiences (Pargament & Exline, 2021) and an important part of human development within the RSM framework. Ruptures in relating to the sacred or anxious struggles with existential predicaments (e.g., death and loss) in life can be incredibly painful and dysregulating, but in some cases spiritual struggles also lead to new meaning making and developmental growth. The RSM highlights the importance of understanding clients' meaning frameworks and their personal understanding of suffering in order to work clinically from within their worldview. While many clients want efficient symptom relief, the systemic orientation of the RSM suggests it is often important to understand the implicit meanings and assumptions "beneath" the symptoms and the ways those symptoms might intensify during periods of destabilization preceding developmental shifts (Gelo & Salvatore, 2016).

The crucible is a key metaphor in the RSM used to represent this intensification process of second-order change moving toward developmental growth. Numerous spiritual writers and psychotherapy theorists have employed the crucible metaphor to represent a process of transformation that initially heats up with the anxiety and ambiguity of primal existential and spiritual themes (e.g., abandonment, engulfment) and requires wrestling with core values and identity commitments. In the RSM, a crucible process might be shaped by dilemmas related to one's own integrity, for example, a person realizes they deeply love someone of another religious faith despite prohibitions against interreligious marriage in their own family and community. But crucibles can also be formed within relationships where each partner has an interlocking dilemma, such as an atheist couple where one converts to a religious faith and now wants to raise their child in that faith. Will the other partner support this and even participate in religious activities related to their child? Can they collaborate across these differences?

A key determinant of whether spiritual, religious, and existential crucible experiences of clients can lead to healing and growth or chronic dysregulation involves the quality of relational experiences surrounding the persons involved and ways relational figures interface with the developmental systems (i.e., attachment, differentiation, intersubjectivity) referenced previously. Therefore, a key assumption of the RSM is that the therapeutic alliance is a primary source of gain in psychotherapy (Wampold & Imel, 2015), as therapist–client interactions need to provide new experiences of attachment, differentiation, and intersubjectivity over time. However, my colleagues and I also assume there are often numerous sources of potential relational influence in clients' lives (e.g., family, friends, partners, coworkers, clergy, other clinical providers, clinical administrative staff), and it is valuable to assess this wider relational ecology and consider interpersonal and systemic intervention strategies that follow from that assessment.

This whole set of relational assumptions above reflects my communitarian values and my theological belief that ultimate reality involves a differentiated web of relations (i.e., differentiated relational ontology; Sandage & Brown, 2018). The developmental systems orientation of the RSM means I view attachment, differentiation, and intersubjectivity (defined below) as three aspects of human development that are typically necessary for collaborative couple relationships, and these developmental constructs integrate readily with the virtues and ideals of many spiritual and religious traditions (Sandage et al., 2020). In addition to symptom alleviation, I also value working toward relational well-being and flourishing with clients (Jankowski et al., 2020), and most couples have relational goals that go beyond simply reducing anxiety and conflict. However, I need to recognize these relational development goals can diverge from the goals of some clients, and this raises challenges for my own differentiation in seeking to relate sensitively with clients who hold more individualistic perspectives or other ideals about relational development.

This challenge to relate sensitively across differences speaks to the importance of spiritual and religious competence (Vieten et al., 2016), as well as other aspects of diversity competence, which combine with social justice commitment as core values within the RSM (Sandage et al., 2020). Spiritual and religious competence involves capacities to relate effectively across spiritual and religious differences in ways I will describe below (see also Morgan & Sandage, 2016). It is important to note the systemic isomorphism or parallel between couples who are trying to relate across differences and their experiences as clients with a therapist who seeks to respectfully engage clients' worldview beliefs and practices across whatever differences exist in the client–therapist relationship.

COUPLE THERAPY PROCESS

An RSM approach to couple therapy has been described in several publications (Sandage et al., 2019, 2020; Worthington & Sandage, 2016), so I will briefly summarize contours of this approach but tailor the focus here to couples struggling with religious differences in the case illustrations that follow. I find it helpful to think of the couple therapy process as roughly following an iterative four-phase model. By *iterative*, I mean a nonlinear process where certain phases might get revisited. This process includes (a) forming an attachment and working alliance with a couple, (b) coconstructing a developmental crucible, (c) processing grief and disappointment, and (d) cultivating and extending collaboration.

Forming an Attachment and Working Alliance

Attachment and alliance building can be more challenging with couples than with individuals as a couple therapist needs to pace two differing personalities and competing sets of concerns, and the attachment styles of the partners are also frequently different (Johnson, 2015). This tests my own differentiation as a therapist, particularly my capacities to (a) self-soothe anxiety and (b) efficiently frame-shift to understand and communicate empathy for the differing perspectives of the two partners. The relational ethic of multidirectional partiality and justice requires I try to position myself in the couple system with balance and fairness to each partner's concerns, unless safety concerns require a more protective stance (Grunebaum, 1987). It would be impossible for me to cultivate or sustain this relational ethic and balanced positioning without a professional community of colleagues who help me metabolize my countertransference reactions to cases.

Coconstructing a Developmental Crucible

As mentioned previously, a developmental crucible involves a set of core dilemmas for an individual or couple that brings together crucial threads of personal narrative and powerful existential or spiritual themes that frame the need for developmental growth. I say "coconstructing" because I believe clients and therapists typically construct this kind of framing together through the relational process. The articulation of common couple treatment goal might be something like "improving the couple's communication." A crucible formulation around communication might start with a question to a client like "I am wondering if your unwillingness to talk to him [husband] about your spiritual differences is a sign of your anxiety or your integrity?" This might prompt the client to ask for clarification, which could give the therapist an opportunity to tie in narrative threads and other themes, for example:

> Well, I was thinking how you described that painful but pivotal episode during college when you were home and your dad tried to convince you that you were not gay and that God could deliver you from those "lies." You said you knew your truth at that moment and that it made no sense to keep arguing with him, and you decisively moved forward with your own sense of identity and sexuality at that point. So, I know that stepping away from a painful difference can be integrity for you. But I also know this marriage means a lot to you. And your own faith commitments mean a lot to you. So I wonder if it feels anxiety provoking to explore these kinds of differences that sometimes result in losing a relationship.

This anxiety-versus-integrity contrast is a common one in Schnarch's (2009) crucible therapy, and ideally the therapist would also be able to coconstruct an interlocking crucible for the partner in this particular couple. This might start by probing the partner's source of courage to voice their RS differences and to advocate for communication about it within their relationship, perhaps as a developmental progression arising within their own narrative. Depending on how each partner responds and the particular themes they identify, this might move toward the coconstruction of a shared couple crucible formulation on something like "finding the courage to explore their spiritual differences and points of common ground" as more nuanced and developmental than simply improving communication.

Crucibles can be coconstructed for couples on a variety of powerful and poignant themes, such as the risk of loving someone you might lose, learning to collaborate versus "going it alone," parenting a partner but then wanting them to act like an adult, longing for intimacy while constantly hiding, managing people rather than trusting them, entering the dark place with someone rather than trying to rescue them from it, holding onto resentment to avoid the shame of being surprised again, and many others. Effectively coconstructing a developmental crucible with clients serves to intensify the deeper existential and spiritual dilemmas that are larger than a particular problem or conflict. This can also result in a clarity and focus to the growth that is needed and the existential and spiritual choices to be considered.

Processing Grief and Disappointment

Another RSM assumption is that developmental growth frequently comes with the need to process and regulate emotions related to grief and disappointment.

Grief and disappointment are also inevitable experiences in the life cycles of couple relationships and even normal responses as couples move from earlier phases of idealization toward greater familiarity. In my clinical experience, many couples presenting for therapy have not previously found ways to coregulate grief and disappointment, yet these can be vulnerable feelings that can help soften interactions "beneath" anger and other defensive reactions. For example, couples working on attachment might benefit from learning to connect in processing the sadness of grief. Couples working on differentiation might work on distress tolerance for disappointing one another and feeling disappointment while learning to self-regulate those responses and cultivating a greater acceptance of differences. Couples working on intersubjectivity may discover unmetabolized grief and disappointment are protective barriers against the risks of deeper intimacy or the forgiveness of ruptures. Many couples in therapy will eventually encounter some level of grief that they may lack personal models and supporting structures for the kind of relationship they are trying to achieve, and this is certainly true of interreligious couples and many couples negotiating significant diversity factors (e.g., same-sex or polyamorous couples).

Cultivating and Extending Collaboration

Collaboration is a vastly underrated relational skill or virtue, and I think of growth in collaboration outside of sessions as one of the primary goals of couple therapy. This might involve various areas of a couple relationship where some level of collaboration is typically necessary, such as finances, sexuality, parenting, relating with extended family and friends, recreation, and navigating religious and other differences. This emphasis on collaboration in the RSM also reflects my own SERT values, including my theological belief that flourishing for human communities and the planet must come through divine–human collaboration amid differences.

In my view, progress in couple therapy will eventually require helping couples restructure relational interactions in some area requiring collaboration. This typically involves increasing capacities for self-awareness of relational patterns that previously have, and have not, worked and planning alternative patterns of collaboration. I frame this to couples as likely anxiety provoking due to past struggles and the unfamiliarity of new patterns, so we prioritize working on emotion regulation strategies in the initial attempts at new forms of collaboration. That is, we target a goal of self-regulation of anxiety and other emotions during repeated attempts at collaboration while countering perfectionistic expectations of ideal synchrony in early attempts at better collaboration. When couples make progress at collaboration in a particular area (e.g., finances), I seek to extend insights about new relational patterns in application to some other area where collaboration is needed. Once a couple has developed new collaborative patterns in two or three areas of their relationship, they likely have achieved enough sustainable growth (i.e., transformation) to consider therapy termination.

The RSM also highlights the need for clinical interventions focused on three relational development systems: attachment, differentiation, and intersubjectivity. Although these relational development systems are overlapping and interactive, I next illustrate two brief couple therapy case examples with one focusing on differentiation and one on intersubjectivity.

CASE EXAMPLE: DIFFERENTIATION SYSTEM FOCUS–RITA AND JANA

As mentioned earlier, the differentiation developmental system involves self-identity, interpersonal flexibility to facilitate cooperation and collaboration with others, and the self-regulation of emotions, particularly related to anxiety over differences. The following case illustrates ways religious differences can factor into couple challenges in differentiation, and in this particular case, difficulties with differentiation were influencing questions about long-term commitments. Case illustrations are based on composites, and details have been changed to maintain confidentiality.

Rita (African American, cisgender woman, Muslim) and Jana (Jewish American, cisgender woman, Unitarian Universalist) were a same-sex couple who had lived together for 5 years and were considering marriage. They came to couple therapy explicitly struggling with religious differences that intersected with other identity dynamics. When they started their relationship, Rita was not very active in religious practice; however, over the past 3 years she has become involved in a Sufi Muslim community that she found to be a helpful alternative to her more traditional Muslim background. Jana wanted Rita to be part of her Unitarian Universalist community; however, Rita had not found it to be a fit despite some involvement. As they considered the possibility of marriage, Jana felt strongly they should be involved in only gay-affirmative communities and was concerned about how they would raise children in terms of religion given their differences. Rita said she felt accepted by her Sufi community even though that community did not take an official public position on same-sex relationships. This lack of explicit affirmation was objectionable to Jana, as she believed it can mask or enable homophobia and discrimination.

They also had conflict over how to handle family members who were not accepting of their sexual orientation and relationship. Jana's family of origin was largely accepting of their relationship, but she had also directly challenged a couple of family members who were not affirming. Rita chose to take a more accommodating stance with her parents and extended family, who were mostly nonaffirming, purportedly for religious reasons. Rita's parents were glad to have her and Jana visit, but they insisted they sleep in separate rooms. Jana came to feel this violated her integrity and had refused to visit them for the previous couple years.

A key RSM clinical strategy related to the differentiation system with couples involves *negotiating a differentiated alliance* (Sandage et al., 2020, pp. 148–149) with sensitivity to differences and power dynamics, and the therapist–client alliance also activates attachment system dynamics involving safety, trust, and connection. Rita and Jana had researched me online prior to our first session, so despite a positive referral from a friend they came in with questions about my abilities as a White Christian male to understand their relationship and the challenges they faced given these differences in experience. I have found it helpful at the outset of therapy to typically invite clients to ask me questions about myself and to discuss the role of my religious identity, gender, race, and other diversity issues in my approach to therapy. The information itself is rarely the key issue, but rather the relational dynamic of openness and the sharing of power that comes from transparency can reduce the understandable attachment anxiety of trusting someone who is barely known. From a social justice perspective, those of us who are clinicians have tremendous power in relation to clients, and it is reasonable for clients to want some information to determine whether our worldviews and experiences seem like a potential fit for the trust required in the therapy process. I will set boundaries about some areas of personal information but find clients rarely probe into those domains.

In this case, the initial work was also for me to convey empathy and understanding to both Rita and Jana related to their primary concerns, which were rooted in their differing relational spiritualities and contexts. We came to understand that for Jana, personal and family involvement in spiritual communities that affirm same-sex relationships not only was a core justice issue but also felt like a key to existential survival. It was helpful to surface these parallel levels of meaning, which Rita had not really grasped previously. For Rita, connection to both her family of origin and a stream of the Muslim tradition carried sacred significance as both an expression of the value of loyalty (key for Rita) and also existential survival as a person of color in the United States (i.e., part of her racial identity). In my own differentiation-based approach to religious faith, this kind of uncovering of layers of personal, social, and existential meaning is a sacred process that both requires and potentially cultivates numerous relational virtues of dialogue such as humility, curiosity, honesty, patience, and compassion (Waring, 2016).

This process of actively exploring differences that trigger conflicts is anxiety provoking, and a key clinical strategy for making differentiation work productive is to explicitly facilitate clients' capacities for self-regulation. I noted to this couple that differences can generate anxiety and we would need to find ways they could each self-soothe anxiety as these differences surfaced. I asked, "Are there ways, for each of you, that your spirituality might help you self-soothe the anxieties that come up when these differences come online?" Like most clients, Jana and Rita were initially surprised by the question in a couple of ways. First, it is new for most clients to be intentional about self-regulation amid relating to their partners on conflicts. Ironically, our capacities for self-awareness and self-regulation are vital for effective communication during interpersonal conflicts, yet it is so easy to lose oneself in a focus on the other person (and often how they are "wrong" about something). Second, it was a novel idea for both to draw on their own spiritual beliefs and practices amid these relational conflicts over religious differences. Like most couples, they had often fallen into the implicit view that spirituality was somehow "offline" in their relationship during these times they were focused on points of disagreement. I say "implicit view" because, upon reflection, neither really believed they were unable to access their own spirituality amid their differences; it was more of an unconscious process that promoted the temporary "exile" of their sources of spiritual grounding. Differentiation theorists refer to this as *fusion*, where members of a couple might lose themselves in the anxious pursuit of self–other sameness (Schnarch, 2009). Growth in differentiation is required to practice a relational spirituality that includes self-regulation while also trying to remain open to understanding one's partner in their similarities and differences. Rita readily identified a Sufi meditative mantra and breathing practice she could use to stay connected with God and move beyond her ego (Sufi theology) during these dialogues with Jana. Jana did not have a particular meditative practice, but she developed a practice of calling to mind and savoring images of an older woman from her Unitarian Universalist congregation she admired and was close to who led programs in social activism. In these ways, Jana and Rita were able to draw on strengths of their own traditions for self-regulation to help them stay in conversations longer and with less reactivity.

However, staying in conversation longer can also lead to deeper encounters with differences within a couple. During a very intense session, I had been probing the options Rita had considered on Jana's desire for Rita to push back against her family's lack of acknowledgment and acceptance of their relationship. Rita suddenly became uncharacteristically angry, turning to Jana and saying through tears,

> You know what? You want to tell my family how to think and tell me how I am supposed to back them in a corner to accept us "or else," but you have no idea what Black families are up against. You will never really understand why we need to stick together or why I remain loyal to them. Your version of justice is all about your own benefit!

This was a complicated moment when several sensitive things were unfolding. Rita, in my view, may have been partially defending against the anxiety-provoking track I was pursuing by asking about her options for negotiating some space for her relationship with Jana in her family system. But she did not seem to change the topic to divert; instead, she opened up a new level of transparency about the deeper existential dilemma beneath her seeming avoidance of taking on her family. After a few long moments of silence and some deep breaths, I said something like "Rita, I know you are afraid Jana won't understand your place in this set of issues . . . but I wonder if you are open to us taking a shot at it."

From an RSM approach to therapy, it is valuable to surface, name, and reflect upon these kinds of existential issues that can shape interlocking integrity dilemmas. In this case, we were able to coconstruct an understanding of their couple crucible on the themes of acceptance, identity, commitment, and working against oppression. Rita's place in the crucible was intensifying a deep dilemma that took this form: *Why should I risk losing my family's acceptance and causing them more suffering by fully committing to someone [Jana] I am not sure really accepts all of me?* Jana's place in the crucible arose from a combination of her strength advocating for her own dignity and liberation combined with her sincere commitment to Rita, yet she found herself in the ironic position of trying to navigate relational differences using the dogmatism and judgmental attitude that were antithetical to her own core religious values. And she also needed to more fully own realities of race in their relationship and wider society. Her differentiation dilemma took this form: *How can I hold onto myself and my own values while also communicating respect and understanding for Rita and the concerns she is holding?*

For both Rita and Jana, these formed what Schnarch (2009) called *integrity dilemmas* that can promote growth in differentiation, and we used the relational process of couple therapy to clarify and probe these dilemmas. I again invited each to consider what her respective religious tradition might offer in considering these kinds of dilemmas. Doing this work in the presence of one another was initially somewhat difficult, but over a series of sessions the honesty about their real underlying struggles was combined with a growing resilience for sitting in the anxiety of their differences. Paradoxically, they each voiced dilemmas they did not initially know how to resolve, but as they gained deeper empathy and acceptance for each other they became more committed to figuring out a way forward. Differentiation is achieved not by avoiding differences but by moving into them in new and less reactive ways. This was a multiyear therapy process with numerous twists and turns, but this differentiation-based work was key to their growth as a couple and their eventual decision to get married. They had not figured out all the interreligious implications of future family life, but they each made adjustments that deepened their mutual trust and commitment amid their differences.

CASE EXAMPLE: INTERSUBJECTIVITY SYSTEM FOCUS–AJAY AND LAN

The intersubjectivity system involves relational and power dynamics between persons that can activate and maintain ruptures of conflict and misunderstanding or move toward intimacy, mutual recognition, and the repair of ruptures through more balanced and attuned relating. Like the other couple cases above, the following case involves challenges of attachment and differentiation, but I will focus here on difficulties of intersubjectivity that were contributing to chronic unresolved conflict and increasing levels of estrangement that worked against intimacy and collaboration.

Ajay (age 51; Indian American, cisgender man, Hindu) and Lan (age 48; Chinese American, cisgender woman, "spiritual but not religious") had been married for 6 years in a second marriage for both. They came to couple therapy reporting that their first year of marriage had been very positive; with Lan on sabbatical from her teaching position, she was able to travel quite freely with Ajay for his work. Religious differences had seemed unimportant when they fell in love after meeting at an academic conference, and they married the following year. However, they had started experiencing significant conflicts over various issues (including religion and spirituality) since that time and currently felt unable to negotiate most differences. Lan complained that Ajay had very "traditional" or even "sexist" views of marriage and seemed to expect her to largely support his "every need" and be available sexually whenever he wanted. Ajay was offended by the charge of sexism, and his version of the problems in their marriage focused on Lan's sister Ming coming to live with them 3 years prior following her own marital separation and divorce. He said, "Ming is a very bitter person and takes Lan to all these esoteric meetings and retreats that pull her away from our relationship." Lan countered, "Ming is not bitter. She has been working through the abuse she experienced in her marriage and finding her own voice. Ajay, you just don't like it when women have a voice, and you don't care about feelings . . . *or spirituality*. You live in your head." Ajay retorted, "She just needs to forgive and move on or she will continue to have all kinds of problems . . . and she will continue to pull us down with her."

In contrast to Rita and Jana, whose struggles with religious differences provoked questions about getting married, Lan and Ajay experienced religious conflicts after a relatively smooth start to their marriage. In this case, Lan and Ajay managed to overlook religious differences during the honeymoon period of their relationship, but problems intensified over time as they move deeper into marriage and needed to negotiate various forms of collaboration as a couple, including the emergence of Ming as a "third party" in their relational system. Ajay had not been particularly active in Hindu religious practice for many years, but his religious beliefs about marriage, gender, interpersonal conflict, and many other things became activated as they settled into married life together. He had started attending some services and events at a Hindu temple in the area with friends, and this also contributed to the reemergence of his particular form of relational spirituality, which focused on a sense of duty and a desire for peaceful harmony through structure and self-discipline. He had stopped drinking and began engaging in daily prayer. Lan had been practicing a "portable" spirituality when they first married; this involved meditation, yoga practice, and reading about Buddhism during her sabbatical. But in recent years, she and her sister had become more socially connected to an informal spiritual community through a local yoga center that offered classes, retreats, and discussion groups that focused on themes like mindfulness, self-compassion, and balancing energies. Religious and spiritual social networks are an important influence on the relational spirituality dynamics of couples, and for Ajay and Lan their social networks had been evolving in different directions.

A key function of the intersubjectivity system is recognition and attempted repair of the ruptures (Eubanks et al., 2018) or breakdowns in subjective understanding that are common in couple relationships. Rupture-repair processes are crucial in couple relationships because the chronic lack of repair of conflicts and misunderstandings leads to some combination of resentment, emotional cutoff, and ineffectual debate. The frequent conflicts between Lan and Ajay also regularly took the form of what Benjamin (2018) calls "complementarity" or "one-up/one-down" relational stances of power imbalance and lack of shared understanding. In the text above, Ajay positions himself as the powerful "knower" of how Ming should handle her past hurts through forgiveness after also labeling her as "bitter," and he casts the alternative outcome to his prescription as resulting in victimization for both Lan and him. Some highly shame-prone partners might respond to this power move by accepting a one-down position and deferring to Ajay's view, and it had sounded as if this might have been a common response in his first marriage. However, Lan was sufficiently empowered to push back against Ajay's perspective about Ming before offering her own diagnosis of him as sexist, averse to spirituality, and excessively cognitive. As a clinician, I am often struck that couples suffering breakdowns into complementarity are often voicing such important, complex, and sensitive themes where they differ (e.g., forgiveness, emotions, spirituality, gender). These areas would be vital to discuss in ways that could lead to mutual understanding, yet the relational power dynamics combine with intense emotional reactivity to generate further alienation and deeper levels of resentment.

There is no easy technique for these situations, but I generally try to interrupt cycles of escalating conflict in session by inserting myself to (a) help create boundaries to restructure space for deeper understanding and (b) draw out more information and reflection from each partner. For example,

> I'd like us to slow down here. This is obviously a place where powerful differences are at play in your relationship, but I need to better understand each of your perspectives. And I am not sure how well you are understanding each other.

This line of intervention can temporarily slow down reactivity and make space for each person to speak without interruption, while also (hopefully) introducing the idea that they may not actually understand each other's perspectives. This typically requires a series of relational moves and reflective questions over several sessions. In this case, I started by engaging Ajay in dialogue about a set of issues that allowed Lan some room to self-regulate and listen for a few minutes. I probed what he meant by "forgiveness" and the notion that if Ming did not forgive her abusive ex-husband, then he and Lan "would be pulled down with her." I learned this reflected his Karmic worldview and the Hindu belief that we all have a duty to practice virtuous actions (*dharma*) like forgiveness to avoid negative consequences and live in spiritual harmony. I checked in with Lan during this dialogue and confirmed this was new information to her. She began to protest that it was "unfair" and "arrogant" for him to impose his beliefs on her and Ming since they did not hold those beliefs about suffering. Internally, my valuing of diversity and differentiation pulled for sympathy toward Lan's complaint about the problems of imposing religious views. However, I have learned these kinds of interreligious dynamics can be complex and tried to remain open to understanding both sides and the various layers of this conflict. I also tried to help contain the affect level at this point in order for the three of us to tease apart a set of issues that were emerging: (a) Ajay was very anxious about the spiritual suffering Ming was experiencing and the possible impact on Lan and him; (b) Ajay believed, based on his religious worldview, that he could offer a moral and spiritual solution to this problem; and (c) Lan and Ming did not believe in a Karmic worldview, so they were working from different RS assumptions about suffering and healing than Ajay. All of these were important issues to consider, but the intersubjective space to do so had previously collapsed amid their intense reactivity.

Like many distressed couples, Lan and Ajay had become used to reacting to one another, so I had to be quite active in intervening during sessions to reduce the number of verbal and nonverbal slights they exchanged and to keep the focus on (a) gaining understanding amid their differences and (b) starting to build their distress tolerance for these differences (i.e., differentiation system work). Over a series of sessions, Lan and Ajay gained awareness of both similarities and differences in their relationship. For example, it became evident that, like Lan, Ajay was concerned about Ming's well-being; however, this was masked by his judgments, proposed solutions, and jealousy over Lan's prioritizing that relationship over their marriage. It proved helpful to draw out their shared concern for Ming, which created some emotional softening in their interactions, while also honestly noting their different views on how to be helpful to her.

Forgiveness became another topic for working on intersubjective awareness of similarities and differences, as we discovered they both valued forgiving others but held different beliefs about the process. Rather than inviting each to comment on the other person's disclosures in ways that might be evaluative (e.g., "Lan, what do you think of what Ajay just said?"), I used questions that fostered intersubjectivity (e.g., "Ajay, how do you understand Lan's perspective on forgiveness?"). This was very difficult for both at first, since they each felt considerable hurt and resentment over their differences in ways that manifested as judgment and contempt during arguments.

As noted in the psychotherapy research literature (Eubanks et al., 2018), those of us who are therapists often experience ruptures with clients also, and I experienced a rupture with Lan and Ajay fairly early in couple therapy. During one of the sessions when we were surfacing their different perspectives on forgiveness, Lan protested (with tears),

> Steve, you and Ajay both act like this is an academic topic! But Ming has suffered abuse and could have died! I don't feel like either of you understand that . . . so this discussion is very painful to me.

Lan's challenge drew out several important issues of awareness for me, but at an emotional and spiritual level I would describe it as a *convicting awakening*. In that moment, I felt a mix of guilt and grief for neglecting to name ways issues of gender and power might be affecting their differing perspectives. These are issues I have written about and discussed with many clients, and I might have tried to defend myself that we were early in the conversation on that topic. But I realized Lan was correct; I had lapsed into finding their respective views to be interesting without conveying much empathy for the gravity of the issues at stake for Ming. And in the triangle of our working relationship in couple therapy, this probably seemed to Lan to place me closer to Ajay than to her. So her move to reinsert Ming into the conversation could be viewed as a balancing move, and this might be part of what motivated Ajay to defend me by responding, "I don't think Steve is being academic. He is just asking us to think about different considerations."

I was now quite embedded or triangulated into the intersubjective matrix of this couple system with the push and pull for allegiance. Benjamin's (2018) concept of third space speaks to the possibility of opening more differentiated awareness in a relational dyad that has collapsed into a power struggle of complementarity where one person will win and one will lose. This differentiated awareness can lead to mutual recognition or subject-to-subject relating that marks healthy intersubjectivity, where each person can convey understanding and acceptance for the other amid differences in subjectivity. In this case, I needed to take responsibility for my part in the rupture with Lan and to seek repair, which required me to quickly metabolize the guilt I felt about the ways I had missed connecting with her on the existential and gender justice issues she was holding. I do not remember my exact words, but I said something like,

> Lan, I appreciate you telling me I am missing you on this and approaching it like an academic. I'm sorry. What you are saying registers with me. And I am an academic who can get pretty cognitive at times. In fact, I have been finding your different perspectives interesting, and in trying to understand each of you I can sense I haven't yet communicated that I feel the life-and-death danger and gravity of these issues for you and for Ming.

This was not a magical moment in the therapy process, as Lan seemed to accept my apology but retain some skepticism about me, and Ajay seemed a bit confused and disappointed by my response and the way it positioned me vis-à-vis his attempt to defend me. In a rather concrete way, I was obviously bringing a third perspective into the couple system, which can prompt ongoing tension for each partner about how my personhood and perspectives fit within their struggles as a couple. With couples who are as conflicted as Lan and Ajay were at that point, my "thirdness" is usually experienced with confusion and ambivalence for some period of time following this kind of rupture-and-repair move. This often challenges my own relational spirituality and attachment security with respect to my ability to maintain faith in the relational process of therapy and to tolerate the ambiguity that is inherent in these kinds of liminal stages. I can find it tempting to either grope for some heroic intervention to rapidly transform the situation or pull back into the safety of emotional distance. Yet my core spiritual values call me to try to keep my heart alive for each partner and the dilemmas of their relationship and to stay within the process of exploring pathways toward healing and growth as long as that seems productive.

In this case, entering into the topic of forgiveness and the many associated dynamics put this couple's differences in the center of our work for much of the first year. Their relational spirituality differences were multifaceted and intersected with their beliefs, values, and relational approaches in a variety of areas. We came to realize they were moving (or seeking) in different directions. Ajay was longing to recover some of the structure, social connection, and sense of religious duty he found stabilizing earlier in his life. In contrast, Lan was drawn to a spirituality promoting mindful relating with her body, the warm and supportive presence and empowerment of other women, and an emphasis on sacred kindness and acceptance. After surfacing these differences and their experiential roots in some depth over several months, I began to invite them to awareness of the pain and anxiety they each felt about these growing differences. The pain was deep, and it became easy to see their conflicts as anxious attempts to either change the other person to be more suitable for their own changes or push the other away to defend against feelings of loss. They each lost a family member to death during that first year of therapy, which allowed us to also work on attachment dynamics and ways they could support each other in grief even amid their different meaning systems and practices. Each made genuine efforts at offering support despite their lingering conflicts and limited intimacy.

Midway through their second year, Lan realized that, despite the decreasing intensity of their conflicts and reduced resentment, she did not want to stay married to Ajay. This seemed to come from a more differentiated place in her compared with her consideration of divorce at the outset of therapy, and she voiced her decision in session with tears of grief and a concern for Ajay's well-being, as well as her own. It struck me as less a stance of rejection of Ajay and more a move toward the acceptance and compassion that was central to her spirituality. Ajay flared up with defensive anger for a couple sessions, but the relational dynamic between them had shifted, and he mobilized his own emerging capacities to cope with anxiety and grief. He was sad about Lan's decision, but he eventually credited her with the courage to face a reality about their relationship that he recognized as true. Differentiation is a complicated developmental process in couples, as growth in differentiation typically moves them toward greater closeness and improved collaboration. Yet in other cases like this one, a reflective and nonhostile decision to divorce may also represent movement toward differentiation.

Both agreed they would like to see if they could be supportive friends on the other side of divorce (i.e., nonromantic attachment), and we spent a series of sessions helping them move toward the decoupling process. I find it personally gratifying to witness couples build more healthy collaboration, but it is also very meaningful to work with couples who find peaceful and forgiving ways to bring closure to their relationship as intimate partners. Lan, Ajay, and I worked out a ritual of closure for our final session together where they each read a brief letter expressing words of hope for good things for the other in their future journey, followed by a moment of silence. They hugged as we closed and said goodbye.

CONCLUSION

Religious differences in couples presenting for couple therapy can be sources of strength, disinterest, or conflict that manifest in a variety of ways. An RSM-based approach to religious differences and other SERT dynamics in couple therapy can focus clinical attention on the ways relational development systems (attachment, differentiation, intersubjectivity) interact with the couples' differing ways of relating to the sacred across the life cycle. This relational approach requires those of us who are clinicians to cultivate ongoing self-awareness related to the intersecting influences of our own SERT journeys and to seek to practice the humility necessary for growth in diversity competence.

REFERENCES

Ammerman, N. T. (2020). Rethinking religion: Toward a practice approach. *American Journal of Sociology, 126*(1), 6–51. https://doi.org/10.1086/709779

Benjamin, J. (2018). *Beyond doer and done to: Recognition theory, intersubjectivity, and the Third.* Routledge.

Caffaro, J. (2011). Fundamentalism and the search for divinity: The varied role of religion in interfaith couples. *Journal of Family Psychotherapy, 22*(4), 328–343. https://doi.org/10.1080/08975353.2011.627796

Chinitz, J. G., & Brown, R. A. (2001). Religious homogamy, marital conflict, and stability in same-faith and interfaith Jewish marriages. *Journal for the Scientific Study of Religion, 40*(4), 723–733. https://doi.org/10.1111/0021-8294.00087

Cila, J., & Lalonde, R. N. (2014). Personal openness toward interfaith dating and marriage among Muslim young adults: The role of religiosity, cultural identity, and family connectedness. *Group Processes & Intergroup Relations, 17*(3), 357–370. https://doi.org/10.1177/1368430213502561

Eubanks, C. F., Muran, J. C., & Safran, J. D. (2018). Alliance rupture repair: A meta-analysis [Supplemental material]. *Psychotherapy, 55*(4), 508–519. https://doi.org/10.1037/pst0000185

Gelo, O. C., & Salvatore, S. (2016). A dynamic systems approach to psychotherapy: A meta-theoretical framework for explaining psychotherapy change processes. *Journal of Counseling Psychology, 63*(4), 379–395. https://doi.org/10.1037/cou0000150

Glenn, N. D. (1982). Interreligious marriage in the United States: Patterns and recent trends. *Journal of Marriage and the Family, 44*(3), 555–566. https://doi.org/10.2307/351579

Gordon, S., & Arenstein, B. (2017). Interfaith education: A new model for today's interfaith families. *International Review of Education/Internationale. Zeitschrift für Erziehungswissenschaft, 63*(2), 169–195. https://doi.org/10.1007/s11159-017-9629-2

Greenstein, D., Carlson, J., & Howell, C. W. (1993). Counseling with interfaith couples. *Individual Psychology: Journal of Adlerian Theory, Research & Practice, 49*(3/4), 428–437.

Grunebaum, J. (1987). Multidirected partiality and the "parental imperative." *Psychotherapy, 24*(3S), 646–656. https://doi.org/10.1037/h0085763

Hill, P. C., & Pargament, K. I. (2003). Advances in the conceptualization and measurement of religion and spirituality: Implications for physical and mental health research. *American Psychologist, 58*(1), 64–74. https://doi.org/10.1037/0003-066X.58.1.64

Jankowski, P. J., Sandage, S. J., Bell, C. A., Davis, D. E., Porter, E., Jessen, M., Motzny, C. L., Ross, K. V., & Owen, J. (2020). Virtue, flourishing, and positive psychology in psychotherapy: An overview and research prospectus. *Psychotherapy, 57*(3), 291–309. https://doi.org/10.1037/pst0000285

Johnson, S. M. (2015). Emotionally focused couple therapy. In A. S. Gurman, J. L. Lebow, & D. K. Snyder (Eds.), *Clinical handbook of couple therapy* (5th ed., pp. 97–128). Guilford Press.

Morgan, J., & Sandage, S. J. (2016). A developmental model of interreligious competence. *Archiv für Religionspsychologie, 38*(2), 129–158. https://doi.org/10.1163/15736121-12341325

Pargament, K. I., & Exline, J. J. (2021). Religious and spiritual struggles and mental health: Implications for clinical practice. In A. Moreira-Almeida, B. P. Mosqueiro, & D. Bhugra (Eds.), *Spirituality and mental health across cultures* (pp. 395–412). Oxford University Press.

Parsons, R. N., Nalbone, D. P., Killmer, J. M., & Wetchler, J. L. (2007). Identity development, differentiation, personal authority, and degree of religiosity as predictors of interfaith marital satisfaction. *The American Journal of Family Therapy, 35*(4), 343–361. https://doi.org/10.1080/01926180600814601

Pew Research Center. (2015). *America's changing religious landscape.*

Putnam, R. D., & Campbell, D. E. (2012). *American grace: How religion divides and unites us.* Simon & Schuster.

Rupert, D., Moon, S. H., & Sandage, S. J. (2019). Clinical training groups for spirituality and religion in psychotherapy. *Journal of Spirituality in Mental Health, 21*(3), 163–177. https://doi.org/10.1080/19349637.2018.1465879

Sahl, A. H., & Batson, C. D. (2011). Race and religion in the Bible Belt: Parental attitudes toward interfaith relationships. *Sociological Spectrum, 31*(4), 444–465. https://doi.org/10.1080/02732173.2011.574043

Sandage, S. J., Bell, C. A., Moon, S. H., & Ruffing, E. G. (2019). Religious and spiritual problems in couples. In L. Sperry, K. Helm, & J. Carlson (Eds.), *The disordered couple* (2nd ed., pp. 305–321). Routledge. https://doi.org/10.4324/9781351264044-19

Sandage, S. J., & Brown, J. K. (2018). *Relational integration in psychology and Christian theology: Theory, research, and practice.* Routledge. https://doi.org/10.4324/9781315671505

Sandage, S. J., Rupert, D., Stavros, G. S., & Devor, N. G. (2020). *Relational spirituality in psychotherapy: Healing suffering and promoting growth.* American Psychological Association. https://doi.org/10.1037/0000174-000

Schnarch, D. M. (2009). *Intimacy and desire: Awaken the passion in your relationship.* Beaufort Books.

Shults, F. L., & Sandage, S. J. (2006). *Transforming spirituality: Integrating theology and psychology.* Baker Academic.

Singh, R. (2017). Intimate strangers? Working with interfaith couples and families. *Australian and New Zealand Journal of Family Therapy, 38*(1), 7–14. https://doi.org/10.1002/anzf.1197

Van Niekerk, J., & Verkuyten, M. (2018). Interfaith marriage attitudes in Muslim majority countries: A multilevel approach. *The International Journal for the Psychology of Religion, 28*(4), 257–270. https://doi.org/10.1080/10508619.2018.1517015

Vieten, C., Scammell, S., Pierce, A., Pilato, R., Ammondson, I., Pargament, K. I., & Lukoff, D. (2016). Competencies for psychologists in the domains of religion and spirituality. *Spirituality in Clinical Practice, 3*(2), 92–114. https://doi.org/10.1037/scp0000078

Wampold, B. E., & Imel, Z. E. (2015). *The great psychotherapy debate: The evidence for what makes psychotherapy work* (2nd ed.). Routledge/Taylor & Francis Group. https://doi.org/10.4324/9780203582015

Waring, D. R. (2016). *The healing virtues: Character ethics in psychotherapy.* Oxford University Press. https://doi.org/10.1093/med/9780199689149.001.0001

Worthington, E. L., Jr., & Sandage, S. J. (2016). *Forgiveness and spirituality in psychotherapy: A relational approach.* American Psychological Association. https://doi.org/10.1037/14712-000

12

AN INTERCULTURAL APPROACH TO SPIRITUALLY ORIENTED PSYCHOTHERAPY OF MILITARY MORAL INJURY

KATHRYN L. BARRS AND CARRIE DOEHRING

The concept of military moral injury (MMI) emerged from therapy with veterans whose posttraumatic stress included lasting moral conflicts about harm caused by themselves, fellow service members, or those in authority. In this chapter, after defining MMI and spiritually oriented therapies, we describe evidence-based treatment approaches that respect the unique values and beliefs of veterans, and their intrinsically meaningful ways of experiencing goodness and recovery. We highlight the importance of identifying our beliefs and values about suffering arising from trauma, military service, and combat. Body-aware practices that alleviate stress, widely used with clients in many trauma therapies, are also helpful for clinicians. We describe how such practices connect us with hope and help us search for life-giving beliefs about suffering using an intercultural approach that builds trust by listening for and respecting what is unique in the ways persons search for meaning and experience transcendence.

Spiritual care in religiously diverse community, medical, military, educational, and prison contexts needs to be intercultural, evidence based, and grounded in psychological research focused on how aspects of religion

https://doi.org/10.1037/0000276-013
Spiritual Diversity in Psychotherapy: Engaging the Sacred in Clinical Practice,
S. J. Sandage and B. D. Strawn (Editors)

and spirituality may help or harm people seeking whole selves. The spiritual struggles of moral injury often shake people to the core of their being, making the need for wholeness more compelling and complex (Kusner & Pargament, 2012). An extensive case study with a Vietnam veteran illustrates the use of spiritually oriented cognitive processing therapy (CPT) and acceptance and commitment therapy (ACT). As clinicians and chaplains step into the story of this veteran, they might consider what spiritual practices help them feel hopeful and grounded. They could contemplate how this particular veteran's emotional pain prompts them to search for meaning in the face of terrible suffering, while also clarifying the values that ground their vocations of care.

WHAT IS MILITARY MORAL INJURY?

In the 1990s, psychiatrist Jonathan Shay (2014) realized that his Vietnam veteran patients diagnosed with posttraumatic stress disorder (PTSD) struggled with what he called *moral injury*—"a betrayal of what's right by someone who holds legitimate authority (e.g., in the military—a leader) in a high stakes' situation" (p. 183). Shay used the Greek warriors Achilles and Odysseus in Homer's ancient Greek epic poems *Iliad* and *Odyssey* to understand how lament over moral culpability in combat is as old as Greek tragedies (Shay, 1992, 2002). Shay initially describes betrayal-based moral distress. Since then, research has expanded to explore differences between betrayal-based and perpetration-based MMI. Feeling responsible for lethal use of force in ambiguous situations is often a liability in "nontraditional forms of combat, such as guerrilla war in urban environments" (Litz et al., 2009, p. 696), that require quick decisions about use of lethal force that may generate moral anguish, and "emotional, spiritual, and psychological wounds" (Drescher et al., 2011, p. 8). Military training focuses on the mission of one's unit, often compelling military personnel to set aside their own needs until trauma and moral injury cause overwhelming stress (Nash, 2019).

Who is responsible for harm—oneself or another—generates different emotional responses (Schorr et al., 2018, p. 2207). Perpetration-based MMI is associated with (a) guilt, shame, and sadness; (b) reexperiencing symptoms and numbness (Stein et al., 2012); (c) beliefs about being unlovable, unforgivable, or incapable of moral decision making; and (d) self-sabotaging and acting out behavior. Betrayal-based MMI, which may include witnessing morally distressing events, is associated with anger, outrage, and frustration (Stein et al., 2012), as well as moral disgust, mistrust of others, and revenge fantasies for the responsible person(s) (Currier et al., 2017). For many clients, these moral and psychological dynamics related to MMI arise from spiritual struggles, which we consider below.

SPIRITUALLY INTEGRATED THERAPY OF MMI

Psychologist of religion Ken Pargament (2007) elaborated a model of spiritually integrated psychotherapy based on extensive research on how aspects of religion and spirituality may promote spiritual wholeness and/or transitional/chronic brokenness. His model may be integrated into MMI treatment models in two ways. First, therapists need to be familiar with research on spiritual struggles and the role of meaning making and spiritual practices in supporting or undermining health and spiritual wholeness. Second, therapists use an intercultural approach to spirituality and religion that respects the complex, distinctive ways that values, beliefs, coping, and spiritual practices are shaped by interacting cultural systems, especially military training and culture. A central concept in research on psychology of religion, and in Pargament's approach, is understanding the role of moral orienting systems. An orienting system

> consists of habits, values, relationships, belief and personality. . . . [and] contains both helpful and unhelpful attributes, resources, and burdens. . . . Spirituality is one aspect of the general orienting system [that] contributes to the individual's framework for understanding and dealing with the world. (Pargament et al., 2006, p. 130)

The values, beliefs, practices, emotions, and relationships of orienting systems shape how and whether spiritual and moral struggles/injury lead to wholeness or brokenness (Pargament et al., 2016, p. 379).

Orienting systems include both *global* beliefs and values about suffering, hope, and the purpose of one's life and *situational meanings* about, for example, potential/actual moral stressors like harm caused in combat. Orienting systems are multilayered, with formative values, beliefs, and coping practices from childhood, family, peer, and cultural systems forming a bedrock orienting system that is often reenergized emotionally under acute/traumatic stress (Doehring, 2015a, 2015b), either by emotions like love and compassion that connect people with goodness in their bodies and relational systems or by shame and guilt that make people feel judged (particularly by God) and/or potentially shunned.

Spiritually integrated psychotherapy uses somatic practices like mindfulness meditation not simply as calming practices but also as part of a search for meanings. Intrinsically meaningful practices that help veterans experience goodness will likely reveal new values and beliefs about suffering and hope that can be incorporated into a veteran's search for meanings. This inter-relationship between intrinsically meaningful spiritual practices and searching for meanings is described by Sandage and colleagues (Shults & Sandage, 2006) as an "unfolding through dialectical processes of spiritual dwelling and seeking" (Tomlinson et al., 2016, p. 64).

STAGES AND MODELS OF TRAUMA TREATMENT USED IN THIS CASE STUDY

The case study reviewed in this chapter, naturally aligned with Judith Herman's three phases of trauma treatment, focuses on the following stages in a sequential order (while also recognizing that individuals do not always move through these stages in a linear fashion): safety and stabilization, mourning and processing, and community reintegration (Herman, 1992). When clinically indicated, I (Barrs) often follow the structure of this sequentially staged treatment model when the client is presenting with a history of repeated interpersonal and/or combat traumas that lead to long-term changes in self-esteem, identity, emotion regulation, distress tolerance, physiological regulation, spirituality, and sense of safety and trust.

Herman's (1992) model indicates that safety and stabilization is the first stage of trauma treatment for those who have experienced complex trauma. This stage of treatment entails treating acute and debilitating symptoms that are interfering with functioning, while also learning stress management, distress tolerance, body regulation, and emotion regulation skills. The client learns about the effects of trauma, how to ask for support, and how to manage and prevent crises. After the individual has developed the skills that will assist them in effectively coping with the next phase of treatment, they move into the remembrance and mourning stage where they process the trauma memories, engage in exposure-based work, and experience the grief and loss associated with what they have survived. In the final stage, reconnection, the individual is learning to live a life where trauma takes up less space, their identity as a survivor versus victim is strengthened, they engage in more meaningful activity, and they practice acceptance. During this phase, the individual works to develop a stronger support system while fostering deeper connection to the community and oftentimes a higher power. Herman's model seemed to be especially relevant to the case study presented in this chapter and is directly in line with the veteran's experience, therapeutic goals, and recovery.

It is important to note that some evidence-based trauma treatments tend to naturally align with the stages of Herman's (1992) model. For example, stress inoculation (Meichenbaum, 2019), dialectical behavior therapy (Linehan, 2014), and seeking safety (Najavits, 2002) are often referred to as Stage 1 trauma treatments because they focus on developing a sense of safety, setting healthy boundaries, learning to calm the central nervous system, asking for help, emotion regulation, interpersonal effectiveness, and distress tolerance. The development and bolstering of these skills often assist individuals in moving to the next stage of trauma treatment where they directly address, confront, process, and reframe their trauma memories, thoughts, emotions, and meaning-making narratives. Stage 2 trauma treatments include such treatments as prolonged exposure therapy (Foa et al., 2019), CPT (Resick et al., 2017), and eye-movement desensitization and reprocessing therapy (Shapiro, 2017). In work with the veteran in this chapter's case study, I (Barrs) used ACT in Stage 3 of trauma treatment, focusing on mindfulness, acceptance, self-forgiveness, identifying values, and engaging in committed action to live in direct accordance with values. Adaptive disclosure is another innovative model of therapy used in treating moral injury in military-affiliated populations (Litz et al., 2016). Although the veteran in the described case study was not treated with adaptive disclosure, it is highly possible that this treatment would also have helped him as the therapy specifically incorporates aspects of military culture, such as warrior ethos, and distinguishes among trauma-related events often experienced by service members (i.e., fear-based stress, loss-related stress, and moral injury). After the type of veteran-specific seminal event is identified, the treatment progresses with a combination of psychoeducation, imaginal exposure, meaning making, and a focus on strengths and recovery.

CTP AND ACT WITH MMI

In the case study presented, I (Barrs) used several evidence-based psychotherapy treatments, including CPT and ACT, to address types of symptoms, facets of moral distress, and phases of trauma treatment. I describe each treatment below before introducing the case study.

CPT is a manualized, evidence-based treatment for PTSD (Resick et al., 2017; Resick & Schnicke, 1992) often used with military-affiliated populations. Pearce et al. (2018) elaborated on the mechanisms of this form of cognitive-behavioral therapy, stating,

> CPT uses cognitive restructuring and behavioral exercises to help individuals change the way they think about the trauma. These cognitive changes allow individuals to better process their emotions, contextualize the event, and integrate the experience in a more positive or adaptive way into their lives. (p. 1)

The identification and challenging of stuckpoints is a primary component of CPT. *Stuckpoints* are defined as automatic thoughts or thinking patterns that interfere with the natural recovery from trauma, leading to symptoms of PTSD and psychological distress (Resick et al., 2017; Resick & Schnicke, 1992). Nieuwsma et al. (2015) elaborated on this concept when they stated, "Beliefs around guilt, shame, responsibility, and culpability are key targets for cognitive processing therapy, as these are the domains in which cognitive errors or beliefs may proliferate" (p. 195).

CPT also uses Socratic dialogue to assist clients in the self-identified realization of certain insight or knowledge through guided but gentle questioning by the therapist (Resick et al., 2017; Rutter & Friedberg, 1999; Rutter et al., 1999). Although the therapist initiates and facilitates the discussion, the conversation is conducted in a balanced and mutual manner in which the therapist is not experienced as the expert or the holder of specific knowledge that he or she is imparting to the client. For example, in the case study described below, I (Barrs) gently assist the client in understanding that he killed in combat due to a wide variety of reasons, including sleep deprivation, fatigue, grief/loss, trauma, and disillusionment with the government. I did so by asking him clarifying questions regarding his mental and physical state at the time of combat, the types of experiences he had in Vietnam, and his experience of the U.S. government as having abandoned him and his comrades.

An additional and optional component of CPT includes the writing and reading of the impact trauma or the traumatic event that is leading to the most amount of distress, difficulty functioning, and/or suffering. The CPT-plus account intervention (CPT+A) was used in the case study that is presented in this chapter. Through the writing of the trauma account, clients recall all memories, emotions, thoughts, bodily sensations, and sensory details (sights, sounds, smells, and physical sensations), along with a chronological account of the actual details and content of the traumatic event. They then read it daily in between sessions and also read it out loud to the therapist in session several times. The CPT theory behind this intervention is that by reading the impact trauma account, individuals feel the natural emotions associated with the event, the distressing emotions will decrease over time, and they will be able to move forward. When describing this intervention, the authors of the CPT manual state, "As emotions decrease, individuals become more receptive to other points of view and acceptance of the traumatic event" (Resick et al., 2017, p. 88).

Although some researchers have supported the use of spiritually integrated CPT with MMI (Pearce et al., 2018), others have indicated that this evidence-based therapy can only go so far in terms of causing lasting change and decrease in MMI-related symptoms (Farnsworth, 2019; Gray et al., 2012). One criticism of the use of CPT with MMI suggests that this particular treatment model focuses on decreasing generalized fear and uses a learning model that does not adequately or thoroughly treat the moral and spiritual injuries that occur in the context of war (Gray et al., 2012; Maguen et al., 2010; Nash, 2007).

The use of ACT, which is a type of psychotherapy grounded in behaviorism theory (Hayes et al., 1999, 2012), seems to be particularly useful when treating spiritually or religiously related psychological or emotional struggles, such as moral injury (Santiago & Gall, 2016). ACT has also been shown to be an effective treatment for PTSD as it focuses on decreasing experiential avoidance, living according to values, acceptance, and mindfulness (Walser & Westrup, 2007). Although literature regarding the use of ACT is relatively new, there seems to be growing consensus in the field that this evidence-based therapy is well suited to the treatment of MMI (Farnsworth, 2019; Nieuwsma et al., 2015). Santiago and Gall (2016) stated,

> ACT is a value-driven therapy that involves facilitating transcendence of physical, mental, and emotional experience to alleviate human suffering; as such, ACT shares common ground with the domain of spirituality. Approached as a spiritually integrated therapy, ACT can help clients to access spiritual resources and create life meaning as well as aid in the resolution or transformation of spiritual struggles. (p. 239)

Symptom reduction and the challenging and restructuring of thoughts are not the primary therapeutic outcomes on which the ACT therapist focuses. Instead, ACT interventions target the increase of psychological flexibility, identification of values, decrease of avoidance-based behaviors, and engagement in values-based living. ACT also focuses on present-centered living and incorporates the use of mindfulness and acceptance into the treatment of a variety of types of psychological and medical ailments (Hayes et al., 2012). A key tenet of ACT suggests that the struggle to control and avoid inner experiences (i.e., experiential avoidance), such as those associated with trauma and moral injury, further perpetuates and sustains such symptoms (Walser & Westrup, 2007). Nieuwsma et al. (2015) commented,

> Positive change is not measured by feeling better but by engagement in personal values and a renewed sense of vitality, by being able to flexibly respond to the current environment in a healthy way. This change goes hand-in-hand with a willingness to experience emotions and thoughts, including sadness, guilt, shame, and other apparently life limited events, as well as life-enhancing internal events such as joy and love. (p. 195)

ACT explores clients' values as a motivation for change. This orientation to values makes ACT compatible with spiritually oriented approaches to therapy, which also explore spiritual practices for alleviating trauma symptoms and grieving loss, as well as values that motivate life-giving changes.

MORAL AND SPIRITUAL ORIENTING SYSTEMS OF THOSE PROVIDING VETERAN CARE

Intercultural care of veterans raises questions for clinicians about suffering arising from military service and combat. In order to not be overwhelmed by the stress of stepping into a veteran's trauma and moral injury, clinicians may need to find and use their own body-aware spiritual practices. Spiritual self-care, such as mindfulness meditation, personal and communal prayer, exercise, and experiences immersed in nature and beauty, fosters hope when clinicians experience goodness in their bodies, relational webs, humanity, and nature. When clinicians regularly practice spiritual self-care, they can use momentary practices when they step into the suffering of a veteran's story. A mindful breath, phrase from a prayer, positive affirmation, or memory of beauty may help them experience hope and clarity in the face of a veteran's trauma. An intercultural approach to spiritual self-care helps clinicians identify their spiritual practices, and their beliefs and values about care of veterans, in order to self-differentiate their own religious, spiritual, and moral struggles from the effects of their clients' military service and combat. Spiritual self-differentiation helps clinicians resist the subtle, sometimes-unconscious temptation to convince clients that spiritual practices, beliefs, and values that help clinicians find hope will "heal" or "save" a veteran. Spiritual self-differentiation is the foundation for intercultural spiritual care that truly respects the particular ways a veteran finds hope, meaning, and value.

For example, I (Doehring) use personal practices of listening to sacred choral music and communal practices of attending Episcopal worship to connect with goodness and beauty. Similarly, I (Barrs) rely on a consistent yoga practice, social interaction, and walks in nature to remain grounded and connected to the world. While these practices have helped us trust others in searching for meanings about suffering, we would not assume that others would find these particular practices meaningful or soothing. Even offering such practices as examples might generate spiritual struggles in clients who feel guilty that traditional religious or spiritual practices are not helpful for them.

We draw upon moral foundations theory and research by moral psychologist Jonathan Haidt (2002, 2008) to identify our foundational values about care of veterans. Clinicians and chaplains might begin to identify values that shape their vocations and therapeutic interventions by identifying more everyday values, such as responsibility/concern for others, compassion, belonging to networks/professions of care, and evidence-based approaches to health and change. Many such values are also identified in professional codes of ethics. In our practice, we find it helpful to describe our foundational values in terms of those common across cultures and studied using moral foundations theory and research (Haidt, 2012). The moral foundation of *caring and doing no harm* is one we embrace, even as it provokes in us a deep sense of lament for the suffering veterans experience and the harm they may cause in following military orders or experiences. We lament the sometimes-chronic moral, spiritual, and religious struggles that may plague veterans for many years after their military service. Vietnam veterans may feel particularly conflicted about seeking help, given antiwar sentiments so prevalent when they returned from military service. Along with lament, our value of caring provokes our own moral struggles as citizens of a country responsible for fighting in the Vietnam War and for not adequately caring for its veterans in its immediate aftermath. Using body-aware practices deepens our compassion for self and others, makes us aware of our own struggles and pain, and clarifies why and how the value of caring for veterans is at the heart of our vocations.

Another foundational value for us is the value of *loyalty* to veterans, who deserve the best evidence-based spiritually oriented care available. A value of *authority* makes us lament experiences of veterans feeling/being betrayed by those in authority—either military or religious authorities—that increase their isolation and fears of being shunned. In addition, psychological struggles often stigmatize veterans, reinforcing societal prejudice that all veterans struggle in this way. Another foundational value of *fairness* makes us question whether those drafted or signing up for military service at the age of 18 can make mindful and informed choices about military service, and whether the responsibilities of military service are equally shared across all social, gender, and racial differences. The value of fairness also makes us grieve for the veterans who did not get the support they needed or deserved from systems or society after they experienced psychological and moral harm during and after their military service. We also feel a sense of moral responsibility for the harm done to veterans, as well as harm caused by complex dynamics during and after military service. Our value of the *sanctity of life* makes us part of a web of caring relationships that seeks to protect life, lament suffering, support recovery, and experience hope together.

Beliefs about the suffering of MMI and possibilities for hope, another part of moral orienting systems, tend to be specific to religious or philosophical orienting systems. Our beliefs and indeed our values about suffering of MMI arise out of personal and communal practices that ground each of us in a sense of goodness—personal, relational, familial, communal, creative, and transcendent goodness. This sense of goodness helps us compassionately understand our stress-based responses to the suffering and resiliency of veterans. Practices grounding us in goodness affirm the life-giving values identified above and evoke the following beliefs about the suffering of MMI.

When we work with service members and veterans, we resist the temptation to valorize individual service members as heroes or diagnose veterans as inevitably wounded and perhaps even condemn them as morally warped. We listen for the ways their stories of combat and war may be tragedies of irreparable human loss that may include posttraumatic growth reverberating across historical, national, family, and personal narratives. Understanding MMI as tragic offers us realistic hope that can be experienced in the here and now, especially through practices—personal and communal—that connect us with goodness:

> Tragedy humiliatingly exposes the limits of our powers, but in thus objectifying our finitude makes us aware of an unfathomable freedom within ourselves. By being newly aware of the boundaries of our being, we sense an eternity of power beyond them. (Eagleton, 2003, p. 122)

We appreciate the tangled ways that agential and receptive moral injury are often intertwined. Indeed, a 21st-century view of creation often uses process philosophies of interconnected power as both agential and receptive. Those searching for a way beyond traditional beliefs about God's omnipotence as wholly agential are often drawn to process theologies of s "the creativity of the universe that makes change and transformation possible. . . . All of reality, including divine and human, are thus part of an interdependent process" (Graham, 2017, p. 51). Process philosophies and theologies of suffering generate a collective rather than individualistic sense of moral responsibility that requires all persons, communities, and nations to work together in caring for those wounded by war.

The following case study illustrates how I (Barrs) put these beliefs and values into practice. Although specific evidence-based CPT and ACT interventions clearly prompted change for the veteran, the relationship of compassion and nonjudgment this veteran had with me and spiritual healers fostered a sharing of receptive and agential power that changed all of them, with change rippling out through their relational webs. It is important to note that the following case study is based on an actual client, but all identifying details have been changed in order to maintain confidentiality.

CASE EXAMPLE: MORAL INJURY—CARL

Carl, a 68-year-old Catholic, cisgender, heterosexual man, is a combat veteran who self-identified as biracial (African American and Caucasian). Carl first decided to pursue individual therapy more than 40 long years after serving two tours of duty in the jungles of Vietnam. He enlisted in the army at the age of 17 after having grown up in a family where his siblings, uncles, and father served in the U.S. military. Much of his family's identity was formed around values of service, patriotism, and sacrifice for the common good. He spoke with pride about a wall of portraits in his mother and father's home where all his male family members who had served were displayed in their uniforms next to an American flag and an ornate painting of the Virgin Mary. When Carl signed on the dotted line, he truly and deeply believed he was going to fight for freedom and democracy along with life, liberty, and the pursuit of happiness. He also talked about being proud of going "to do God's work" and identified deeply with having grown up in a Catholic family.

More than 40 years later, when he initially called in for therapy, Carl reported that he was experiencing overwhelming pressure in his chest, anxiety, self-loathing, and sadness as his daughter refused to allow him to meet his one and only newborn grandchild due to his many years of isolation and avoidance. Carl had spent so many years separating himself from others, physically and emotionally, that his daughter felt chronically abandoned by him and did not want her child to experience the same sense of loss. During his initial call for services, he choked on his tears and expressed deep shame, stating he had avoided calling in for help for many decades but could no longer deal with the chronic sleepless nights, self-hatred, loneliness, and anger he had experienced "since going to that hellhole." He also mentioned several times that he could barely look at himself in the mirror and hated the man he had become.

During his first therapy appointment, Carl spent most of the session trying to catch his breath as he sobbed through pressured speech and clear feelings of tangible shame. He arrived at the clinic a few minutes early and stumbled down the long hallway outside the clinic door to the building bathroom. The hallway was lined with many luscious and tall potted plants leading down the hall to a sterile white bathroom. When I (Barrs) initially walked out to get him from the clinic waiting room, he was clearly disoriented and immediately began stammering, stating repeatedly that he felt as if he was transported back to the jungle in Vietnam while walking down the clinic hallway. He was sweating and commented a few times that he smelled the jungle air, the vegetation, and the rainwater he had become so familiar with during his time in country. It was only when he stumbled into the sterile white bathroom at the end of the hallway that he realized he was back at the clinic in the present day.

After he calmed down and I brought him back to my office, Carl spoke openly about the years he had isolated himself and struggled with the grief and loss surrounding the death of his wife, whom he always referred to as the love of his life. He spent many decades isolating himself in his wood shop in the garage, working on elaborate and beautifully crafted woodworking projects that he noted helped him to "zone out from the world" and remain separate from the stressors of civilian life. His successful woodworking business clearly brought him great pride and satisfaction, intermittently leaving him with a feeling of mastery and purpose.

Carl was raised Catholic and attended Mass periodically throughout his adult life, returning in a much more active manner to his faith community in his later years after the tragic death of his wife from a very aggressive form of heart disease. During the first few years of returning to Mass, Carl often fled the church midservice sweating and in a panic; he often stated that he felt the other members of the congregation knew he was a "murderer." He felt the congregation could see the evil and sin within him, which led to a sense of heightened panic and shame. He deeply desired a connection with God and his church but could hardly stand to sit in "God's house" due to the deep guilt associated with the many lives that he took while in combat.

Even more distressing than actually taking the lives of these enemy soldiers was that Carl remembered enjoying and reveling in the adrenaline he experienced when "killing as many Gooks as possible." He talked about the spiritual, emotional, and physiological effects of taking another human's life, and although killing was initially very distressing for him, over time he became numb and detached from the actual experience and meaning of the act and began to find some solace and a sense of control in killing as he felt he was honoring his best friend, who had died in his arms in Vietnam. Carl talked about the day his best friend was killed as a turning point in him "where something changed inside and the monster was born." The feeling of adrenaline and the rush of killing felt safer than connecting with the grief, loss, helplessness, and sadness he experienced under the surface of the rage.

In therapy, Carl identified deeply with symbolic images that assisted him in conveying the conflict he felt internally between being a kind man who loved his family and God, and feeling he was a "monster or murderer." Carl believed that God no longer loved him and that he was irredeemable. For many years, he refused to look in the mirror in his home and avoided gazing upward when brushing his teeth or shaving as he felt a sense of shame and disgust when looking at himself in the eyes. He often arrived at therapy wearing shirts displaying images of sharks, wolves, and other fiercely predatory animals, commenting that he identified with these animals as he also saw himself as a vicious hunter.

When positive aspects of his identity were highlighted or identified, such as father, grandfather, friend, beloved partner, community member, child of God, and soldier, he immediately dismissed these images of himself and stated that he did not deserve to be associated with these roles. He often commented that if people really knew what a "monster" he was, they would immediately cast him aside and ostracize him. Carl almost seemed to experience some comfort and understanding in his daughter's emotional distance from him as she "must have really seen [him] for what [he] was." Her refusal to allow him to meet his grandchild seemed to serve as the validation he was looking for that he was in fact unworthy of love and connection.

During a more intense period of therapy, he was shopping at a local grocery store when a young teenage cashier welcomed him to the store and proudly stated, "Thank you for your service." Carl ran from the store, cried in his car, and experienced a brief period of reemergence of his severe panic disorder symptoms and nightmares. Although he appreciated the sentiment of this young boy, who was clearly attempting to be respectful, this interaction only further illuminated Carl's deep and entrenched moral injury and the heavy weight of his guilt. He was adamant that he did not need to be thanked for "being a murderer."

Over time through therapy, Carl made significant progress in learning to view himself through a more compassionate and balanced lens. He began to see himself as a more integrated and spiritual human being who had engaged in many behaviors that were strongly against his moral code, religious beliefs, and personal values but who was also a caring partner, family member, and group member.

Sadly, approximately 3 years into therapy, Carl was diagnosed with terminal Stage 4 cancer and died within months of receiving the news. Understandably, this diagnosis dredged up strong feelings of spiritual angst and existential fear in him that increased some of his inner turmoil and reignited the negative feelings and beliefs he had about himself. At the same time, however, he experienced some comfort in knowing he had mostly repaired his relationship with his family, had a relationship with his grandson, felt realigned with God, and had connected with his treatment team and fellow group members. He began experiencing grueling nightmares where Viet Cong soldiers were waiting on the other side to punish him and hold him accountable for their deaths. He spent hours and hours wondering whether he would be sent to hell and sentenced to an eternity of pain and suffering for taking the lives of many "enemy" veterans, whom he had actually begun to see as equal human beings who were simply fighting for their morals and values, just as he was initially when he enlisted.

I continued to meet with Carl every week until he died. He called a few days before his death to thank me for my support and to let me know I had helped him to work toward "feeling whole again." Toward this end, I talked with him several times about possibly allowing his priest to visit him and help him to receive last rites—a Catholic ceremony for the dying that begins with confession, remembrance of baptismal promises, Holy Communion, and a blessing and prayers that include an anointing with oil. Carl refused to ask a priest for this rite due to the shame and fear he felt. Even after having done so much work on self-acceptance and forgiveness, he felt at the end as if he deserved to be held fully accountable for taking the lives of Viet Cong soldiers. He died partially believing his cancer was a physical manifestation of his sin and his punishment for what he had done in Vietnam. Even though his moral and spiritual injuries were still alive and well at the end of his life, Carl died having developed more of a sense of self-compassion and understanding for his behaviors during combat, along with a stronger connection with his family, community, nature, and God.

Summary of the Overall Process of Treatment

The overall process of therapy with Carl aligned with Judith Herman's (1992) three phases of trauma treatment, focusing on the following factors in a sequential order: safety and stabilization, mourning and processing of trauma, and community reintegration. Carl sequentially worked on the following goals and processes in therapy: stabilization of acute trauma-related and panic symptoms, telling his trauma story, changing the narrative regarding his impact trauma and combat-related behaviors, challenging unhelpful and paralyzing automatic thoughts regarding his trauma and moral injury, identifying values and living more consistently with these values, practicing acceptance and mindfulness, working toward self-forgiveness, reintegration with the community, and reconnecting with God and his spiritual identity.

Stage 1 of Treatment: Safety and Stabilization

The initial year of treatment with Carl focused primarily on helping him to establish emotional and physical safety in his life. I worked with him to understand the role and effects that trauma played on his life, his identity, his relationships, his spiritual/religious life, and his body. Therapy targeted acute symptoms of PTSD, panic disorder, insomnia, avoidance, and depression. He learned and practiced specific skills, such as progressive muscle relaxation, sleep hygiene, deep breathing, mindfulness, grounding techniques, positive affirmations, and anger management. He also built prayer and reflection into his daily life, which initially caused more distress because his shame and guilt—so clearly palpable to him at the time—were part of his religious and spiritual struggles with what was likely an experience of God's judgment, a central feature of religious struggles (Exline et al., 2014). Though many aspects of therapy helped him find and use personally meaningful spiritual and religious practices, some practices, like last rites, were irrevocably associated with his sense of spiritual unworthiness.

Carl also agreed to join a support group for Vietnam veterans. He initially dropped out, stating that if the group members knew who he really was, they would not want him there; however, after months of challenging his thoughts about this, he decided to go back, expressed his fears to his fellow veterans, and was accepted back into the group with open arms. With much practice and commitment to his therapy, he clearly internalized the skills he learned and generalized the use of these calming and self-regulating methods to a variety of environments. At the time, however, he reported that he was still not ready to go back to Mass.

Stage 2 of Treatment: Mourning and Processing of Trauma

After Carl's acute PTSD and panic symptoms subsided, a deep sense of depression and sadness seemed to arise from beneath his more palpable symptoms of anxiety and agitation. It seemed his chronic and acute symptoms of PTSD and anxiety had been masking the underlying moral injury and wounds to his identity that he had been struggling with for 40 years. He began to speak openly about the loss of his best friend in combat and how this particular event transformed him from "from good to beast." He discussed feeling extreme guilt, shame, and anxiety about being unable to save his best friend the day that he died in combat.

He became preoccupied with his identity as a "monster" and "murderer" and seemed to want me to confirm that he was indeed a damaged and dangerous human being who was unworthy of love from himself and others. These thoughts were clearly interfering with his willingness and ability to get close to his family and experience any sense of joy in his life. Carl reported that his moral injury was keeping him away from going back to Mass or speaking with a priest as he was too ashamed and afraid to do so—a clear indication of chronic religious struggles with God and religious authorities that are correlated with many negative health and emotional health outcomes (Abu-Raiya et al., 2015). He attempted several times to go back to Mass, but during each service he was flooded with intrusive thoughts about being unable to save his best friend, along with the memories of the many Viet Cong he had killed.

At this point in his treatment, Carl agreed to complete CPT in order to help him make sense of his behaviors in combat, challenge the unhelpful and damaging automatic thoughts that were keeping him stuck in his recovery, experience the natural emotions he had been avoiding for many decades, and decrease self-blame regarding his friend's death.

One of the initial interventions associated with CPT is completing the impact statement, which occurs after Session 1. According to Resick et al. (2017),

> One objective of the Impact Statement is to elicit the client's appraisals about the cause of the traumatic event and to have the client examine the effects the event has had on his or her life in several different areas (i.e., safety, trust, power/control, esteem, intimacy). (p. 102)

When Carl completed his initial impact statement, he identified his primary impact trauma as losing his best friend in combat. He also indicated that he believed the death of his friend was his fault and he should have been able to save him, although it was clear this was not actually the case once he explained the circumstances surrounding the event. Through this exercise and Socratic questioning, Carl was easily able to identify how this loss, along with his experiences of killing, had affected his views of self, others, the world, and God.

As has been found, "moral injury can result in psychological symptoms (e.g., shame, guilt, rage) and spiritual symptoms (e.g., spiritual struggles, moral concerns, loss of meaning, self-condemnation, difficulty forgiving, loss of faith, loss of hope)" (Pearce et al., 2018, p. 2), all of which have proven to be significant barriers to recovery from trauma and improvement of suffering (Shay, 2014). Research on MMI and spiritual struggles demonstrates that when veterans and service members experience ongoing guilt, anger, shame, and disgust about traumatic events that caused harm, they are likely to experience God and those in religious authority as judging them (Evans et al., 2018). Spiritual and religious practices that are used to connect veterans with God and a sense of their own goodness now induce shame and guilt, as Doehring (2019) illustrated in an MMI spiritual care case study. This was clearly the case for Carl, and he began to realize and sit with the profound effect that Vietnam had on his life and spiritual identity.

After writing and reading the trauma account associated with his primary impact trauma, Carl began to allow himself to connect more and more with the natural emotions of grief and loss he felt after the death of his friend. He also began to identify the stuckpoints associated with his PTSD and depression symptoms: "I didn't do enough to save my friend," "I should have done more that day," "I am a murderer," "I am a monster," "I am a disgusting human being," "I don't deserve happiness," "I cannot get better," "I should not be allowed to hold my grandson," and "I cannot find any joy." As he learned to challenge his automatic thinking and create more balanced and realistic thoughts, Carl began to report less of a sense of moral injury, and a decrease in feelings of hopelessness, guilt, shame, and self-disgust. This decrease in moral injury related to thoughts, behaviors, and feelings led to subsequent decreases in symptoms of depression and PTSD, while also increasing his behavioral engagement with his family and community.

Through CPT, Carl and I also worked to help him reframe the circumstances that prohibited him from being able to save his best friend's life in combat. He had been telling himself for 40 years that he was "not a good enough soldier" and that he "didn't do enough"; however, through Socratic dialogue and gentle challenging of his perceptions of the events that day, he was able to see that many factors that were outside of his control had influenced the resulting death of his battle buddy (e.g., spiritual disillusionment, fatigue, malnourishment, chronic insomnia, experiencing an ambush, grief and trauma, and the unpredictable nature of combat). Carl also began to work on challenging and reframing his stuckpoints and automatic thoughts regarding killing. He began to understand more deeply the context of these aggressive behaviors and was able to practice more self-compassion and self-forgiveness. Through therapy, he realized that he "acted as a consequence of the trauma context and not as a premeditated act or with instrumental intent to victimize" (Smith et al., 2013, p. 461).

It is important to note that, after much discussion, Carl finally agreed to meet with a local VA chaplain to discuss some of his spiritual/religious-related stuckpoints, such as "God does not love me," "I am unforgivable," "I should not be allowed at Mass," "I will go straight to hell," and "I will be forever punished for what I did." The combination of being able to challenge his stuckpoints with both a secular therapist and a chaplain seemed to help him reframe not only the objectively challengeable thoughts but also those that were more spiritual and values based in nature. Speaking to the chaplain also allowed him the opportunity to seek religious guidance about how to use prayer, meditation, and confession as tools to reduce the emotional and psychological impact of his religiously oriented stuckpoints. Carl's final CPT impact statement demonstrated the significant growth he made toward reduction of symptoms, understanding the context of his combat-related behaviors, practicing compassion of self, tolerating natural emotions, reconnecting with God, and thinking in a more balanced and nuanced manner about his trauma.

Stage 3 of Treatment: Community Reintegration and Committed Action

After the completion of CPT, I began taking more of an ACT-based approach with Carl because this particular evidence-based treatment focuses more on the identification of personal values, acceptance, mindfulness, cognitive defusion, and living life in the present according to one's values, which is wholly consistent with the treatment of moral injury (Nieuwsma et al., 2015). I also employed a spiritually oriented approach focused on Carl's particular values, beliefs, and religious practices.

Carl began this phase of therapy by identifying his primary core values, including accountability, calmness, compassion, community, contentment, faith, growth, honor, patriotism, and gratitude. He noted with significant insight that his current values were significantly different than the values he held so tightly when he first initiated therapy; these prior values included accuracy, carefulness, predictability, order, and self-control. So much of his life had been filled with experiential avoidance and compulsive attempts to control his inner experience (i.e., thoughts, memories, bodily sensations, and feelings related to the trauma), which paradoxically assisted in the maintenance and reinforcement of his symptoms.

For Carl, experiential avoidance in the context of trauma and moral injury included the avoidance of the following: religious practice, spending time with family, emotional intimacy, and social interaction. In addition, he had a long history of working more than 15 hours per day. Over time, Carl began to understand that during combat the act of killing also served as a form of experiential avoidance for him as this behavior temporarily served to distance him from the grief, disillusionment, rage, helplessness, and sense of meaninglessness he experienced in Vietnam.

Not only did Carl become more aware of his values and more accepting of his internal experiences, but he also began to live his life more engaged in mindful and intentional committed action. ACT defines *committed action* as a "values-based action that occurs at a particular moment in time and that is deliberately linked to creating a pattern of action that serves the value" (Hayes et al., 2012, p. 328). For Carl, attending therapy, spending time in nature, repairing his relationships, getting to know his grandson, praying, attending Mass, and giving back to his community demonstrated his strong dedication to committed action.

Carl benefited tremendously from learning and practicing mindfulness, which for most of his adult life he had avoided, other than in the context of his carpentry, during which he could intently focus for hours on end. A core component of ACT is a focus on present-centered living instead of a focus on rumination about the past or worry about the future, which this veteran worked on diligently before his death. Over the last year of his life, he formed a strong connection with nature and animals and spent hours walking in the woods, studying plants, smelling flowers, and marveling over insects. He often brought in pictures he had taken of beautiful leaves or interesting bugs to share with me and would talk about the way in which mindfully petting and walking his dog soothed his soul.

He also began to practice mindfulness and intentionality during prayer and while in Mass, which led to him being less carried away by intrusive memories, along with feelings of guilt and shame. Carl became more and more comfortable sitting in Mass, and one Veterans Day he even spoke to the congregation about his experience as a combat veteran and how God and therapy had helped him to work toward forgiveness and self-acceptance. He developed a strong relationship with his daughter and grandson, who began attending therapy and church with him.

Although he worked on decreasing guilt, shame, and self-hatred for much of his therapy, it was clear that Carl continued to experience much distress, as killing was still directly in conflict with his core values of compassion, community, and faith. It is essential to note that the goal of ACT in the context of moral injury is not to fully take away an appropriate sense of guilt for having engaged in a behavior that is considered morally or spiritually in conflict with one's values, morals, and/or religious beliefs. Nieuwsma et al. (2015) addressed this:

> Whatever may be the true state of human beings' agency, there is some danger in adopting a therapeutic stance that entirely precludes the very possibility of culpability. If a wrong (perceived or actual) has been committed, there may be need for a process of forgiveness (of self and/or others). (p. 201)

Carl began to focus on self-compassion and self-forgiveness, which he came to understand to be a nonlinear, spiritual, and ongoing process. As he began to practice forgiveness of self, he realized that giving back to the community and his church would allow him to begin to experience some sense of restitution. He began to do some volunteer work at church, which seemed to provide him with a sense of meaning and purpose. He began to see himself as a more integrated and spiritual human being who had engaged in many behaviors that were strongly against his moral code, religious beliefs, and personal values but who was also a caring partner, family member, and community member. He became more and more comfortable looking at himself in the mirror for sustained periods of time, and even as a symbolic gesture toward acceptance and forgiveness of self, he allowed a photographer to take a picture of his face, which he enlarged and hung up as a way to practice his commitment to self-compassion and his personal journey of change and recovery.

In one session after learning of his cancer diagnosis, I shared "The Veteran's Prayer" by Hugh Scanlen with him. He had been working on acceptance, mindfulness, committed action, present-centered living, cognitive defusion, self-forgiveness, and compassion, all processes that seemed to be highlighted in petitions of this prayer:

> May I accept who I am now. . . .
> Help me to remember and to dim—
> not forget—the tragic past. . . .
> Give me the strength to face the time I have left here
> to reconnect with humanity. (Tick, 2014, p. 235)

He was also working to reconnect with God and to let go of some of the religious and spiritual struggles he had held onto for 4 decades. When he read this prayer aloud for the first time in therapy, he immediately began weeping, looked up at the therapist, and simply and adamantly stated, "This is me." Carl kept this prayer by his bed and read it nightly; he reported that it gave him deep comfort and that he felt it was written just for him.

During the last few months of his life, Carl was clearly living in a manner that was more consistent with his values, and he was actively engaged in more intentional committed action in his life. He worked toward practicing acceptance that he could not change his past or his future, but he could change the quality of the moments he had left with his family, himself, God, and nature. Although he was terrified of what would happen after he "crossed over" and faced God, he also experienced some comfort in knowing he could only focus on living life according to his values in the present moment. This provided him with a sense of freedom and release that most likely helped him live more fully, mindfully, and intentionally in his final moments.

CONCLUSION

An intercultural approach to spiritually oriented psychotherapy helps clinicians identify the layers in their own religious, spiritual, or moral orienting systems that shape the care they want for veterans like Carl. Our spiritual practices grounded us in goodness and hope as we entered Carl's story of suffering. Our values of *care and doing no harm* provoked a deep sense of lament for not only the suffering Carl experienced and the harm he caused at such a young age but also his chronic moral, spiritual, and religious struggles over 40 years. We lamented the terrible suffering arising from combat done in the horrendous conditions Carl experienced. Spiritually oriented care is not just about caring for persons; it's about social justice that challenges life-limiting and destructive systems that exacerbate suffering (Graham, 2017). We are grateful that Carl was able to accept a referral to a chaplain who did represent a caring religious authority, even though Carl could not permit himself to receive last rites. We see this as a tragic outcome of his deep sense of being unworthy, which we might describe as an irreparable soul wound or sense of desecration of humanity— of Carl, his buddy who died, and those he killed—that comes when the foundational value of sanctity of life is trespassed.

We experienced hope in the ways that Carl's therapy brought about such radical transformation and posttraumatic growth, enabling him to connect with goodness through this therapeutic relationship and with his departed wife ("the love of his life"), his daughter and grandchild, his religious rituals and prayers, and his joy in nature. The goodness he experienced was, we believe, a sign of the goodness he entered into upon death and the goodness that lives on, among those who read and ponder this case study and the ways it evokes values, beliefs, and practices of caring for veterans like Carl.

REFERENCES

Abu-Raiya, H. I., Pargament, K., & Exline, J. (2015). Understanding and addressing religious and spiritual struggles in health care. *Health & Social Work, 40*(4), e126–e134. https://doi.org/10.1093/hsw/hlv055

Currier, J. M., Farnsworth, J. K., Drescher, K. D., McDermott, R. C., Sims, B. M., & Albright, D. L. (2017). Development and evaluation of the Expressions of Moral Injury Scale—Military version. *Clinical Psychology & Psychotherapy.* https://doi.org/10.1002/cpp.2170

Doehring, C. (2015a). *The practice of pastoral care: A postmodern approach* (Rev. ed.). Westminster John Knox.

Doehring, C. (2015b). Resilience as the relational ability to spiritually integrate moral stress. *Pastoral Psychology, 64*(5), 635–649. https://doi.org/10.1007/s11089-015-0643-7

Doehring, C. (2019). Military moral injury: An evidence-based and intercultural approach to spiritual care. *Pastoral Psychology, 68*(1), 15–30. https://doi.org/10.1007/s11089-018-0813-5

Drescher, K. D., Foy, D. W., Kelly, C., Leshner, A., Schutz, K., & Litz, B. (2011). An exploration of the usefulness of the construct of moral injury in war veterans. *Traumatology, 17*(8), 8–13. https://doi.org/10.1177/1534765610395615

Eagleton, T. (2003). *Sweet violence: The idea of the tragic.* Blackwell.

Evans, W. R., Stanley, M. A., Barrera, T. L., Exline, J. J., Pargament, K. I., & Teng, E. J. (2018). Morally injurious events and psychological distress among veterans: Examining the mediating role of religious and spiritual struggles. *Psychological Trauma: Theory, Research, Practice, and Policy, 10*(3), 360–367. https://doi.org/10.1037/tra0000347

Exline, J. J., Pargament, K., Grubbs, J. B., & Yali, A. M. (2014). The religious and spiritual struggles scale: Development and initial validation. *Psychology of Religion and Spirituality, 6*(3), 208–222. https://doi.org/10.1037/a0036465

Farnsworth, J. K. (2019). Is and ought: Descriptive and prescriptive cognitions in military-related moral injury. *Journal of Traumatic Stress, 32*(3), 373–381. https://doi.org/10.1002/jts.22356

Foa, E. B., Hembree, E. A., Rothbaum, B. O., & Rauch, S. A. (2019). *Prolonged exposure therapy for PTSD: Emotional processing of traumatic experiences.* Oxford University Press. https://doi.org/10.1093/med-psych/9780190926939.001.0001

Graham, L. K. (2017). *Moral injury: Restoring wounded souls*. Abingdon Press.

Gray, M. J., Schorr, Y., Nash, W., Lebowitz, L., Amidon, A., Lansing, A., Maglione, M., Lang, A. J., & Litz, B. T. (2012). Adaptive disclosure: An open trial of a novel exposure-based intervention for service members with combat-related psychological stress injuries. *Behavior Therapy, 43*(2), 407–415. https://doi.org/10.1016/j.beth.2011.09.001

Haidt, J. (2002). The moral emotions. In R. J. Davidson, K. R. Scherer, & H. H. Goldsmith (Eds.), *Handbook of affective sciences* (pp. 852–870). Oxford University Press.

Haidt, J. (2008). The emotional dog and its rational tail: A social intuitionist approach to moral judgment. In J. E. Adler & L. J. Rips (Eds.), *Reasoning: Studies of human inference and its foundations* (pp. 1024–1052). Cambridge University Press. https://doi.org/10.1017/CBO9780511814273.055

Haidt, J. (2012). *The righteous mind: Why good people are divided by politics and religion*. Pantheon/Random House.

Hayes, S. C., Strosahl, K. D., & Wilson, K. G. (1999). *Acceptance and commitment therapy: An experiential approach to behavior change*. Guilford Press.

Hayes, S. C., Strosahl, K. D., & Wilson, K. G. (2012). *Acceptance and commitment therapy: The process and practice of mindful change*. Guilford Press.

Herman, J. (1992). *Trauma and recovery: The aftermath of violence from domestic abuse to political terror*. The Free Press.

Kusner, K. G., & Pargament, K. (2012). Shaken to the core: Understanding and addressing the spiritual dimension of trauma. In R. A. McMackin, E. Newman, J. M. Fogler, & T. M. Keane (Eds.), *Trauma therapy in context: The science and craft of evidence-based practice* (pp. 211–230). American Psychological Association. https://doi.org/10.1037/13746-010

Linehan, M. (2014). *DBT skills training* (2nd ed.). Guilford Press.

Litz, B. T., Lebowitz, L., Gray, M. J., & Nash, W. P. (2016). *Adaptive disclosure: A new treatment for military trauma, loss, and moral injury*. Guilford Press.

Litz, B. T., Stein, N., Delaney, E., Lebowitz, L., Nash, W. P., Silva, C., & Maguen, S. (2009). Moral injury and moral repair in war veterans: A preliminary model and intervention strategy. *Clinical Psychology Review, 29*(8), 695–706. https://doi.org/10.1016/j.cpr.2009.07.003

Maguen, S., Lucenko, B. A., Reger, M. A., Gahm, G. A., Litz, B. T., Seal, K. H., Knight, S. J., & Marmar, C. R. (2010). The impact of reported direct and indirect killing on mental health symptoms in Iraq war veterans. *Journal of Traumatic Stress, 23*(1), 86–90. https://doi.org/10.1002/jts.20434

Meichenbaum, D. (2019). Stress inoculation training: A resilience-engendering intervention. In B. A. Moore & W. E. Penk (Eds.), *Treating PTSD in military personnel: A clinical handbook* (pp. 136–150). Guilford Press.

Najavits, L. M. (2002). *Seeking safety: A treatment manual for PTSD and substance abuse*. Guilford Press.

Nash, W. P. (2007). Combat/operational stress adaptations and injuries. In C. R. Figley & W. P. Nash (Eds.), *Combat stress injury: Theory, research and management*. Routledge.

Nash, W. P. (2019). Commentary on the special issue on moral injury: Unpacking two models for understanding moral injury. *Journal of Traumatic Stress, 32*(3), 465–470. https://doi.org/10.1002/jts.22409

Nieuwsma, J. A., Walser, R. D., Farnsworth, J. K., Drescher, K. D., Meador, K. G., & Nash, W. P. (2015). Possibilities within acceptance and commitment therapy for approaching moral injury. *Current Psychiatry Reviews, 11*(3), 193–206. https://doi.org/10.2174/1573400511666150629105234

Pargament, K. (2007). *Spiritually integrated psychotherapy: Understanding and addressing the sacred.* Guilford Press.

Pargament, K., Desai, K. M., & McConnell, K. M. (2006). Spirituality: A pathway to posttraumatic growth or decline? In L. G. Calhoun & R. G. Tedeschi (Eds.), *Handbook of posttraumatic growth: Research and practice* (pp. 121–135). Erlbaum.

Pargament, K., Wong, S., & Exline, J. (2016). Wholeness and holiness: The spiritual dimension of eudaimonics. In J. Vittersø (Ed.), *The handbook of eudaimonic wellbeing* (pp. 379–394). Springer International. https://doi.org/10.1007/978-3-319-42445-3_25

Pearce, M., Haynes, K., Rivera, N. R., & Koenig, H. G. (2018). Spiritually integrated cognitive processing therapy: A new treatment for post-traumatic stress disorder that targets moral. *Global Advances in Health and Medicine: Improving Healthcare Outcomes Worldwide, 7.* https://doi.org/10.1177/2164956118759939

Resick, P. A., Monson, C. M., & Chard, K. M. (2017). *Cognitive processing therapy for PTSD: A comprehensive manual.* Guilford Press.

Resick, P. A., & Schnicke, M. K. (1992). *Cognitive processing therapy for rape victims: A treatment manual.* SAGE Productions, Inc.

Rutter, J. G., & Friedberg, R. D. (1999). Guidelines for the effective use of Socratic dialogue in cognitive therapy. In L. VandeCreek, S. Knapp, & T. L. Jackson (Eds.), *Innovations in clinical practice* (Vol. 17, pp. 481–490). Professional Resource Press.

Rutter, J. G., Friedberg, R. D., & VandeCreek, L. (1999). *Innovations in clinical practice: A source book.* Professional Resource Press.

Santiago, P. N., & Gall, T. L. (2016). Acceptance and commitment therapy as a spiritually integrated psychotherapy. *Counseling and Values, 61*(2), 239–254. https://doi.org/10.1002/cvj.12040

Schorr, Y., Stein, N. R., Maguen, S., Barnes, J. B., Bosch, J., & Litz, B. T. (2018). Sources of moral injury among war veterans: A qualitative evaluation. *Journal of Clinical Psychology, 74*(12), 2203–2218. https://doi.org/10.1002/jclp.22660

Shapiro, F. (2017). *Eye movement desensitization and reprocessing (EMDR) therapy: Basic principles, protocols and procedures* (3rd ed.). Guilford Press.

Shay, J. (1992). *Achilles in Vietnam: Combat trauma and the undoing of character.* Scribner.

Shay, J. (2002). *Odysseus in America: Combat trauma and the trials of homecoming.* Scribner.

Shay, J. (2014). Moral injury. *Psychoanalytic Psychology, 31*(2), 182–191. https://doi.org/10.1037/a0036090

Shults, F. L., & Sandage, S. J. (2006). *Transforming spirituality: Integrating theology and psychology.* Baker Academic.

Smith, E. R., Duax, J. M., & Rauch, S. A. M. (2013). Perceived perpetration during traumatic events: Clinical suggestions from experts in prolonged exposure therapy. *Cognitive and Behavioral Practice, 20*(4), 461–470. https://doi.org/10.1016/j.cbpra.2012.12.002

Stein, N. R., Mills, M. A., Arditte, K., Mendoza, C., Borah, A. M., Resick, P. A., Litz, B. T., Belinfante, K., Borah, E. V., Cooney, J. A., Foa, E. B., Hembree, E. A., Kippee, A., Lester, K., Malach, S. L., McClure, J., Peterson, A. L., Vargas, V., & Wright, E. (2012).

A scheme for categorizing traumatic military events. *Behavior Modification, 36*(6), 787–807. https://doi.org/10.1177/0145445512446945

Tick, E. (2014). *Warrior's return: Restoring the soul after war.* Sounds True.

Tomlinson, J., Glenn, E. S., Paine, D. R., & Sandage, S. J. (2016). What is the "relational" in relational spirituality? A review of definitions and research directions. *Journal of Spirituality in Mental Health, 18*(1), 55–75. https://doi.org/10.1080/19349637.2015.1066736

Walser, R. D., & Westrup, D. (2007). *Acceptance and commitment therapy for the treatment of post-traumatic stress disorder and trauma-related problems: A practitioner's guide to using mindfulness and acceptance strategies.* New Harbinger.

13
SPIRITUALITY, SELFHOOD, AND SOCIAL CLASS IN PSYCHOTHERAPY

NEIL ALTMAN

As the title of this chapter suggests, there is a complex and multidimensional matrix at the intersection of psychology, religion, spirituality, and social class. In a context of specialized academic disciplines, these aspects of human life tend to be considered in isolation from each other. However, social class, interacting with culture, religious affiliation or the lack of same, and a variety of other factors, influences help-seeking behavior, how people feel helped, and the way they interact with helpers. For example, in general, people of upper middle class and above, around the world, are relatively likely to turn to secular mental health professionals, whereas people of lower middle class and below are relatively likely to turn to ministers, priests, rabbis, or imams as counselors, or to a spiritual healer in their community (Chalfant et al., 1990). Our experience is holistic, however, and all these facets continually interact. Before attempting the integration of these various threads, highlighting social class, let me bring you in on some of my own development to date at this confluence of identities and commitments.

https://doi.org/10.1037/0000276-014
Spiritual Diversity in Psychotherapy: Engaging the Sacred in Clinical Practice,
S. J. Sandage and B. D. Strawn (Editors)

PERSONAL SOCIAL CLASS AND SPIRITUAL HISTORY

I grew up in a Reform Jewish family in Minnesota. My parents sent me to Sunday school, which I dutifully attended. I had a Bar Mitzvah. There was no soul to it all. Looking back, I see that I noted subliminally that my parents rarely went to the synagogue except on the High Holy Days of Rosh Hashana and Yom Kippur and that there was no discussion of religious matters, or observance of religious rituals, at home. None of my parents' friends taught in the Sunday School. Religious education was entirely outsourced; I heard my father joking that the rabbi made sure Saturday morning services ended in time for him to make his tee-off time at the country club. I observed him once myself surreptitiously glance at his watch as the time approached 1:00 p.m. one Saturday. I went through a brief period of being terrified that I would not be written in the Book of Life if I didn't attend Yom Kippur services from morning until night and did so for exactly 1 year when I was 10. Some seeds must have been planted, however, because years later, having become a father, I became a fairly active member of a Conservative synagogue in New York City as a family matter, then finding myself very identified with Israel and anguished about Middle Eastern politics for some years. It took 3 decades for my Jewish identity to assert itself, a sort of "time bomb" in Paul Cowan's (1983) vivid words.

Meanwhile, Eastern religion captivated me from age 15. I read Alan Watts's (1957) *The Way of Zen*, enthralled, while on vacation with my parents in Miami Beach. I followed J. D. Salinger's (1981) book about the Glass family, raptly, with close attention to the role of Buddhism in their faintly Jewish lives. I attended the University of California at Berkeley from 1964 through 1968 and lived in Haight-Ashbury in 1967. Eastern spirituality was in the atmosphere and pervaded my consciousness. After college, I went to the Peace Corps, making sure my placement was in India. I lived in a rural South Indian village of 5,000 people for nearly 3 years. After India, I began following Swami Chinmayananda on his visits to New York, studied Vedanta, gradually discovering that Hindu philosophy was folk wisdom among "uneducated" (in Western terms) village people, Hindus and some Muslims (Sufi Islam was and is a strong thread in the Indian context).

As an undergraduate I discovered psychoanalysis in a class called "The Psychology of the Unconscious" taught by one Professor William McKinnon who dressed in a suit and tie while propounding the most radical and fascinating ideas about the mysteries at the core of the human psyche and soul. Psyche and soul have remained linked for me, forming a deep connection between Eastern religion and the healing world of psychoanalysis, which has long formed my professional identity.

I had no clue, until recently, that the preoccupations I just described were those of an upper-middle-class person who did not have to worry about where the money was going to come from. Among the "privileges" of my social class status was the opportunity to remain oblivious to the sublime disdain in which I held material concerns. Having become more aware of my own social status, I have learned something about the way social class structures affect people's lives in the United States and elsewhere. I have learned that the United States is supposed to be the land where social class doesn't matter, where fixed class positions don't exist, and where upward mobility is available to everyone. This myth originated among European immigrants who were seeking freedom from the imprisonment of hereditary class positions. We have been slow, across the centuries, to recognize how core social class remains in the lives of people in the United States, sometimes precisely because social class status is not fixed at birth but must be earned. In this chapter, we look at some of the ways social class infiltrates psychotherapy and other forms of healing practice in the United States and in other countries, as well as some of the ways social class intersects with culture in the domain of emotional and psychological healing.

Although I refer frequently in this chapter to *psychoanalysis*, I mean thereby to include a wide variety of psychotherapies. I do not subscribe to a narrow definition of psychoanalysis based on frequency of sessions, use of the analytic couch, the attempted abstinence or anonymity of the therapist, the restriction of interventions to interpretation of unconscious sexual and aggressive impulses, or other such factors. My use of the term *psychoanalysis* refers to any psychotherapy that focuses on the unconscious (broadly defined) level of the patient–therapist emotional interaction. By this definition, there is no reason in principle to exclude therapies that are cognitively or behaviorally or systemically or interpersonally oriented. Likewise, there is no reason to exclude putatively psychoanalytic treatments in which the focus is sometimes, or frequently, focused on such factors.

To further complicate matters, social class and culture are intertwined in ways that are difficult to disentangle when either is considered in relation to people's religious and spiritual lives. Social classes have cultural correlates, cultural locations, and ways of being that feel comfortable and natural to people based on their social status and sometimes race and ethnicity as well. (Bourdieu, 1984; Layton, 2004) These social-class-linked locations include religious and spiritual places, activities, and ways of being. Think about who feels at home in a yoga class? Who feels at home in a Pentecostal church?

SOCIAL CLASS INFLUENCES AND EMOTIONAL DISTRESS

Sennett and Cobb's 1972 book pointed out and documented that when social class is not inherited, when upward mobility is supposed to be available to all, lower class status is likely to be attributed to personal failure. Lower socioeconomic status leads to low self-esteem. I thought of this point in my work with Mr. D, whom I saw in psychotherapy in the aftermath of the Wall Street crash of 2008. Mr. D was depressed, frantic really, after being laid off from his well-paying job as a banker. For 1 year, he had been diligently looking for work. At first, few jobs were available in the banking industry, then as some positions began opening up, he never quite made the final cut. There were too many people in his dire position applying for the same jobs. Mr. D's savings were dwindling. He had a big mortgage on a big house in an affluent suburb where he lived with his wife, who did not work outside the home, and three children. The family had, for a year, maintained their "standard of living" in material terms by drawing down their savings nearly to the vanishing point. Mr. D., increasingly depressed as one job after another slipped out of his grasp, began to believe that a depressed demeanor, or a positivity that felt forced, was responsible for his failure to do well in his interviews. Each failed job application only reinforced his depression. Periodically, I asked Mr. D whether he felt anger about his situation, about the unsustainable financial structures that had fallen on him like a house of cards, about the expectations of his social network that ruled out his ability to envision a downsized life, about the anger and disappointment he felt from his family about his failure to land a job. This question led nowhere. Mr. D was trapped in his self-blame and his depression, until he finally got a job with a salary on which he felt he could just scrape by, at which point he felt better and terminated our psychotherapy. I had to face the limits of my influence on Mr. D's superego; much as I tried to broaden the sources of his self-esteem, or lack of same, there was nothing like a good job and a respectable salary to make him feel good about himself.

THE POVERTY OF AFFLUENCE OR THE SPIRITUAL POVERTY OF AFFLUENCE

From the other end of the socioeconomic spectrum, Ava was a 14-year-old girl from an affluent section of New York City. Her parents both worked long hours in Wall Street firms, so that a caregiver had most of the childrearing responsibilities since early childhood for Ava, an only child. Ava ran with a fast crowd, did middling well in her private school, and was slated to go to a boarding school for high school. She had a plan to go to a top business school after completing high school, so she knew that she needed to work hard and improve her grades, but it was difficult for her to focus on things beyond her physical appearance and her social status in the popular group in her elite school. I will focus here on one particular interaction with her parents around Ava's wish to spend the summer before high school in a resort area in the South of France where one of her friends was going to be living with a rotation of parents and other caregivers. Ava's mother opposed this plan, thinking that she really only wanted to party without adult supervision, while Ava maintained that she needed a carefree and fun summer before buckling down to work hard in high school. She thought it was ridiculous and demeaning for her mother to think that all she cared about was partying and boys and alcohol, when in fact she had such serious plans for herself and would not do anything so self-destructive as what her mother imagined.

In one session, I asked Ava how she thought she could convince her parents that she was not simply out to have fun, as her mother seemed to believe. She hemmed and hawed a bit, until I asked her what she *really* cared about in life. Why did she want to go to a top business school?

AVA: Money.

NEIL: Why do you want money?

AVA: I don't know, everyone wants money, to have nice things, I guess.

NEIL: Your parents have a lot of money. Why do you think they want money?

AVA: (*Thoughtfully, after a pause*) I think he [her father] likes to take care of his family, us, but also his parents and brother and sister.

NEIL: Would that be one reason you want money too, to be able to take care of your family, the children you might have some day, other people in your family?

AVA: (*Brightening up*) Yes! I want to have money so I can do what my father does.

NEIL: I think that if you explained that to your parents, they'd be less likely to think that all you want is to party.

I found myself, in this interchange, probing for, or trying to get Ava to formulate, a value system that goes beyond pleasure or social status, that gets closer to something one might call spiritual or religious, something that goes beyond the self. As I spoke to her, I remember thinking, as perhaps a 10-year-old, that my grandfather's purpose in life seemed to center on buying my grandmother mink coats. My grandmother had five of them, and I think I was on to something. It was a moment of clarity, although I could not have articulated the significance of what I was perceiving. I group this moment of clarity about human motivation in the same category as the insight that dawned on me when, as a 12-year-old riding my bike, it suddenly became clear to me that most of what people did was about sex.

My search for a transcendent value system in Ava's hedonistic and narcissistic presentation of self, not entirely atypical for a 14-year-old, reflected the sense of meaning that I find in being a psychotherapist, that is, in being able to attune myself to the feelings of other people and to work with them to sort out their conflicts and their suffering. It seems that, for me, and I believe for many other people, meaningfulness emerges from self-transcendence, from caring about and for others. This value system, to be found prominently among the values animating religious and spiritual traditions generally is not easy to reconcile with the unbridled and self-centered greed and hedonism that is front and center in a secular capitalistic value system. But it must be acknowledged that matters are not so black and white. Religious communities contain more than their share of self-centered individuals such as charismatic cult leaders intent on aggrandizing power and money. More to the point, narcissistic concerns are undercurrents in most if not all individuals, groups, and movements in which other-centered, religious and spiritual values are in the foreground.

On the other side, where self-aggrandizement and narcissistic inflation are in the foreground, there is sometimes to be found an undercurrent of love and devotion to others. To me, the argument in supply side economics (an outgrowth of the Protestant ethic, after all) that unbridled acquisitiveness ultimately benefits everyone seems contrived and self-serving, yet it cannot be denied that some of the most ruthless and greedy individuals and families have been also among the most generous philanthropists. The auto industry, in my view, is not particularly socially responsible, yet I must acknowledge, with appreciation, that the Ford Foundation did choose to fund generously a conference on prejudice and racism on which I was working.

Where are the boundaries between what is called *greed* and what is called *acquisitiveness*? When it comes right down to it, why should it be more virtuous to be greedy, or acquisitive, in the service of one's family, or one's religious group, or one's nation, than to be greedy or acquisitive in the service of self, narrowly defined? And how to balance altruistic generous and philanthropic impulses with narcissistic and greedy impulses in the same people? People have multiple and contradictory aspects, undermining efforts to categorize them in one dimensional terms. There are few people who unequivocally would have as much chance to enter heaven as a camel would have to pass through the eye of a needle, or who would have a reserved seat in heaven due to their spiritual or religious commitments, their selfless devotion to the poor as God's children. In this way, perhaps, we can avoid dismissal of other people as essentially evil or hypocritical, or as essentially good and devoted.

In the end, as a psychotherapist to Ava and her parents in this particular case, my goal seemed to have been to help them all connect around shared transcendent values. Her parents cared about her, she cared about them. Her parents loved money and social status, and so did Ava. Ava's parents infused her with the materialistic and hedonistic values that then underlay the behavior ("partying," substance abuse, and cultivation of sex appeal) that worried them and they deplored. The community in which the parents and Ava lived supported these values, unlike traditional religious communities in which caring for others might be more prominent. It took some probing for me to locate where Ava might sense a transcendent set of values in her parents, and in herself, via which she could connect with them in a way that I thought might be durable, beyond the transient impulsivity of adolescents and the anxieties of their parents. After all, adolescents are also famously values-driven, sometimes rigidly so, but inspiring to their parental generation if their elders are open to listening. At this historical moment as I write, adolescents are taking the lead of action to address climate change, both for the self-centered reason that they will live with the consequences of global warming but also because they care about their Mother Earth. Their mothers (and fathers) at home have to be resonating with those concerns at some level.

The relationship between social class and religion/spirituality is complicated in this family, as in all families, beyond any simplistic categorization of people and classes. My therapeutic goal in this particular case was to try to bridge the gap between these people by focusing with Ava, on how money must be *for* something, sometimes hedonistic and narcissistic, and sometimes transcendent, thus linking her with concerns that could link her psychically with her parents. I suggest that Ava's parents' worries about her behavior reflected a subliminal awareness that there was an emptiness in herself that arose from the one-sided pursuit of money for its own sake, potentially leading to a form of self-destructiveness that might take concrete form in partying with its ultimate hangovers, if not overdoses. (See Altman, 2005, for an elaboration of this dynamic.)

SOCIAL CLASS INFLUENCES WHERE PEOPLE GO FOR HELP

From the affluent precincts of Manhattan's Upper East Side to the economically impoverished South Bronx can be a 20-minute trip on the subway. My career has spanned both extremes, so near in physical distance, yet so far in socioeconomic status. When I worked at a Community Mental Health Center in the Bronx, I saw an African American boy whom I called "Thomas" in a previous publication (Altman, 2010). I saw Thomas as he was placed in a series of foster homes while his biological mother fought for custody in court over a period of years but failed to show up for scheduled visitation. At last, the court terminated Thomas's mother's parental rights, and he was adopted by the African American foster family with whom he had last been placed.

Thomas's adoptive parents were conservative Christians; their lives were centered on the church. As their foster child, Thomas resisted going to church and acted up when he was there, but nothing seemed to disturb the solid commitment of this family. I met regularly with the foster mother, who came dutifully to the sessions and reported on some of Thomas's activities but did not seem very attuned to his feelings. Her husband came for the first session to meet me. He said little and never came again. I would call him from time to time to get his observations of Thomas.

After the judge terminated Thomas's mother's parental rights and he was adopted, his behavior changed dramatically. He became much calmer, less provocative, more thoughtful and reflective, and related better with me in the sessions. In contrast to his previous behavior, he was now less frenetic, no longer desperately seeking food, more willing to leave at the end of sessions with a sense that there would be another session soon. Thomas also suddenly became an enthusiastic member of his family's church. A few months after the adoption became final, Thomas, his family, and I agreed that it made sense to terminate the treatment. At our last session, Thomas invited me to come to Sunday services at his church. I was moved by his invitation and happy to accept. A few weeks later, I found myself in the pews of a conservative Christian church in the Bronx, listening to the preacher and contemplating what life would be like to feel that one could be transformed through faith at any moment. Being in this church exposed me to a sense of purpose and inspiration that I had not often encountered sitting in a clinic in the South Bronx. Especially, I was impressed by the men. I had seen many women of strength and determination who brought their children to the clinic. Men were too often conspicuous by their absence. In the church, I saw men at the pulpit and in the congregation who could give a boy something to look forward to in growing up to be a man. I was grateful to Thomas for inviting me to see what kind of life he was entering.

Thomas seemed exceptionally responsive to the commitment and stability provided by his adoptive family. Religion seemed to offer a structure that assisted this family in containing the feelings that Thomas tended to induce in them, so that they could steadfastly maintain their commitment to him in the face of all manner of provocation. Once Thomas felt secure with them, he adopted the church as his own containing structure. Transcending my own class-based secular worldview, I learned from Thomas and his family that healing does not occur only in the clinic.

Why this divergence in help-seeking? Of course, the cost of mental health services in the private sector is one crucial factor; alongside economics is culture. The roots of the cultural divergence on which I will focus is to be found in the history of a bifurcation of science or reason from religion or faith, with roots in the European Enlightenment. In general, science, and education based on science and reason, became the province of the middle classes, whereas faith and religion remained the province of the relatively lower classes (Van Dulmen, 1992). Let us look at this history in more detail, ultimately to see if there is a potential resolution to this split, an integration that would benefit both ostensibly science-based psychotherapy, and ostensibly faith-based spiritual healing.

REASON VERSUS FAITH

George Makari (2015) tracked the evolution of Western conceptions of mind from an earlier conception of soul, in parallel with a move from faith to reason in European epistemology. The soul belonged to the transcendent realm of spirituality that was the domain of the Catholic Church, a mystery that was accessible only to priests. The mind became an empirical phenomenon, a thing among other things in the world that was accessible to ordinary people—to all those who had access to reason. This democratization of knowledge was a central aspect of the Enlightenment and the Protestant Reformation. The priest was downgraded to minister in terms of privileged access to knowledge, as ordinary individuals were empowered to think for themselves and even critique the secular power of the Church. Some of the mystique of the priest was transferred to the special powers of the scientist, while the mystique of the priest remained intact in large segments of society. Freud was a central and bridging figure in this evolution as psychoanalysis developed a conception of the mind as having a transcendent element (the unconscious). The psychoanalyst, a scientist but with special knowledge of the unconscious, became a kind of secular priest, one with privileged access to mysteries of the mind (see Hoffman, 1998, for a discussion of the potential therapeutic impact of the mystique of the psychoanalyst). From this point of view, the cognitive-behavioral therapist represents a demystification of the therapist, a downgrading of the role to technician who follows an evidence-based, scientific, manualized procedure.

Although there have been recent efforts to integrate science with traditional spiritual practices for healing purposes (e.g., there is an evolving science-based program of neuroanatomical studies of the potentially therapeutic effects of meditation and other forms of mindfulness practice, supported by the Dalai Lama; Davidson & Goldman, 2017), the replacement of faith with reason, however, has never taken hold fully even in Europe and North America, not to mention the rest of the world. In large parts of the world a European-style enlightenment did not occur (although the values of the Scientific Revolution were imported and imposed on much of the non-European world via colonialism). Therefore, the move from soul to mind is the province of a scientific self-nominated elite, a circumstance which leads me to wonder how the domain of psychotherapy would look (or, indeed, looks) if faith and reason were not (as they are not in many quarters) so segregated from each other in this domain.

My experience is that, in Europe and North America, there is a strong and complex interaction between the prevalence of a post-Enlightenment, science-based approach to psychotherapy and social status. As a split between reason and faith took hold, with science winning the status of elite among epistemologies, healing methods based on religion and faith increasingly were to be found in the churches, mosques, and street front botanicas of working-class suburbs and lower class inner-city neighborhoods. This trend was moderated by the dominance in the public sector of government-financed hospital-based mental health clinics in the aftermath of the Community Mental Health movement of the 1960s. Payment for mental health services came to depend on a *Diagnostic and Statistical Manual* diagnosis and a correlated "evidence-based" treatment model. The insurance industry, too, required a diagnosis-based treatment plan for reimbursements on which working-class and middle-class people depended to access mental health services in the private sector. Only the most affluent who could pay out of pocket were able to afford psychological treatments outside the scientific, medical-model based system, where faith-based healing methods morphed into a new elite composed of "new age," "alternative" forms of practice, often promoted in the media by celebrities.

CONVERGENCE OF SOCIAL CLASS, CULTURE, AND SPIRITUALITY

In the 1970s and 1980s I was a psychologist in public sector mental health clinics in economically impoverished areas of the Bronx. The clinics where I worked were government-funded and required diagnoses and treatment plans based on a medical model. The professional staff, psychiatrists, psychologists, social workers, and psychiatric nurses had been trained in a scientific model mostly in medical settings. The clientele was predominantly of Afro Caribbean origin, largely from Puerto Rico and the Dominican Republic, and African American, as were the paraprofessionals who were bilingual and bicultural. The clientele and the paraprofessionals (along with the clerical staff) were familiar with spirit possession theories of dysfunction based on *espiritismo* and *santeria*, and traditional healing methods from their cultures of origin, designed to ward off or exorcise evil spirits with the aid of saints derived from both the Catholic tradition and African deities. In the wake of the 1960s, the Community Mental Health movement sought to moderate the elitism of medical hierarchies with the participation of local bicultural paraprofessionals. However, in the 1970s and 1980s, federal funding for the community mental health centers was phased out; local governments and agencies mostly failed to pick up the slack. The movement faded, along with the counter-elitist, culturally attuned values that had animated it.

Many of our patients had already consulted *espiritistas* who worked out of storefront *botanicas* in the neighborhood. Others hedged their bets by simultaneously working with the espiritistas and the psychiatric staff at our center. Although there was an occasional nod to education of the professional staff about espiritismo and santeria, the local practitioners of these healing methods remained marginal to our work at best. I knew enough to inquire during initial intakes about the patient's history, perhaps ongoing, with traditional healing methods, but I never went so far, as advisable as it would have been, to collaborate with espiritistas down the block. I think this reticence reflected both cultural and religious prejudices on my part; thus, the split between scientific and faith-based approaches to healing was reinforced. This outcome demonstrates how good intentions—to be attuned to local cultures in the provision of mental health services—needs continual reinforcement at the level of supervision and clinic leadership.

More recently, I have embraced a more integrative approach to psychotherapy, working in the well-to-do precincts of Manhattan in private practice, less impeded by cultural and socioeconomic prejudice. I sometimes draw on my knowledge of mindfulness meditation practices and suggest that patients look into that tradition to get a handle on anxiety and driven, obsessive thinking. I note the prevalence of holistic healing approaches, derived from Eastern spiritual traditions and bringing together nutrition, cognitive retraining, mindfulness meditation, and Hatha yoga.

My own explorations of psychotherapy outside a European-style split between faith and reason, or between spirituality and science, have taken place in India. Psychoanalysis took root in India in 1922 when Girindrashekar Bose established the Indian Psychoanalytic Society, a branch of Freud's International Psychoanalytic Association. Bose promptly took issue with the centrality of the Oedipus Complex in Freud's theory as it applied to India (1929/1999), in a series of communications with Freud, Bose argued that because masculinity and femininity were not so sharply split off from one another in India as they were in the West, castration anxiety as Freud framed it was not a central concern in Indian psychic development. Freud quickly grew tired of Bose's cross-cultural challenge, and the dialogue ended almost before it began. The next encounter between India and psychoanalysis occurred when Erik Erikson went to India to do the research that led to his writing of *Gandhi's Truth* (Erikson, 1969). Erikson brought a version of psychoanalysis with a psychosocial focus to India, opening the door to cross-cultural considerations. In the end, however, his verdict on Gandhi was rather critical from a fairly conventional psychoanalytic point of view, arguing that Gandhi's work was distorted by sexual repression. Sudhir Kakar (1982), who studied with Erikson early in his career, carried forward the work of developing a version of psychoanalysis that respectfully engaged with Indian culture. Kakar studied traditional healing methods in India and took account of the specific structures of the Indian family, such as the intergenerational joint family and the intense tie between Indian men and their mothers, as it influenced psychic development in Indian people. Kakar is a novelist as well as a psychoanalyst; his work follows Freud's in being empirically based on case studies presented in a literary form, while not attempting to conform to a controlled experimental model. Meanwhile, psychoanalysis developed along fairly conventional Kleinian and Freudian/ego psychological lines in various urban centers under the auspices of the International Psychoanalytic Association.

Kakar's work was carried forward by his student, Ashok Nagpal, in collaboration with Honey Oberoi Vahali (see her valuable overview of the history of psychoanalysis in India; Vahali, 2010), first at Delhi University, then at the School of Human Studies (SHS) of the Ambedkar University of Delhi. SHS brought a psychoanalytic sensibility together with a commitment to community-based clinical work. In 1995 (revised in 2010), I had written *The Analyst in the Inner City: Race, Class, and Culture Through a Psychoanalytic*

Lens (Altman, 1995, 2010; see also Altman, 2015), describing and reflecting on my own efforts to learn about how psychoanalysis could enable and enrich high-quality psychological work in the public sector. Since 2004, I have visited SHS approximately once a year to teach and learn and to share ideas about bringing psychoanalysis to community-based work. I have been fascinated by the form taken by psychoanalysis as it has emerged in India, outside the private practice model, for the most part, and with a larger sector of society less hidebound by the faith-reason split imposed by the enlightenment. Following is but one example of the experiences I had in India that opened my eyes to how psychoanalysis might be conceived outside the Euro-American context.

PSYCHOANALYSIS AT A SUFI SHRINE IN NEW DELHI

Friday evenings at the Nizamuddin mosque in New Delhi, people who are thought to be possessed by spirits (perhaps "mentally ill" in a Western medical context) are brought to a healing shrine, the Hazrat Nizamuddin Aulia Dargah, generally by family members. With the students in a class I was teaching at SHS, along with some faculty, I planned to attend the Muslim sabbath services at the mosque to experience, and then perhaps to understand, the healing process at a gathering of the possessed.

The approach to the mosque this Friday at dusk consisted of a tangle of crowded narrow streets buzzing with life, conversation, shop owners and customers transacting business. To my mind, the scene was reminiscent of any crowded bazaar in India, or perhaps the Old City of Jerusalem. Hundreds, thousands, of worshippers threaded their way through the bazaar on their way to the mosque.

At the entrance, one checked one's sandals and proceeded through a gate, swept along by the rush of people trying to reach, before sunset, the large assembly hall where prayers were taking place. By prior arrangement, we met a woman, our guide, who was the mother of a young man who had been possessed by a spirit and who was in the habit of attending Friday services at the shrine.

She took us into a fenced off area filled with people shouting, or grabbing onto the chain link fence surrounding the space, or with heads down silently in various postures of depression, despair, perhaps sleep. The scene reminded me of visits I had made, decades earlier, to mental hospitals in the days before Thorazine and other major tranquilizers brought a measure of quiet and order to psychiatric units in hospitals.

We proceeded through the assembly hall, where the prayers had turned into *qawwalis*, devotional hymns amplified via loudspeaker. On the far side of the hall was a young man who seemed to be engaged in a strange ritual. Bare-chested, he would take a running leap onto the concrete floor, slide along its moistened surface, get up, return to his starting point, and begin the process again, over and over. Eventually, another man blocked his way and asked him to stop. The first man asked permission, in a high-pitched voice, to perform the ritual one more time. He did, and we moved on.

The next day, in class, one of the students informed the rest of us that this man was possessed by a snake-spirit, which was manifest in the slide along the floor, and a woman, manifest in his high-pitched voice. In class discussion, the student informed us that the goal was not to exorcise the spirit but for the spirit to have an opportunity to come out, to have a space for expression. I thought: *This is psychoanalysis*, in which the goal of the ritual is to provide a space for the possessing spirit, otherwise known as the neurosis, the transference, to manifest itself. Healing is connected with expression, not necessarily with exorcism. Suddenly, the strange had been rendered familiar, the familiar strange.

With this experience in mind, I undertook a study of the prestages of psychoanalysis in hypnosis and catharsis, the laying on of hands and the instruction to say whatever came to mind so that the unconscious could manifest itself in free associations and dreams (Freud, 1900/1966). Psychoanalysis, given the context of Freud's scientific and medical aspirations, had to address itself not simply to expression but to exorcism, as it were, to the removal of symptoms. I became aware also of the way that theories of spirit possession and exorcism survive, to this day, in the Catholic Church. There is, in fact, a Church-sanctioned manual for the exorcism of demons and other spirits. I watched *The Exorcist* and other such movies, finding that scientific medicine coexists with more faith-based approaches to mental illness and spirit possession in the "enlightened" West.

On a visit occasioned by the baptism of the child of friends in South Texas, I had a conversation with a Mexican American Catholic priest about some of these issues. At the reception after the baptism, attended by observant Catholic people of mostly upper middle class, I asked him if he had much contact with people who might be considered mentally ill. He launched eagerly into the following story: A woman once came to him saying that the house she lived in was haunted. He agreed to come to her house to investigate.

He then asked me: "Has your hair ever stood up on end?" I said yes, probably so. He then recounted that her house, as it happened, was built on a Native American graveyard. As he stood in her living room, leaning against the wall, he felt the wall moving against his back, and the hair on the back of his neck stood up on end.

Reflecting on this story, I noted how a "symptom," delusional from a modern scientific standpoint, had acquired different meanings from the point of view of a priest with his faith-based approach to life and with his Mexican American heritage. Why is his ethnic background relevant? Because whatever was haunting this house, and this woman, and this priest, had to do with the Native American graveyard on which they stood. The original inhabitants of this land have not been properly buried; they persist as ghosts. In the United States, these ghosts have been largely ignored, the history of the genocide has been swept under the rug. In Mexico, it is my impression that native history is more alive, more acknowledged in the official narrative of Mexican history. This Catholic priest did not relegate his parishioners' "symptom" to a *DSM* category, there to be "treated" in some "evidence-based" way. He answered my question about mentally ill people with an answer that drew on a traumatic and dissociated history of place, the place on which we stood. I don't know what further steps the priest thought were advisable in this case, whether some form of exorcism, dismissal of the ghosts, or addressing of the ghosts, some way to lay them to rest, if that were possible. Whatever the end of that story, I recount it here to show how one's perspective on the world, on symptomatology from a medical point of view, can open up when faith and reason are not so sharply differentiated. This integration of faith and reason is partly a matter of culture, but also of social class, as the group of upper middle class people of Mexican American cultural background, seemed relatively comfortable tacking back and forth between a faith-based and a scientific perspective on the priest's anecdote.

LOCATING MYSELF

This is perhaps the place to try to further locate myself historically and culturally as a participant-observer interacting with the Indian Muslim and Mexican American Catholic people, with the culturally situated phenomena I observed and experienced. I say "try" to locate myself because I believe that our most impenetrable blind spots form around our own biases and perspectives. In some ways, you, the reader are better positioned to locate me culturally than I am myself. Nonetheless, I can note that what is most visible to me is that, as a Jew, as a child of the 60s, and a middle- to upper-middle-class American, I am both imbued with and inclined to skepticism about mainstream points of view. By mainstream, I mean perspectives derived from the Euro-North American Enlightenment and the ensuing Scientific Revolution, as well as the feeling of superiority based on science and technology in relation to the rest of the world that justified and rationalized colonial violence. As a member of the professional-managerial class, I was nonetheless educated and imbued with the ideology of science. I am open to the possibility that there are Oedipal roots to this skeptical attitude that informs a hostile undercurrent to my attitude toward the mainstream, as well as denial of the degree to which I myself am shaped by the very attitudes that I deplore in the West; further, I am open to the possibility that I idealize the mysticism and emotionality that I perceive in the non–Enlightenment-bound East and in the first peoples of the Americas. I am convinced, nonetheless, that my skepticism toward the mainstream has been illuminating and productive in raising my consciousness about my own cultural location and the biases that I bring to my encounters with people whose cultural and subsequent class backgrounds differ from my own.

A CAVEAT ABOUT MULTIPLICITY

Stereotypes seem inevitable when discussing various cultures and the philosophical inclinations within them. For example, "Western" and "Eastern" cultures each consist of numerous subcultures, not to mention that there are global "Southern" cultures, that, literally speaking, include countries as diverse as Brazil and Australia. The diversity within countries and cultures, North and South, East and West, is at least as great as the diversity between countries and cultures. Likewise, when discussing the various cultures of healing, while the Enlightenment-based, scientific approach to psychological symptoms may be quite prevalent in the United States, for example, there are also various healing methods based on holistic, "Eastern"-influenced, methods: from acupuncture, to yoga and meditation, to numerous herbal remedies, to faith-based ideas about healing rooted in various versions of Christianity. These healing methods are often studied and evaluated from a scientific perspective (Davidson & Goldman, 2017), aside from the enthusiastic self-reports of those who practice or use them. To further complicate matters, "Western" science is quite prevalent in India and elsewhere in Asia, especially among the urban middle and upper middle classes, with quite a bit of emphasis on "evidence-based" practices in psychotherapy, standardized and manualized treatments, with plenty of skepticism about faith-based or poorly controlled and unstandardized treatments like psychoanalysis. That said, if one attempted to do justice to the diversity within categories, one would be continually tangled up in caveats. One might then miss the ways in which there are trends within cultures and subcultures and class that can be usefully identified and discussed, as long as these caveats are kept in mind.

FORKS, AND CONFLUENCES, IN THE ROAD

Let us return to the experiences I described at the Hazrat Nizamuddin Aulia Dargah at the Nizamuddin Mosque in New Delhi and to my conversation with the Catholic priest in Texas. In both cases, one could say that a translation was occurring between the medically based language of mental illness and the spiritually based language of possession. What difference does it make which language we use in speaking about the underlying phenomena? In what ways does the translation effect a transformation, and in what ways does the translation allow us to shuttle back and forth between cultural worlds in addressing comparable phenomena?

At the descriptive level, it appears that there is a family resemblance, as it were, between the behaviors being referred to, whether in terms of illness or possession. Behaviors such as repetitive sliding along the floor like a snake are unusual, defying widely shared norms of human behavior, and are dysfunctional in terms of ordinary life, especially from a Western scientific perspective. Other people tend to feel frightened, perhaps intrigued, as their most basic assumptions of what a human being is, and what a human being does, are called into question by the behavior of what otherwise looks like a fellow human. With our fundamental categories questioned in this way, we resort to thinking that the person in question is sick, or perhaps possessed, to make sense of this otherwise profoundly confusing behavior. Likewise, experiencing one's house as haunted calls into question the very notion of home, the idea that home is a place where one can feel safe, "at home" as is said, a place where things are predictable, not a place where wildly unexpected things, like walls moving out of the blue, occur. Again, if we think that the person in question is sick or possessed by an alien spirit, perhaps we can allay the panic and confusion that we would otherwise feel. There is a complex interaction between culture and social class in the cases I describe, but in the end, there is transcendence of the bifurcation of reason and faith.

The evolution of psychoanalysis shows us one way in which the language of illness, based in science, has evolved from the language of spirituality and faith, via notions of spirit possession. I suggest that these are different languages for referring to common phenomena. I say *common*, not *identical* partly because the way these behaviors are understood influences specific manifestations. Following are some of the ways I have come to understand commonalities underlying conceptual frameworks that have come to diverge sharply between psychoanalysis and spiritual interventions in the context of social class and cultural differences.

1. Transcendent spaces: Psychoanalytic theory, and the theory of spirit possession, both make reference to spaces that transcend ordinary phenomenal reality. In psychoanalysis, such a space is referred to as the *unconscious*— a timeless realm in which reside presences from the past—ghosts, as it were—and where ordinary logic does not apply. In spiritual language, transcendent spaces are the realm of spirits, especially ancestors, usually with unfinished business from ordinary life, or with newly unfinished business from failure to honor properly the memories of ancestors. Loewald (1979) memorably referred to psychoanalysis as a process of turning ghosts into ancestors by laying them properly to rest. In Chinese traditional healing (Tseng, 1978), spirit possession often occurs when the graves of ancestors are not properly cared for.

2. Influence of the past: In psychoanalysis, the past remains alive, or comes alive, through transference, the reproduction of the past in the present relationship with the analyst. Also, in psychoanalysis, the past remains alive in the unconscious in the form of *internal objects* and *internal object relationships*. In spiritual language, internal objects are comparable to ghosts, or to the interaction between spiritual reality and ordinary reality that takes place via possession. In psychoanalytic language, this interaction takes place via dissociation in which two realities coexist side by side, with the person shuttling back and forth in what appear to be radical transformations. Hindu philosophy refers to the influence of the past via karma, the influence of past lives on the present. In the timeless unconscious, of course, it is a matter of insignificance whether the past is understood as a past life, or as a life in the past. It is also a matter of insignificance whether there is thought to be continuity across lives, across the death–birth gap, or whether there is thought to be continuity across different self-states in a single lifespan.

3. Relationship to the healer or guide: A personal relationship between healer and sufferer is a commonality between psychoanalysis and most, if not all, traditional spiritual healing methods. Psychoanalysts frame this relationship as "transference," which can be seen, in part, as the investment of the analyst with a mystique (Hoffman, 1998), which makes the facilitation of radical life changes possible. Irwin Hoffman made a special point of retaining the therapeutic benefit of rituals in the psychoanalytic process as a way of summoning a *mystique* (a less science-unfriendly word

derived from the spirit-friendly word *mystic*) similar to the mystique, the special powers, of parents, in the eyes of the young child. This special power, in the case of the analysand, accounts for the attachment of the adult to the experiences of childhood. According to Hoffman, the analyst needs a comparable social power to dislodge that ongoing presence in the unconscious of the analysand. The use of the couch, the recumbent posture of the analysand, the injunction to say whatever comes to mind without self-censorship, all derive from hypnosis, a way of bridging gaps of dissociation, bringing self-states together. Part of Freud's historical significance derives from his way of bridging the gap between traditional healing methods and the purportedly science-based method of psychoanalysis, via rituals such as those mentioned.

The hypnotist is not generally a spiritually invested figure, though one could claim that hypnoid states are part of many spiritually intense experiences often involving a charismatic leader or guide. The Hindu guru, on the other hand, like the psychoanalyst, is invested with a special significance that derives from knowledge and experience of a transcendent realm. The comparison here requires us to make a translation back and forth between the spiritual experience of enlightenment and the psychoanalytic experience of insight. Meditative practices entail an inner-directed sight, as well as an openness to the flow of thoughts and feelings through consciousness, a kind of free association, with the facilitation of a guide. The guru in the Hindu conception, on the other hand, is not generally seen as a figure deriving from the personal history of the spiritual seeker, and the guru is not generally seen as a guide to the overcoming of personal difficulties in living, or psychological symptomatology. The purpose of the guru is, in fact, to facilitate transcendence of the entire self-centered or ego-centric realm in which such personal difficulties arise and exist.

Emmanuel Ghent (1990, 1992) bridged the gap between the psychoanalytic and the Hindu–Buddhist notions of transcendence with his conception of transcendence via "surrender" of "false self." In adopting and recontextualizing D. W. Winnicott's (1960/1965) concept of false self, Ghent brought to light a linkage between spiritual and medical/scientific worlds that had been sundered by the polarization of these worlds in the Enlightenment.

In Winnicott's (1960/1965) conception, false self is a psychological structure with roots in personal history (i.e., in the parent–child relationship). "True self," by contrast, is not seen as a structure by Winnicott but rather as process, or flow. The flow of true self is interrupted and blocked by the need to attend to the parent's needs as imposed upon the child. False self manifests in later life as a self organized around an overriding need to adapt to impingement from others by compliance or resistance. Because Ghent, following Winnicott, viewed others as potential sources of impingement upon the flow of true self, he, like Winnicott, saw the analyst as a background, facilitating figure, rather more like a guru-guide to meditation than a partner in an intersubjective interaction. Winnicott (1958) referred to the capacity to be "alone in the presence of another" as a marker of true self living, in childhood and in the analytic situation. Because Ghent followed Winnicott in this respect, he was disinclined to give up the "one-person psychology" of classical psychoanalysis, in favor the more interactive "two-person psychology" that was arising in psychoanalysis in the United States. Ghent's version of relational psychoanalysis emphasized the "one person" factor in a two-person context, as occurs when one is alone in the presence of an unobtrusive other (Grossmark, 2018).

Ghent imported the notion of "surrender" from Eastern religion, recontextualizing it in contrast to "submission." Surrender he saw as a one-person process, the surrender of the structure of false self. Submission, for Ghent, meant compliance with the will of another in a dominant–submissive setup, precisely the interactive configuration that gives rise to, and reinforces, false self. It is of utmost importance, then, that the spiritual seeker be seen as surrendering ego (in the Hindu or Buddhist sense) not as surrendering *to* the person of the guru. The guru is thus seen as a vehicle for the facilitation of surrender, rather than as requiring submission. Requiring submission, for Ghent, would be the ultimate perversion of the process.

CONCLUSION

In this chapter, I have tried to sort out some of the complexity that arises at the junctions of social class and culture, science, and religion/spirituality, with each other and in relation to psychotherapy. I have suggested that fault lines between reason and faith, between science and spirituality, have influenced the development of healing methods, including psychotherapy. Intellectual and socioeconomic elites gravitated toward science-based approaches; faith-based approaches persisted outside that self-nominated elite. Taking as a starting point the evolution of healing methods outside this Enlightenment-sponsored split, I have tried to envision how commonalities in healing methods might become more apparent in a more integrative, less elitist framework.

Freud set psychoanalysis and psychotherapy on this path as he tried to bring healing techniques from the "dark" ages of faith, personal influence and suggestion, to the "light" of elite medical science and objective study. Thus, the need for this volume to do its part to heal the splits underlying the development of modern psychotherapy and to reclaim the connection to spirituality that constitutes one of the major babies often thrown out with the bathwater.

A recent emphasis on mindfulness, contemplative methods, and holistic healing demonstrates an ongoing felt need for the spiritual element. In the context of the development of psychoanalysis, the tools for the reclamation of spirituality, in my view, turns out to have been provided by Winnicott, with this notion of true and false self (itself an artificial polarity) and the link provided by Ghent between false self and the Eastern ego. For Ghent, surrender of ego/false self is the route to healing, to the reclaiming of true self, viewed as process as opposed to structure (another artificial polarity). At the time of his premature death, the psychoanalyst Stephen Mitchell, in collaboration with Ghent, was beginning to develop this tantalizingly integrative contribution of Winnicott: the notion that false self interrupts "ongoing being," the flow of true self. Perhaps it is not too much to intuit that Winnicott, with roots in colonial British culture, was channeling a healing potential in the British fascination with India that had been perverted into the dominant–submissive framework of empire and elitism based on social status.

Finally, I offer a few practical suggestions for psychotherapists who wish to enhance their skills working with social class issues:

- Think about your own social class background and that of your family. Ask yourself: When did you first become aware of your social class status? What memories stand out in which social status became salient in your life? Was social class salient in school? Do you think that your family's social status was reflected in your religious education or practices? If you are honest with yourself, can you think of ways in which you have idealized or denigrated attitudes toward people based on social status?

- Think about the social class makeup of your practice. Are you aware of varying feelings about your patients based on their social status? Have any of your patients ever expressed the feeling that your feelings about them reflect prejudice? Ask yourself how you feel about the religious and spiritual lives of your patients and how these feelings might reflect feelings about social status.

- Make an effort to be open to patients' feelings that you have attitudes toward them, positive or negative, based on social class. Ask yourself: Do patients seem to present themselves to you in ways that might plausibly reflect their anxiety about how you might feel about them based on social status? Do you think your patients believe that you have feelings and attitudes about their religious and spiritual lives?

- Finally, think about your spiritual and religious life and how you associate your religious beliefs, or your religious community, with a particular class position that you feel you occupy or to which you aspire.

REFERENCES

Altman, N. (1995). *The analyst in the inner city: Race, class, and culture through a psychoanalytic lens.* Routledge.
Altman, N. (2005). Manic society. *Psychoanalytic Dialogues, 15*(3), 321–346. https://doi.org/10.1080/10481881509348833
Altman, N. (2010). *The analyst in the inner city: Race, class, and culture through a psychoanalytic lens* (2nd ed.). Routledge.
Altman, N. (2015). *Psychoanalysis in times of accelerating cultural change: Spiritual globalization.* Routledge. https://doi.org/10.4324/9781315719337
Bose, G. (1999). The genesis and adjustment of the Oedipus wish. In T. G. Vaidyanathan & J. J. Kripal (Eds.), *Vishnu on Freud's desk* (pp. 21–38). Oxford University Press. (Original work published 1929)
Bourdieu, P. (1984). *Distinction.* Harvard University Press.
Chalfant, H. P., Heller, P. L., Roberts, A., Briones, D., Aguirre-Hochbaum, S., & Farr, W. (1990). The clergy as a resource for those encountering psychological distress. *Review of Religious Research, 31*(3), 305–313. https://doi.org/10.2307/3511620
Cowan, P. (1983). *An orphan in history: Retrieving a Jewish legacy.* Bantam Bros.
Davidson, R., & Goldman, D. (2017). *The science of meditation: How to change your brain, mind, and body.* Penguin.
Erikson, E. (1969). *Gandhi's truth: On the origins of militant nonviolence.* Norton.
Freud, S. (1966). The interpretation of dreams. In J. Strachey (Ed. & Trans.), *The standard edition of the complete psychological works of Sigmund Freud* (Vols. 4–5). The Hogarth Press. (Original work published 1900)
Ghent, E. (1990). Masochism, submission, and surrender: Masochism as a perversion of surrender. *Contemporary Psychoanalysis, 26*(1), 108–136. https://doi.org/10.1080/00107530.1990.10746643
Ghent, E. (1992). Paradox and process. *Psychoanalytic Dialogues, 2*(2), 135–159. https://doi.org/10.1080/10481889209538925
Grossmark, R. (2018). *The unobtrusive relational analyst.* Routledge. https://doi.org/10.4324/9781315708096
Hoffman, I. Z. (1998). *Ritual and spontaneity in the psychoanalytic process: A dialectical constructivist view.* The Analytic Press.
Kakar, S. (1982). *Shamans, mystics, and doctors: A psychoanalytic inquiry into India and its healing traditions.* Knopf.
Layton, L. (2004). This place gives me the heebie jeebies. *International Journal of Critical Studies, 10,* 36–50.
Loewald, H. (1979). The waning of the Oedipus Complex. In *Papers on psychoanalysis* (pp. 384–404). Yale University Press.
Makari, G. (2015). *Soul machine: The invention of the modern mind.* Norton.
Salinger, J. D. (1981). *Franny and Zooey.* Little Brown.
Sennett, R., & Cobb, J. (1972). *The hidden injuries of class.* Vintage Books.

Tseng, W. (1978). Traditional and modern psychiatric care in Taiwan. In A. Kleinman, P. Kunstadter, E. R. Alexander, & J. Gates (Eds.), *Culture and healing in Asian societies: Anthropological, psychiatric, and public health studies* (pp. 311–328). Schenkman Publishing Co.

Vahali, H. O. (2010). Landscaping a perspective: India and psychoanalytic vista. In G. Misra (Ed.), *Psychology in India: Vol. 4. Theoretical and methodological developments* (pp. 1–99). Pearson Publications.

Van Dulmen, R. (1992). *The society of the Enlightenment: The rise of the middle class and Enlightenment culture in Germany* (A. Williams, Trans.). Polity Press.

Watts, A. (1957). *The way of Zen*. Pantheon Books.

Winnicott, D. W. (1958). The capacity to be alone. In *The maturational processes and the facilitating environment* (pp. 29–36). International Universities Press.

Winnicott, D. W. (1960/1965). Ego distortion in terms of true and false self. In *The maturational processes and the facilitating environment*. International Universities Press.

CONCLUSION

Summary and Future Directions

BRAD D. STRAWN AND STEVEN J. SANDAGE

In this volume, we have attempted to contribute to the literature on spiritual diversity in clinical practice in two primary ways. In the first half of the book, authors were invited to reflect on their personal spiritual, existential, religious, and theological (SERT; Rupert et al., 2019) traditions and values as well as the related impact on their approach to spiritually integrated psychotherapy (SIP) as demonstrated in clinical material. In the second half of the book, authors engaged a similar task but focused on ways particular diversity issues can intersect with religion and spirituality in psychotherapy. In the introduction to this book, we cited a meta-analysis of studies on SIP by Captari et al. (2018), a body of research showing that such treatments are typically effective but also calling for greater attention to diversity among both clients and therapists in this area.

Throughout this book, we have sought to encourage a pluralistic and inclusive approach to the meaning of SERT orientations (including atheist, humanist, and other orientations toward these constructs that may not posit a "sacred" dimension) while we have also promoted in-depth attention to the unique features of a diverse array of SERT traditions. We hope this volume aids the

https://doi.org/10.1037/0000276-015
Spiritual Diversity in Psychotherapy: Engaging the Sacred in Clinical Practice,
S. J. Sandage and B. D. Strawn (Editors)

development of spiritually integrated psychotherapies by extending and deepening intersectional awareness of diversity and the associated interpersonal processes between clients and therapists in psychotherapy. As editors, we noticed several themes emerging from these contributions that we highlight in this conclusion along with suggested areas for future research. We also appreciate the ways these chapters reveal aspects of the personal narratives of this diverse group of clinical scholars. We go on to summarize some points for further reflection from the combined insights of these contributors to offer next steps for clinicians wanting to grow in spiritual and religious competence (SRC).

PERSON OF THE THERAPIST

The authors in this book have courageously allowed us into their minds and personhood—not just as clinicians but as clinicians of intersectional diversity, including SERT diversity—reminding us that clinicians are, first of all, people with their own personal histories. They have risked displaying not simply their countertransference in response to clinical situations but who they are as individuals embedded within in SERT backgrounds, traditions, and values. They have demonstrated how these traditions and values shape their thinking and theorizing, their sense of self, why they do what they do (i.e., vocation), and how all of this impacts the way they understand personhood, clinical work, and respect for diversity. The uncommon nature of this task was clearly stated by Pargament (see Chapter 2), a leading international scholar in the psychology of religion and spirituality for decades. He said no one had ever asked him to reflect on his own SERT tradition and how that impacted what he does. We realize some clinicians are not particularly interested in SERT issues on a personal level, but we hope a growing number of clinicians will help with retrieving attention to the person of the therapist that has been a central value within many psychotherapy traditions.

Before summarizing some of the themes of this book, we also want to explicitly recognize the obvious point that the themes might be relatively idiosyncratic to the authors who were invited to contribute. The themes could be expanded, deepened, or challenged by engaging a different set of authors with other combinations of clinical and SERT orientations. Yet that "limitation" serves to reinforce the larger point that, like all psychotherapy, SIP involves diverse intersecting dynamics of the person of the therapist as they seek to relate in skillful ways with diverse groups of clients seeking healing and growth.

TEN THEMES FROM THIS BOOK

We now turn to illustrating a number of themes that have emerged from the chapters. While there are many themes one might note, we focus primarily on those related to the overall focus of the book: SERT-related concepts.

Theme 1

Acknowledging one's own SERT traditions and values as a clinician does not mean imposing those traditions and values on clients. These chapters demonstrate that clinician awareness can facilitate openness, prevent countertransference dominance, and foster generous hospitality toward difference. It is often a lack of self-awareness that can lead to covert colonialism in clinical practice (Dueck & Reimer, 2009). Yet we need further research on processes that are associated with growth in the development of SRC (Vieten & Scammell, 2015; Vieten et al., 2016) among clinicians over time as well as research that identifies factors (e.g., spiritual grandiosity, religious authoritarianism, religious trauma history) that might impede clinician progress in SRC.

Theme 2

Acknowledging one's SERT influences can sensitize clinicians to interest in the particular traditions and values of their clients. Reflecting on and owning how one's own worldview, meaning making, and moral and ethical decision making can be influenced by specific traditions and values facilitates the clinician to do the same for the client. This may free up the clinician to work within the client's SERT traditions, when desired, and make use of their rituals, practices, and ethical worldview in ways consistent with the client's culture(s) and values (see Chapter 5 by Khan). It may also help when working across differences (i.e., when therapist and client's frameworks are different; see Chapter 4 by Sheppard and Chapter 6 by Strawn). This roughly corresponds to the roles of cultural openness and comfort in the multicultural orientation model, which suggests that therapists who grow in openness and comfort with engaging cultural issues will tend to be more clinically effective (Davis et al., 2018; Owen et al., 2016). To work more openly, comfortably, and effectively with the diversity and wholeness of our clients, we may need to first own and attend to the diversity and wholeness within ourselves (Cooper-White, 2011). However, we note the obvious point that the narratives in this volume are authored by clinicians, and further research is needed on client experiences and narratives about ways SERT diversity dynamics are negotiated in various approaches to psychotherapy.

Theme 3

SERT issues and challenges emerge in relation to a wide variety of clinical issues (e.g., anxiety, depression, relational problems, trauma). Often the presenting problem is not framed by clients as SERT related, yet SERT dynamics emerge as relevant over time (see Chapter 7 by Starr). In other cases, clients deliberately seek out SIP; however, this seeking might be communicated with the varying of verbal explicitness or through symbolic means (e.g., bringing a Bible to sessions; see Chapter 4). A body of research on individual differences in preferences for engaging spirituality and religion in therapy shows that most would prefer engagement (Harris et al., 2016; Rose et al., 2008; Sandage et al., 2022). Yet very little of this research is with actual therapy clients, so we need to learn much more about the preferences of clients representing diverse SERT orientations and at various points in the treatment process. We also need more research on preferences related to SERT dynamics in couple, family, and group treatment modalities in which there is always some level of SERT diversity among the clients (see Chapter 11 by Sandage; see also Sandage et al., 2020; Walsh, 2019).

Theme 4

Reading this book with a systemic or sociological lens can lead us to see that therapists sometimes provide a relational space for engaging SERT issues for clients who may have found it difficult to do so in traditional religious communities (e.g., see Chapter 9 by Hopwood, Chapter 10 by Moon, and Chapter 13 by Altman). The authors in this volume are not suggesting that therapy should take the place of other religious or spiritual communities; rather, at times, therapy may provide an alternative sense of community for those going through periods of SERT transition, seeking refuge from social or religious oppression, or trying to heal from traumatic disasters and crises (e.g., see Chapter 5). There is room for further interdisciplinary research and reflection on the various ways different clients navigate their SERT community and therapy involvements. For example, do clinical settings provide a sense of community for some clients yet come up short in that way for others? Can group modalities of treatment be helpful for clients specifically negotiating SERT conflicts, struggles, and transitions while feeling socially isolated?

Theme 5

For particular issues, certain spiritual and religious traditions have been overtly opposed to specific psychological understandings and practices. Case in point: Some religious communities have condemned certain sexual and gender orientations as sinful or unnatural, and subsequently resisted psychological understandings or interventions that support them (see Chapters 9 and 10). Some SERT communities do not support interreligious marriage (see Chapter 11). These kinds of intersectionality challenges can potentially be difficult for both client and therapist. The balance of respecting a client's beliefs while opening up new possibilities is fraught with certain ethical sensitivities. The examples put forth in these chapters suggest ways of working with clients that are welcoming and affirming of both individual persons and their SERT traditions and values while also making space of exploration. Clients may move away from, "re-tradition" (i.e., begin to reformulate their understanding of the tradition's beliefs and practices while choosing to remain within it), or join new SERT communities or orientations based on their work in therapy. Whatever the outcome, this work is highly idiosyncratic to each set of therapy relationships, and, therefore, great care and attention must be paid to all the SERT orientations in the room. There is also a need for further research and interdisciplinary reflection on the ways clinicians and clinics can and do navigate the ethical and relational complexities of, for example, communicating a social justice stance on specific issues while serving clients of various sociopolitical and SERT orientations.

Theme 6

Some critics of spirituality and religion have noted that people of faith may be dogmatic, prejudiced, and exclusionary toward others who are different from them. Although this can certainly be true, the chapters in this book suggest alternative outcomes from SERT commitments. The authors located places *within* their own traditions that explicitly make space for practicing hospitality across diversity (e.g., see Chapter 1 by Tummala-Narra; Chapter 3 by Jennings; and Chapters 5, 6, and 11). At the same time, we acknowledge that the authors selected to contribute to this volume value diversity and seek to practice with SRC. Therefore, to understand the impact on clinical practice, it would be useful to have qualitative studies exploring client experiences of spiritual or religious bias with therapists or to interview counselors and therapists who voice more exclusivist stances toward SERT issues. We believe in and want to promote the sacred value of diversity competence, yet we do not want to be idealistic about the ways SERT issues are actually handled by clinicians of various orientations.

Theme 7

The psychological effects of SERT traditions are on a continuum. A clinician may have a tradition that includes regular involvement in religious/spiritual communal and individual practices (e.g., see Chapter 6; see also Chapter 8 by Tisdale), or the tradition may operate in more subtle off-line ways, nevertheless influencing the clinician's worldview, morals, and ethics (e.g., see Chapters 3 and 7). While the authors of these chapters were encouraged to demonstrate more overt influences from SERT traditions, many clinicians are influenced by SERT and other philosophical or cultural dynamics in more subtle and implicit ways. Living in a radically pluralistic and "postreligious" time, many people have also been raised without any overt reference to SERT traditions or may have adopted a hybrid set of SERT influences. This can make it difficult for some people to recognize that they may have some level of SERT influence or values operating within their clinical orientation and practice. As we noted in the Introduction, interacting with Browning and Cooper's (2004) work, we believe that it is difficult for clinicians to completely avoid internalizing some set of values or ideals from surrounding cultural, philosophical, and SERT influences. Some clinicians might try to claim a completely neutral personal stance toward SERT issues, yet this approach risks the minimization of SERT diversity and the neglect of resources that might be useful for clinical work (Sandage et al., 2020).

We recommend clinicians become curious about the range of factors influencing their particular SERT-related assumptions and values, wherever that exploration takes them (including negative views of SERT traditions). As Pargament stated in Chapter 2, it is important for therapists to move their influences from implicit to explicit. We would also like to see more research on training modules and exercises that can help clinicians gain awareness of these influences.

Theme 8

Despite some arguable ongoing prejudice in the psychological field against religion and the actual damage that some religious communities have inflicted on others, all authors of this volume identified positive psychological aspects of spirituality and religion. Although correlations between indices of psychological health and spirituality and religion have been noted in empirical research, these studies have typically studied religion in relatively monolithic and general ways (Captari et al., 2018). The chapters in this volume can contribute to fairly unique and nuanced understandings of specific positive psychological aspects of spirituality and religion across different SERT traditions and within clinical settings that can contribute to client's healing and well-being.

We are enthusiastic about more research integrating positive psychology and SERT dynamics in psychotherapy. At the same time, we also recognize the place for a cultural appropriation-type critique when clinicians regularly apply concepts like mindfulness, forgiveness, or hope in generic ways that are stripped of any historical, semantic, or conceptual associations with cultural or SERT traditions and practices. This is one of the reasons we want to affirm the diversity value of a "thicker" awareness of cultural and SERT traditions and resources as well as promote clinician awareness of the sociocultural and class contexts that shape our assumptions and epistemologies about suffering and healing (see Altman, Chapter 13).

Theme 9

We noticed a recurring theme of resonance between the goals and desired outcomes of psychotherapy and some of the goals of SERT traditions (e.g., see Chapters 2, 3, 5, 6, 7, and 9; see also Chapter 12 by Barrs and Doehring). Both psychotherapy and SERT dynamics were conceptualized as teleological in nature and headed toward goals, such as overcoming oppression of various kinds and achieving health and wholeness, restoration and justice, and even the recovery of the capacity of love.

Theme 10

Professional therapists can work effectively with clients' SERT traditions and values while still prioritizing mental health treatment goals. Good therapists always seek to work from within their client's worldview and social location, which may include various diversity dynamics. This is consistent with findings from the aforementioned meta-analysis (Captari et al., 2018), which found that spiritually integrated psychotherapies were equal to secular treatments on mental health outcomes but often were superior on spiritual outcomes. The chapters in this book illustrate differing ways spiritually integrated treatment processes can potentially achieve positive spiritual and psychological outcomes (e.g., see Chapters 6 and 8). At the same time, we affirm the reality that, like other psychotherapies, spiritually-integrated psychotherapies do not heal all forms of suffering or relational and spiritual struggle (see Chapters 11 and 12). We agree with Captari et al. (2018) in calling for further attention to both (a) spiritual processes and outcomes and (b) spiritual well-being and spiritual struggles in psychotherapy research in a variety of clinical practice settings.

These considerations also bring us back to questions we considered in the Introduction about the reasons a therapist might be tempted to avoid working with a client's SERT tradition. It may be that some therapists who explicitly or implicitly understand the meaning and power of clients' SERT traditions knowingly or unknowingly separate the psychological from SERT dimensions. They may fear that working with SERT dynamics could result in undercutting a client's faith, thus leading to either premature termination or an overall negative therapeutic outcome (Sorenson, 2004). Or, therapists may correctly worry that they are terribly underqualified to work with issues of such grave importance. These are valid concerns and call for ongoing training, supervision, and consultation on SERT issues. Continued research and volumes like the present one are important as are peer consultation and collaboration with spiritual and religious leaders from the client's tradition. Thankfully, a growing number of excellent book-length resources are available for working clinically with spiritual and religious issues (see Griffith & Griffith, 2003; Pargament, 2011)

While there are undoubtedly additional themes that the reader may glean from these chapters, we must note that sometimes SERT traditions are unknowingly overlooked. That is why we encourage readers to engage in the practice of exploring the potential influence of SERT traditions on their work with clients. Without doing so, important elements of a person's identity may simply remain unavailable to therapeutic work. For example, at the end of a presentation one of us (B.D.S.) did on religion and psychotherapy, a member of the audience commented, "I can talk to my patients about sex, anger, and even their finances, but I wonder why we never talk about religion?"

For those interested in further training on SERT dynamics in therapy, we point to (a) the many books and articles cited throughout this volume (particularly SIP models cited in the introduction); (b) an excellent online training program developed by Pearce, Pargament, and colleagues (Pearce et al., 2019); and (c) free videos available on The Albert & Jessie Danielsen Institute website (see https://www.bu.edu/danielsen/). Readers interested in further resources for enhancing their capacities to work with spiritual and religious diversity might also access Richards and Bergin's (2014) *Handbook of Psychotherapy and Religious Diversity* and Vieten and Scammell's (2015) *Spiritual and Religious Competencies in Clinical Practice*.

REFLECTION QUESTIONS

We now turn to reflection questions as takeaways or practical aids for those clinicians desiring to work on their own SERT awareness and skill in SRC. These questions are designed to spark reflection and imagination in therapists hoping to explore new SERT terrain and might be useful for training or consultation conversations in clinical settings. Rupert et al. (2019) outlined a reflective group process approach to clinical training and consultation in SERT dynamics, which has received some preliminary research evaluation (Crabtree et al., 2021).

Clinicians and SERT Dynamics

Again, SERT stands for spiritual, existential, religious, and theological dimensions (Rupert et al., 2019), and we have also suggested how various cultural and philosophical traditions (broadly interpreted) can affect our perspectives and identities as clinicians. Some clinicians identify with specific SERT traditions through either a particular religious framework (e.g., Hindu, Jewish, Islam) or in broader philosophic categories, such as humanism, pantheism, feminism, Afrocentrism, and many others. For some clinicians, identifying their SERT framework will be relatively simple because they may have been raised in or continue to practice within a specific spiritual or religious tradition. As suggested earlier, SERT identifications can also take hybrid or combined forms, such as a clinician who identifies as Jewish, Buddhist, and a social justice progressive. For others who have not previously identified a particular set of frameworks or values with which they identify, this can be more challenging and may require tolerating some ambiguity as one begins to explore these issues. It is possible for SERT-related beliefs and values to function in conscious or more unconscious ways.

Here are a few questions for reflecting on SERT influences and commitments:

- Is there any history of SERT involvement in your extended family system? And if so, how have those SERT dynamics influenced you in positive, negative, or mixed ways? Hodge (2001, 2005) offered guidelines for doing a spiritual and religious genogram or ecogram, and it can be useful to notice (a) intergenerational and contextual transitions in SERT involvements and (b) ways SERT diversity has been handled in your family history.

- Are there key values, morals, or implicit ethical systems that pervade the cultures or SERT traditions that have influenced you? These might be organizing principles at varying levels of specificity that shape your views

354 • *Strawn and Sandage*

of meaning in life, obligations, and relationships (e.g., the need to care for others, the need to be authentic, the value of questioning authority, the primacy of family, the virtue of hard work, the sacred value of nature). How do these values or ethics shape your approach to your clinical work and your overall sense of vocation? Do you notice times they help you understand certain clients? Do you notice other times you feel provoked when clients express alternative values and ethics?

- Here are a few questions you might ask yourself to dig deeper into your own implicit SERT framework:
  - What are your images or working definitions of "mental health," "well-being," "normality," and the "good life"? Do these reflect SERT traditions or values? Other cultural or philosophical values?
  - How do you believe humans are to treat one another? What do you consider core values in life or what humans are obliged to do? How do these issues emerge in your work with clients?
  - How do you go about making ethical decisions? What are the key themes and sources of moral influence? (See Chapter 12 for a helpful set of themes from moral foundation theory.)
  - Do you have a sense of "the transcendent"? And if so, what role does it play in your ongoing life?
  - Do you have a sense of the sacred? What do you consider ultimate or what do you ultimately value? What factors have influenced your view of the sacred or the ultimate? If the term "sacred" does not fit for you, is there another term that represents what is ultimately important to you?
  - Are there particular diversity dynamics that have intersecting influences on your SERT and ethical orientations (e.g., example, race, ethnicity, gender orientation, sexual orientation, social class, region)?

Clients and SERT Dynamics

Clients are often influenced by or identify with SERT traditions and values at various levels. The available research cited earlier has found most individuals would prefer to discuss SERT issues in therapy if they felt their therapists were open and respectful of those issues (Harris et al., 2016; Oxhandler et al., 2018; Sandage et al., 2022). As mentioned throughout this volume, client orientations toward SERT dynamics can come in a myriad of forms and include commitments to SERT traditions, open exploration of SERT dynamics, painful struggles with SERT dynamics and communities, and disinterest in SERT issues. Therefore, working therapeutically with SERT traditions requires clinician flexibility and respect for complexity as part of SRC. It can be useful to engage these reflection questions:

- What have been some of my prior clinical experiences with SERT dynamics with clients? How have these experiences influenced my approach to these issues? What are some of the diverse expressions of SERT dynamics I have seen among clients?

- What do I know about the SERT traditions and values of some of my current clients?

- How do I feel about asking clients about their SERT traditions and values? One approach from Tan (1996) is to explicitly ask clients during intake if they have spiritual or religious commitments and whether they see those commitments as relevant to the work in therapy. However, these questions might be complemented by interest in clients' SERT-related questions and inquiring when that seems clinically relevant (Sandage et al., 2022).

- Do I have particular anxieties or concerns about asking clients about SERT dynamics? If so, what are those anxieties and concerns? Do I know clinical colleagues I might approach who seem to have more comfort or competence in this area to learn how they handle those issues?

- Can I envision possible ways of integrating SERT dynamics into therapy when clients desire that goal? If not, can I identify clinicians for consultation? Am I open to asking clients for help in co-constructing that kind of integration?

- Am I open to engaging SERT issues with clients who are devout as well as those who are hurt by or questioning specific SERT traditions? Do I know my own countertransference vulnerabilities in this area?

- Can I recognize individual differences even *within* SERT traditions? Every major SERT tradition will have diversity, and individuals will bring their own subjectivity to SERT beliefs and practices. Is there a particular tradition I want to better understand through reading, conversations, or attendance at services? Do I know anyone who might be willing to help me learn about diversity within that tradition?

- Am I open to asking clinical colleagues if SERT dynamics might be relevant when they are presenting a case in a staffing, training, or consultation meeting in which those dynamics have not been considered? Can I voice concern when I hear a colleague enact a spiritual or religious microaggression or bigoted comment? Is my clinical context a safe environment for expressing SERT diversity?

• The *E* in SERT stands for "existential," and this can invite questions about various existential themes that might be relevant to clinical practice (Sandage et al., 2020). From this vantage point, clinicians can listen for clients' struggles or ways of making meaning in the face of existential dilemmas and predicaments related to death, loss, choices, guilt, fate, feelings of meaninglessness, and the like (Yalom, 1980). These may first appear as quiet echoes but, nevertheless, have a deep enduring influence on how a client experiences struggles or tries to make sense of the world. Yet those of us who practice therapy often have chronic exposure to suffering, so it can be important to also reflect on our own existential struggles related to clinical practice.

These questions, takeaways, or practical aids are clearly inexhaustible. We encourage readers to continue to reflect and ask questions of themselves, their clients, and their clinical approaches in the hope of expanding openness to the importance of SERT traditions and values in psychotherapy. The aforementioned research has demonstrated that not only may SERT dynamics be of central importance to some clients, but their incorporation into therapy may be highly valued and may even contribute to positive outcomes (Captari et al., 2018). This volume provides one set of approaches to what it might look like clinically to take spiritual diversity seriously. Our hope is that this project might promote ongoing research and clinical reflection that ultimately benefits clients, therapists, and our wider communities.

REFERENCES

Browning, D. S., & Cooper, T. D. (2004). *Religious thought and the modern psychologies*. Fortress Press.

Captari, L. E., Hook, J. N., Hoyt, W., Davis, D. E., McElroy-Heltzel, S. E., & Worthington, E. L., Jr. (2018). Integrating clients' religion and spirituality within psychotherapy: A comprehensive meta-analysis. *Journal of Clinical Psychology, 74*(11), 1938–1951. https://doi.org/10.1002/jclp.22681

Cooper-White, P. (2011). *Braided selves: Collected essays on multiplicity, God, and persons*. Cascade Books.

Crabtree, S. A., Bell, C. A., Rupert, D. A., Sandage, S. J., Devor, N. G., & Stavros, G. (2021). Humility, differentiation of self, and clinical training in spiritual and religious competence. *Journal of Spirituality in Mental Health, 23*(4), 342–362. https://doi.org/10.1080/19349637.2020.1737627

Davis, D. E., DeBlaere, C., Owen, J., Hook, J. N., Rivera, D. P., Choe, E., Van Tongeren, D. R., Worthington, E. L., & Placeres, V. (2018). The multicultural orientation framework: A narrative review. *Psychotherapy, 55*(1), 89–100. https://doi.org/10.1037/pst0000160

Dueck, A., & Reimer, K. (2009). *A peaceable psychology: Christian therapy in a world of many cultures*. Brazos Press.

Griffith, J. L., & Griffith, M. E. (2003). *Encountering the sacred in psychotherapy: How to talk to people about their spiritual lives*. Guilford Press.

Harris, K. A., Randolph, B. E., & Gordon, T. D. (2016). What do clients want? Assessing spiritual needs in counseling: A literature review. *Spirituality in Clinical Practice, 3*(4), 250–275. https://doi.org/10.1037/scp0000108

Hodge, D. R. (2001). Spiritual genograms: A generational approach to assessing spirituality. *Families in Society, 82*(1), 35–48. https://doi.org/10.1606/1044-3894.220

Hodge, D. R. (2005). Spiritual ecograms: A new assessment instrument for identifying clients' strengths in space and across time. *Families in Society, 86*(2), 287–296. https://doi.org/10.1606/1044-3894.2467

Owen, J., Tao, K. W., Drinane, J. M., Hook, J., Davis, D. E., & Kune, N. F. (2016). Client perceptions of therapists' multicultural orientation: Cultural (missed) opportunities and cultural humility. *Professional Psychology, Research and Practice, 47*(1), 30–37. https://doi.org/10.1037/pro0000046

Oxhandler, H. K., Ellor, J. W., & Stanford, M. S. (2018). Client attitudes toward integrating religion and spirituality in mental health treatment: Scale development and client responses. *Social Work, 63*(4), 337–346. https://doi.org/10.1093/sw/swy041

Pargament, K. I. (2011). *Spiritually integrated psychotherapy: Understanding and addressing the Sacred*. Guilford Press.

Pearce, M. J., Pargament, K. I., Oxhandler, H. K., Vieten, C., & Wong, S. (2019). A novel training program for mental health providers in religious and spiritual competencies. *Spirituality in Clinical Practice, 6*(2), 73–82. https://doi.org/10.1037/scp0000195

Richards, P. S., & Bergin, A. E. (Eds.). (2014). *Handbook of psychotherapy and religious diversity* (2nd ed.). American Psychological Association. https://doi.org/10.1037/14371-000

Rose, E. M., Westefeld, J. S., & Ansley, T. N. (2008). Spiritual issues in counseling: Clients' beliefs and preferences. *Psychology of Religion and Spirituality, S*(1), 18–33. https://doi.org/10.1037/1941-1022.S.1.18

Rupert, D., Moon, S. H., & Sandage, S. J. (2019). Clinical training groups for spirituality and religion in psychotherapy. *Journal of Spirituality in Mental Health, 21*(3), 163–177. https://doi.org/10.1080/19349637.2018.1465879

Sandage, S. J., Jankowski, P. J., Paine, D. R., Exline, J. J., Ruffing, E. G., Rupert, D., Stavros, G. S., & Bronstein, M. (2022). Testing a relational spirituality model of psychotherapy clients' preferences and functioning. *Journal of Spirituality in Mental Health, 24*(1), 1–21. https://doi.org/10.1080/19349637.2020.1791781

Sandage, S. J., Rupert, D., Stavros, G. S., & Devor, N. G. (2020). *Relational spirituality in psychotherapy: Healing suffering and promoting growth*. American Psychological Association. https://doi.org/10.1037/0000174-000

Sorenson, R. L. (2004). *Minding spirituality*. The Analytic Press.

Tan, S.-Y. (1996). Religion in clinical practice: Implicit and explicit integration. In E. P. Shafranske (Ed.), *Religion and the clinical practice of psychology* (pp. 365–387). American Psychological Association. https://doi.org/10.1037/10199-013

Vieten, C., & Scammell, S. (2015). *Spiritual and religious competencies in clinical practice: Guidelines for psychotherapists and mental health professionals.* New Harbinger Publications.

Vieten, C., Scammell, S., Pierce, A., Pilato, R., Ammondson, I., Pargament, K. I., & Lukoff, D. (2016). Competencies for psychologists in the domains of religion and spirituality. *Spirituality in Clinical Practice, 3*(2), 92–114. https://doi.org/10.1037/scp0000078

Walsh, F. (2019). Spirituality, suffering, and resilience. In M. McGoldrick & K. V. Hardy (Eds.), *Re-visioning family therapy: Addressing diversity in clinical practice* (3rd ed., pp. 73–90). Guilford Press.

Yalom, I. D. (1980). *Existential psychotherapy.* Basic Books.

Index

C

Calhoun, L. G., 118
Calvin, John, 141
Captari, L. E., 345, 352
Care, inhibition of, 228
Caring, as moral foundation, 305
Catechism of the Catholic Church, 188
Challenging misalignments, 233–235
Change, Roman Catholic perspective on, 199–200
Chinmayananda, Swami, 322
Christianity. *See also* Roman Catholicism; Wesleyanism
and desire, 259–261
fundamentalist, 143–144
and gender identities, 246–247
in history of psychology and psychotherapy, 137–138
truth-telling in, 256–259
types of evangelicals in, 143
Cisgender, 225
Class. *See* Social class
Class positions, as earned, 323
Client focus, 232
Clients
preference of, for engaging in SERT issues, 348
and SERT dynamics, 354–356
Clinical integrative practice, 143
Clinicians
asking about clients' gender identities, 230–231
context of, 225–229
contribution to therapy by, 145
help-seeking with, 321
openness of, 346, 347
reflections on SERT dynamics for, 353–354
self-awareness of, about SERT issues, 350
SERT traditions of, 10–11, 146–148, 146–148, 150–156, 150–156, 276–278, 347, 350
training of, on religion and spirituality issues, 250
values of, 253–254
Cobb, J., 324
Coconstruction, of developmental crucible, 281–282
Cognition, in Sufi Islamic psychology, 117–118

Cognitive processing therapy (CPT), 301–303
Coherence approach, to authenticity, 254, 257–258
Collaboration, cultivating and extending, 283–284
Committed action, in trauma treatment, 313–316
Community Mental Health movement, 331
Community reintegration, in trauma treatment, 313–316
Competence
cultural, 5
spiritual and religious, 5–7
Complementarity, 289–290
Conceptualization(s)
of authenticity, 252–253
of mental illness, and religion, 334–335
in Roman Catholic psychoanalytic approach, 203
Conscious biases, 124–125
Contemplative listening, 201
Contemplative methods, of healing, 341
Contemplative spirituality, 188–190
Conversion therapy, 262
Convicting awakening, 291–292
Cooper, T. D., 9, 350
Core beliefs, uncovering, 235–238
Countertransference
in psychoanalysis, 191
in spiritually integrated clinical practice, 124–125
Couples therapy, 271–294
and definitions of spirituality and religion, 272–273
differentiation system focus in case example, 284–288
intersubjectivity system focus in case example, 288–294
personal SERT journey to, 276–278
process of, 281–284
relational spirituality model of psychotherapy, 278–281
religious differences and couples, 273–276
Courage, 242–243
Course of treatment, in Roman Catholic psychoanalytic approach, 203–205
Cowan, Paul, 322
CPT (cognitive processing therapy), 301–303

M

Makari, George, 329
Matt, D. C., 174
McKinnon, William, 322
McWilliams, Nancy, 144, 202–203
Meaning(s)
   creation of, 235–236
   search for, 299–300
   situational, 299
   of symptoms, 279
Meaningfulness, 326
Meditative practices, in Sufism, 116
Mental health
   religion, spirituality, and, 4, 350–351
   stigma of, in Haiti, 132
Mental illness
   religion and conceptualizations of,
      334–335
   and spirit possession, 337–340
Mercy
   Roman Catholic perspective on,
      196–197, 212–213
   transformation by, 190
Merton, Thomas, 266
Military moral injury (MMI), 297–317
   ACT with, 303–304
   case example of psychotherapy with,
      306–316
   CPT with, 301–303
   defining, 298–299
   moral and spiritual orienting systems
      of those providing veteran care,
      304–306
   spiritually integrated therapy of,
      299–300
   stages and models of trauma treatment
      with, 300–301
Mind
   embedded in interactive field with other
      minds, 165–166
   Roman Catholic perspective on,
      198–199
Mindfulness meditation practices,
   314–315, 331–332, 341
Mirroring, 244–245
Misalignments, challenging, 233–235
Mitchell, Stephen, 165–166, 341
MMI. *See* Military moral injury
Modes of Therapeutic Action (Stark),
   193–195
Mohammed, Mufti Shaheed, 131
Moral injury, 298

Morality
   in psychotherapy, 147–148
   in spiritually integrated clinical practice,
      124–125
   in Wesleyanism, 140, 146
Mother Teresa, St., 189
Motivation, sources of, 198
Mourning, in trauma treatment, 311–313
Multicultural framework
   linking postcolonial framework and,
      121–123
   and multiple aspects of identity, 115
   Sufism in, 120–121
Multiculturalism, pertinence of, 124
Multiplicity, 336–337
Music, spiritual, 243–244
Muslims
   differing experiences of, 114–115, 125
   in Haiti, 131–133
   orientalist opinion of, 122–123
   trauma treatment with Rohingyan
      refugees, 126–130
Mystique, 338–339

N

Nachman, Rabbi, 162
Nafs (self, ego, psyche), 116–118
Nagpal, Ashok, 332
Names, using preferred, 230
Narratives, identities evoked in, 122
Negotiating a differentiated alliance, 285
Neo-evangelicalism, Wesleyan, 144, 150–156
Neutrois (identity term), 224
New Seed of Contemplation (Merton), 266
Nieuwsma, J. A., 302, 303, 315
Noman, N., 255
Nonbinary (identity term), 224
Nontraditional gender identities, 224–225
Nontransgender, 225
Nugent, R., 251

O

Object relations, 192–193
On-up/one-down relational stance,
   289–290
Organismic approach, to authenticity, 254
Orientalism (Said), 122–123
Orienting systems
   and moral injury, 299–300
   of those providing veteran care, 304–306
Outness, authenticity and, 255, 256

P

Pargament, Ken, 9, 273, 299
PDM 2: Psychodynamic Diagnostic Manual (Lingiardi & McWilliams), 202–203
Pearce, M., 301
Perpetration-based MMI, 298
Postcolonial framework, 121–123
Postcolonial psychotherapy, 118–119
Poverty of affluence, 324–328
Powerlessness, 231–232
Privacy, secrecy vs., 257–258
Privilege
  discrimination and invisible, 231–232
  visible, 227–229
Processing, of trauma, 311–313
Psyche, in Sufi Islamic psychology, 116
Psychoanalysis
  and culture, 333–335
  evolution of field, 190–191
  object relations in, 192–193
  related to particular religious traditions, 186
  shift to two-person paradigm in, 163
  and spiritual healing, 337–340
  synthesis of multiple theories into useful methods in, 193–195
  theoretical and clinical constants in, 191–192
  and *tikkum olam*, 161, 162, 175–177. *See also* Kabbalah
  Wesleyan-Christian, 144–146
Psychodynamic Diagnostic Manual: PDM 2 (Lingiardi & McWilliams), 202–203
Psychodynamic psychotherapy, Sufi spirituality and, 118–119, 124
Psychological first aid, following Boston Marathon bombings, 130–131
Psychological Measure of Islamic Religiousness, 121
Psychology, history of Christianity and, 137–138
Psychopathology, Roman Catholic perspective on etiology of, 199
Psychotherapeutic theories
  informing Roman Catholic approach, 190–195
  and SERT tradition elements, 147–148
Psychotherapy
  history of Christianity and, 137–138
  implicit cultures embedded within theories of, 147–148
Purity culture, 259–260

Q

Qalb (heart), in Sufi Islamic psychology, 116, 117
Queer Eye (television series), 255
Queer individuals. *See* LGBQ individuals

R

Reason, faith vs., 329–330
Receptive moral injury, 306
Recitation, in Sufism, 116
Rejection
  by family members, 241
  by religious communities, 236–238
Relational psychoanalytic approach, 145, 161, 163
Relational space, to discuss SERT issues, 348
Relational spirituality, defining, 272
Relational spirituality model (RSM) of psychotherapy, 278–281
Relationships. *See also* Couples therapy
  and development, 280
  with Divine, 239
  healing, 240–244
  for seeking and developing one's truth, 176–177
  between sufferer and healer, 338–339
  in Sufism, 115, 116
Religion(s)
  and assumptions of harm, 229
  clinicians' discomfort in addressing, 120–121
  and conceptualizations of mental illness, 334–335
  contextual variations in, 119
  defining, 272–273
  definitions of, 225
  differences of, in couples, 273–276
  Freud on, 185
  and help-seeking, 328–329
  history of Christianity and, 137–138
  as main marker of difference in today's world, 119
  mental heath, well-being, and, 4, 350–351
  and psychoanalysis, 186
  and questions about gender identities, 246–247
  using nonreductionis framework in addressing, 119
Religiosity, measures assessing, 121

About the Editors

Steven J. Sandage, PhD, LP, is the Albert and Jessie Danielsen Professor of Psychology of Religion at Boston University, Boston, Massachusetts, with a joint appointment in the School of Theology and the Department of Psychological and Brain Sciences. He is director of research and senior staff psychologist at The Albert & Jessie Danielsen Institute and adjunct faculty in psychology of religion at the MF Norwegian School of Theology, Religion and Society in Oslo, Norway. His coauthored or coedited books include *Relational Spirituality in Psychotherapy: Healing Suffering and Promoting Growth* (2020); *Relational Integration of Psychology and Christian Theology: Theory, Research, and Practice* (2018); *Forgiveness and Spirituality in Psychotherapy: A Relational Approach* (2016); *The Skillful Soul of the Psychotherapist: The Link Between Spirituality and Clinical Excellence* (2014); *Transforming Spirituality: Integrating Theology and Psychology* (2006); *The Faces of Forgiveness: Searching for Wholeness and Salvation* (2003); and *To Forgive is Human: How to Put Your Past in the Past* (1997). Dr. Sandage was also featured (with Everett L. Worthington, Jr.) in the American Psychological Association–produced DVD *Forgiveness in Couple Therapy*.

Dr. Sandage practices as a licensed psychologist with clinical specializations that include couple and family therapy, multicultural therapy, and spiritually integrative therapy. The American Psychological Association produced a clinical demonstration of Sandage engaging the dynamics of forgiveness in couple therapy.

Brad D. Strawn, PhD, is the Evelyn and Frank Freed Chair of the Integration of Psychology and Theology in the School of Psychology & Marriage and Family Therapy, Fuller Seminary, in Pasadena, California. His coauthored or coedited books include *Enhancing Christian Life: How Extended Cognition Augments Religious Community* (2020); *Christianity & Psychoanalysis: A New Conversation* (2014); *The Physical Nature of Christian Life: Neuroscience, Psychology, and the Church* (2012); and *Wesleyan Theology and Social Science: The Dance of Practical Divinity and Discovery* (2010). He has also coedited special issues of *Psychoanalytic Inquiry*, the *Journal of Psychology & Theology*, and the *Journal of Psychology and Christianity*.

Dr. Strawn is currently editing a new book series based on the annual Fuller Integration Symposium that addresses psychology and theology. He is a licensed psychologist in clinical practice in Pasadena.